THE BEARABLES BIG BOOK OF SEX

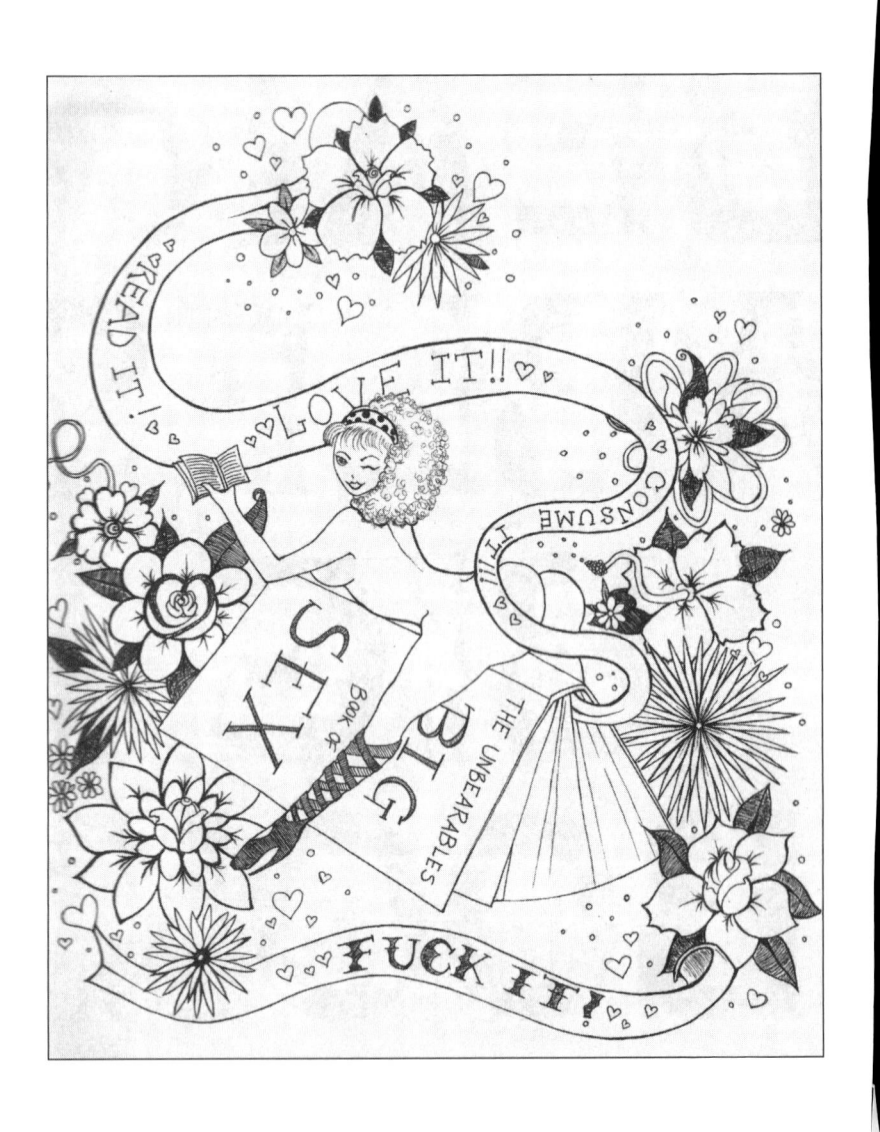

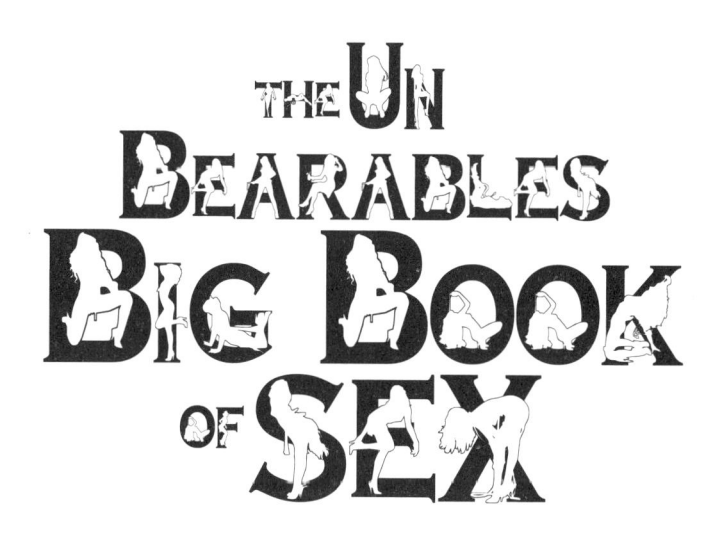

THE UNBEARABLES BIG BOOK OF SEX

EDITED BY

RON KOLM
CAROL WIERZBICKI
JIM FEAST
STEVE DALACHINSKY
YUKO OTOMO
& SHALOM NEUMAN

AUTONOMEDIA / UNBEARABLE BOOKS

ISBN: 978-1-57027-233-2

Donald Breckenridge's piece is an excerpt from his forthcoming novel *This Young Girl Passing* (Unbearable Books/Autonomedia, 2011); Denise Duhamel's 'Or Wherever Your Final Destination May Be' was published in *The Normal School*, Volume 2, Issue 1 (Spring 2009); Susan Mauer's poem was previously published in *The Hollins Critic*; Eve Packer's poem 'at sally's' was previously published in her book *Playland Poems 1994–2004* (Fly By Night Press, 2005); Thad Rutkowski's story was published in his recent book, *Haywire* (Starcherone Books, 2011); Max Blagg's 'Nights in White Satin' appeared in *Ten Men/ Spring Summer* 2010; Ron Kolm's piece was published in *Sensitive Skin Magazine* online; Penny Arcade's text is from the performance piece, *Longing Lasts Longer*; Tsaurah Litzky's story, 'Run-In,' was published in *Got A Minute* (Cleis Press, 2007); Roberta Allen's 'Hot' was published in *The Brooklyn Rail* (Nov. 2007); Heather Austin's piece, 'Five Moments of Marjane,' was published in *Pequin* online (2007); Chavisa Woods' poem appeared in *Danse Macabre* (The Stonewall Issue); John Farris' piece is from his novel, *The Ass's Tale* (Unbearable Books/Autonomedia, 2010); Steve Cannon's piece is excerpted from his novel, *Groove, Bang and Jive Around* (Genesis Press, 1998); Samuel Delany's piece is excerpted from his forthcoming book, *Through the Valley of the Nest of Spiders* (Magnus Books, Oct. 2011); Rami Shamir's piece is from the forthcoming novel of the same name, TRAIN TO POKIPSE; Diane Spodarek's 'Men & Cars' has appeared in several places: *Even More Monologues for Women by Women* (Heinemann Drama, 2001), *Millennium Monologs* (Meriwether Publishing, 2002) and *Young Women's Monologues from Contemporary Plays* (Meriwether, 2004); Jonathan Lethem's 'Man Jet or Eros in Transit' appeared in *Nerve*.com (2000); Sharon Mesmer's poem was previously published in her book, *Annoying Diabetic Bitch* (Combo Books, 2007); Doug Nufer's piece is from *Omo the Only*, an unpublished novel where adjacent words have no letters in common; Lynn Crawfords's story 'Meg' is from a forthcoming book, *Shankus;* Carol Weirzbicki's poem first appeared in *Pink Pages* #10; Wanda Phipps' poems were first published in *Wake-Up Calls: 66 Morning Poems* (Soft Skull Press, 2004); Jerome Sala's poems are from *Look Slimmer Instantly!: Poems* (Soft Skull Press, 2005); Janice Eidus' story first appeared in *The Celibacy Club* (City Lights, 2001); Robert Hershon's poem was published in *Calls from the Outside World* (Hanging Loose Press, 2006); Arthur Nersesian's piece is from his novel, *Suicide Casanova* (Akashic Books, 2005); Mike Golden's 'Pain' is from *Giving Up the Ghost;* Elaine Equi's 'Alien Fantasy' appeared in *The Cloud of Knowable Things* (Coffee House Press, 2003); Anyssa Kim's poem is from *Ovarian Twists: New and Selected Poems* (Fly By Night Press, 2003); Gerard Malanga's poem is from *Three Diamonds* (Black Sparrow Press, 1991); Peter Werbe's piece was in *Fifth Estate;* and Michael Lindgren's 'Femme Fatale' was a review published in the Wilkes-Barre (PA) *Times-Leader Weekender*, 2002.

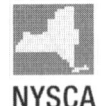

NYSCA

This publication is made possible in part with public funds from the New York State Council on the Arts, a state agency.

Autonomedia
POB 568 Williamsburgh Station
Brooklyn, New York 11211-0568 USA

info@autonomedia.org
www.autonomedia.org
www.unbearables.com

Printed in Canada

Table of Contents

5

Graphics Table of Contents

FROM I'M YOUR MAN
FLOYD SYKES

imes Square early on a summer Sunday is like a sleepy small town in its way; stores that aren't closed are almost deserted, sending music or television noises and the soft, always accented voices of bored clerks out into baking streets and sparse traffic. Those few people who are on the sidewalks by noon are likely to be the addicts desperate enough to come out early to score and dealers small-time enough to take their money. There are the homeless, there are always the homeless. There are the police. There are a few kids from the suburbs who don't know that nothing happens before dark. Any neatly dressed strangers hurrying through at this hour are almost certainly in town for the day from New Jersey or Long Island, heading from the bus or the PATH train to brunch and a matinee.

And Fred is here. About twelve-thirty he leaves his apartment near Ninth Avenue on his usual early Sunday walk. He has money in his pocket and he has his Walkman hooked on his belt, headphones plugged into his ears. He is here but he is not here, the music feeds his head, the music helps keep his feet just off these sidewalks and takes his mind wherever he wants it to be. The music is the score of a life he lives outside the life he lives; the music helps him be someone, somewhere, else. Inside the music he cannot die. Or fail, for long. He makes his own tapes, cannibalizing with obsessive care favorites he's culled from radio programs likely to play what he wants to hear. He will buy a tape for one song, spend hours half-listening to a background of prerecorded radio junk and chatter, waiting for the one uncollected treasure that makes it worthwhile. The right sound — and he has by now hundreds of hours of right sounds — acts like a drug on his mood, lifting him to just where he want to be, cocooned in the music, just above, just beyond, the world. Today he leaves the apartment with the Stones, "Start Me Up" — "If you start me up, I'll never stop..." By the time he reaches Eighth Avenue that's replaced by the Police, "...walk the streets for money, you don't care if it's wrong or right." No order, no sense, only the sound counts, the connection it has to the emotions that keep him just free from reality.

He walks the block, almost empty now, between Forty-third and Forty-second. The peep shows are open, here and on Forty-third; outside one a dirty-looking blond drag queen, eighteen or so — pink Lycra pedal pushers, a man's blue dress shirt tied off above the navel — leans against the wall, the slightly scared look of an addict who doesn't know where her next fix is coming from in her darting, mascaraed eyes. The Koreans whose corner store sells bags, wallets, sunglasses, caps, batteries — cheap goods, always in enough demand — are opening up but in no hurry. The one bar along the block to Forty-second is equally quiet; only drinkers damaged enough to be lost to time and the most self-consciously decadent slummers would be out this early. Fred moves on, past a couple of storefronts selling soda, junk food and drug basics — rolling papers, pipes, cigarette lighters — past the stale grease smell of a fried chicken restaurant, past the subway entrance. He crosses the street to the Port Authority Bus Terminal, where he is most likely to find a trick — that's what he's looking for, a boy, preferably new out here, attractive enough, interesting enough, to let him relax and spend the rest of Sunday doing something other than looking for sex. The Port is also where he's most likely to run into someone he has had and doesn't want again but who will ask for another chance, or at least for money. He dismisses the few early arrivals — no one new, no one interesting, but then no one he has to talk to — and crosses into the newer, uglier of the two buildings that make up the terminal. The effect is of an aging decrepit mall — noisy escalator, cracked yellowing floors, too many empty spaces among too many businesses with too few customers. He takes the escalator up to the second floor and walks down a couple of long hallways to the bowling alley in the older building, its small video game arcade empty at this hour except for the uniformed guard playing something quick, watched by one of the terminal's plainclothes cops. He takes a second escalator down, past the bank of pay phones where half a dozen Mexican youths sometimes hang out, sometimes making themselves available.

No one there either.

He goes up another escalator, making his rounds, as two perfect boys just off a bus from somewhere, baseball caps at tough angles, strong tan legs and arms in summer shorts and tank tops, pass him going down the parallel escalator and head for the exit. They are not part of the life he lives. He regrets them and forgets them. They can't be anything to him. Upstairs two men Fred has seen around for years, two of the dozens he walks among and competes with for the same favors from the same boys, slowly trace this route all of them take regularly, watchful for any likely newcomers. There are none right now; the only one looking to sell instead of buy is a heavy effeminate young man in a blue warm-up suit. He is too old, too gay, too overweight. Fred and the others barely need a glimpse to reject him.

Someone Fred took home once is standing outside the building, leaning back with one foot up on the brick wall behind him, smoking a cigarette. He approaches, embarrassed, ducking his head, not looking Fred in the eye for two seconds at a time, knowing he will be rejected but too needy not to try. Fred must have known his name once but it's lost in a jumble of the half-remembered. Tito? Luis? Something Spanish. Whoever he is he is tall and slender, around twenty, pleasant-looking with long carefully combed curly hair. Fred had been attracted not so much by his nice enough face as by his build, by the long striding walk, purposeful and masculine, the air of confidence. Which turned out to be a lie, so far as this, so far as selling sex was concerned. He was, to begin with, too thin, fat and poorly muscled, with too much body hair. And then he hardly managed to perform at all, rubbing pre-come from the tip of Fred's dick so hard it hurt, squeezing his nipples painfully, mechanically — doing everything too fast, too hard. Unpleasant sexual details attach more firmly than names.

Now he wants to try again, mumbles a few promises including a hurried, eyes-averted, "I do anything with you this time," that is intriguing but Fred shakes his head, gives his usual "Just walking around right now" line and pulls out two of the singles he keeps in folded pairs in his pocket for just these occasions. The young man slinks back wordlessly to lean against the wall and wait some more.

Fred continues his walk, thrown off his hopeful high by this intrusion, uninspired by Boston, "It's been such a long time" — it has, too, since he's found anyone out here worth the time he puts in. He smiles and goes on. He knows that the music is always effortlessly ironic and tells himself this awareness is one of the things that keeps him from falling beyond hope.

Right now there are no other familiar faces for him to cringe at the sight of, no more "no's" and excuses and evasions and crumpled dollar bills to pass out:

"What's up, Fred?"

"Just walking around right now."

"You be back later? I gotta make, you know, not all that much this time. I wanna get out of here."

"Yeah, well, maybe later."

"What time you be back?"

"I don't know. Maybe I won't. Don't know for sure what I'll do."

"You could buy me a slice? And a soda?"

And so on. Always vain attempts to pin down times and turn brush-offs into promises, always silenced with a couple of dollars. Fred has a problem with simple "no's"; feelings might be hurt, hostility awakened. He can find reasons to feel guilty and he can't deal with hostility.

He starts back up Eighth, ready to go home to rest for another round later — there's always later, always hope all out of proportion to what experience has taught will be there and available. Later there may be someone new. And maybe the someone new will be younger and fresher than the usual pack of used-looking, twenty, twenty-five year olds. When he comes back in an hour, not one person he's seen on this first pass might still be around, although more likely, of course, most of them will; chances are the men strolling the halls, the effeminate young man waiting upstairs, Fred's former trick, all will be around for large chunks of the day. As Fred will be himself, moving or standing among the shifting population of regulars and one-timers, sellers and buyers, the compulsive and the merely curious, all looking for the one real right thing, waiting out the heat to feed their Times Square daydreams well into the night.

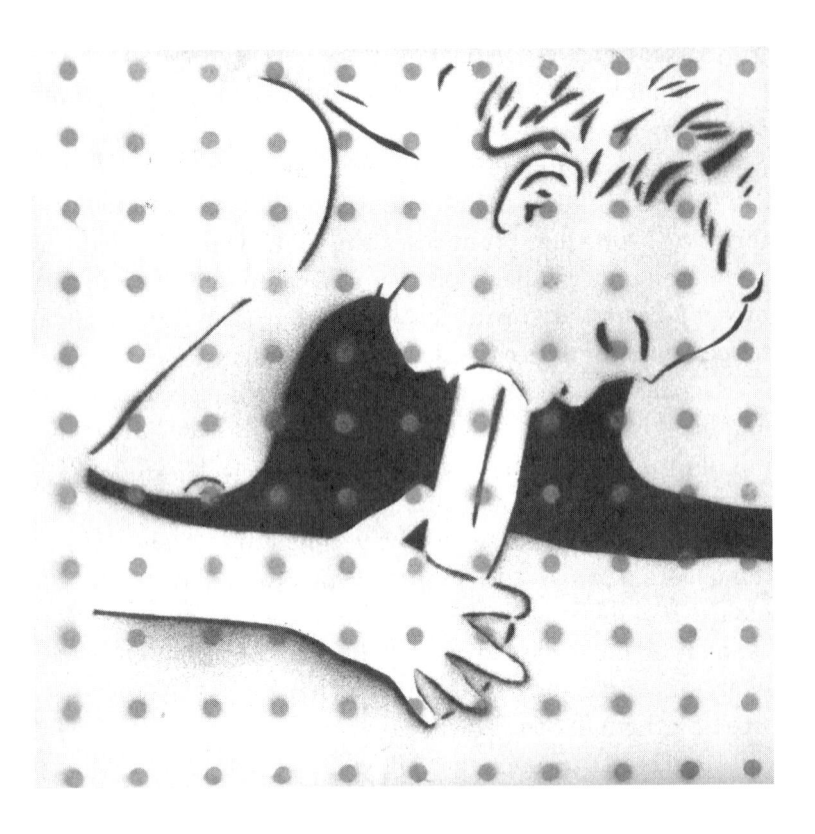

"I GOT YOU"
JILL RAPAPORT

She held Tom's arm as they walked west. In her mind's eye was the sublevel length of pavement where she knew that a wrought iron railing separated the street from the trash cans. She would take him there. Actually the idea was not firm in her mind. It began to jell as they crossed Eighth Avenue.

"Where are you walking me?" he asked in his peremptory baritone, slightly scratchy — which she found exciting.

"I don't know," she said.

They continued west. At that time, there was nothing past Tenth Avenue. It was long before the buildup and the new parks, the dog runs, the esplanades and the innovative condo towers full of angles and colored Pez tiles. It was a seedy outlying area where seedy business types rented rooms in the dilapidated corner building over the "gentlemen's club." She imagined them removing polyester jackets with loose threads hanging from them. Tom would never have been caught dead in a joint like that.

She was hungry and thought with some sharpness about a green apple. Maybe she could find one later in one of the delis. Though most of these fell away this close to the far western avenues. She didn't dare eat much when she was with him. She wanted to preserve what there was of her catlike fitness. He would ask if she weren't hungry and though she was, she'd mutter something about a bad stomach or a fragile esophagus. She did not want him to think she was trying to watch her weight. It spoiled the illusion of carelessness she had fostered from the beginning. His hand on the small of her back began to clutch and she looked up at him (he was very tall and almost dwarfed her, which most of them couldn't, as she herself was tall); he smiled down at her in that moony way that always unsettled her. She was in fact of two minds about it: it put her off in the sense that it defanged him, but on the other hand it also appealed to her in its disarmingness. If he wanted to play the gentle giant, it wasn't the worst thing. Besides, there were ways to take care of that if refanging him was what she wanted to do.

Lucky for her that she had had two drinks before; otherwise, she wasn't sure how she would have thought to brazen him down to the sublevel passage. They were getting near Ninth and the passersby coming toward them were fewer. One man looked at them boldly and she wondered what he was thinking. Maybe that he envied Tom for having her? That he wanted to supplant him and take her away? Or that she was a little too fat or that her hair was messy? That her clothes weren't in fashion? She knew the black boots were past their prime and sort of stupid looking and wished she hadn't ever bought them, but, having bought them, she couldn't afford not to wear them.

The street enveloped them in darkness. But on the other side were lined-up globe lights in front of the whitish townhouses that all looked a little sorry and ramshackle. This was a part of the city that seemed to have gotten stuck in an old decade. Few pedestrians, no shops, and the cars like big moving humps scuttling past.

Soon the passageway came into view. She studied it nonchalantly as they walked, trying to discern where one got in. All the buildings were the same and all had the passageway; it was common to all of them and was where the trash got taken. But it was dark and there was scaffolding covering some of the building fronts. Tom didn't seem perturbed; she did not know what was going through his mind, but she knew she would have to find some way down there before they got to the end of the block.

She thought of her glory. It was about to be left in a heap at the curb. She would take him down below the level of the street, where decorum of some sort still governed, and she would become even if just for a few minutes a base, cheap version of her highborn self. Refuse regina.

Bus and taxis passing. Elderly dog hobbling on its leash, leading a callous "master."

Fleeting sound of a woman's voice: "The baby needs to sleep now." It was one of those squeaky, high voices that she had just started noticing around town, mired in domesticity and ignoble to the core. And here was she, about to go below the level of the street.

She thought she felt a stone in her sock. It kept moving around in there. No doubt the hole in the sock had let it in, and she grieved to think of yet another pair that was no longer good.

Tom was like a big, bony rag doll. He flopped where she made him flop and then wherever else she made him flop. And every now and then he complained about being taken for granted.

They were a block from the next avenue. Soon they'd be all the way over at the wholesale beer dispensary and the disused overpass; a note of panic hit her. Rag doll he might be, but she was finding her pelvis in chaos, her courage awol. She had actually never possessed a lot of that sterling virtue, in spite of the effusions heaped on her by allies and supporters. As she had discovered when first trying to step onto an escalator, the hardest part was the stepping on. Her mother had practically had to carry her onto the moving stair when they went to the Coliseum Gem Show, and this was when she was already nine and nearly taller than either parent (she had outstripped them both by the age of seventeen). The reason was that, where she had come from, it had been so rural that the escalator hadn't been instituted yet, and she had arrived unprimed in the huge city. So it was step, step, step, and with each, the inner shaking grew more pronounced, and that first escalator wasn't even very long or very fast.

He strolled next to her, his angular body inspiring in her a dread mixed with exaltation. My, he was like the nicest of El Grecos, walking lankily (clodhopperishly, really) by her side, not showing fear or uncertainty.

O well-articulated shoulders, O pale-complected birthday suit, O hands that grasped tenderly, high up upon the loftbed of middle resort, amid airs of a procrustean jouissance....

They had met in that narrow old bar that was by fantastic coincidence right next door to the first building she had lived in in New York. She had been away, and was exhilarated and intoxicated with herself for having traveled through a European city alone, if you didn't count useless Emil. They saw each other right away. They tried fitting themselves together using desire for glue. He was certainly beneath her in some aspect of social standing, but he loomed above her in height; and his family undoubtedly had been more successful at attaining status in America. His mom had worked for *TV Guide* or something and his dad taught Greek. And Tom was one of those rabid Mumia agitators, or could have been. No, scratch that, he was too middle-class (or not middle-class enough?) to have been a

Mumia agitator. He had defended himself from bullies in the local grade school and all he'd had to do was use his immense size. They'd picked on him because he was gangly and had intellectual parents and he'd prevailed against them for the same reasons. Had he not come from the prosaic local reservoir, he would have been one of those wooden statues of Spanish martyrs, limbs rising into the air, neck twisting unanatomically, unearthly light source under the skin. But he had come from the reservoir. He drank milk and beer. He watched TV.

He patted her on the butt, fondly, and tenderly spoke corninesses into her ear as she recoiled inwardly, swooned outwardly, doing her own agonized twisting. How could she love a person into whose open cranium she could gaze, like a surgeon or a pathologist? And yet, the way he put those long arms around her torso and with his hands made other moves....

***

A glint of pewter caught her eye and she realized with suddenness that here was an opening. Why she had not seen others was something to be sorted out some other night. The metal cans were lined up in a neat row and all their tops were on. They were fluted and chained together, and the slight smell of raw trash only added to the piquancy and thrill of the tableau. And here was our up-at-heels queen, descending as if with train and retinue and leading him by the hand as, slowly coming aware, he began to expostulate: "Huh... where're we going, babe?" Scratch that: it wasn't he who had used that hokey and proletarian diminutive, it was Keith, left behind five years ago in the ruins of the tiny blue-carpeted cave where they had once lived as a couple. She thought by now he must have packed up and moved to New Orleans, where all the men she liked hanging around with wound up going at some point or other. Tom just called her "you," or sometimes, in a high-lonesome whine, called her by her name. Her cowrie-shell earrings seemed to call to her in an echo of that whine, which in his case came from adenoids and, in the case of the shells, from the African ocean.

"Stand there," she said as she pushed him against the low wall at the top of the ramp, "and tell me if you hear anybody coming."

And then as he watched, incredulously, this lady whom he had held on his lap in the bar, this female who had become like a doll by virtue of spending time with him in his great and superior height, this exemplar of the contra-dictions in the feminine who spoke in opalescent flames about the things she hated and the things that made her furious, among which she sometimes included him, knelt facing him and undid his fly, and with fierce hands and other things gave him several "jobs" the like of which he hadn't had since seeing a prostitute in twelfth grade, when another boy had dragged him along. She disappeared into the mass of shadows folding around his thighs, and he felt his long neck twist back at an unlikely angle as he swooned.

Variation: "Sex"

Can't discuss it in detail with the upbringing I had, but I took Clovis by the hand one night and escorted him to the railing on the shadowy street where the lower level ran for the trashcans and out of view (just barely) of the street. Took him by the hand down to the lower level and faced him, then got down low and undid his belt. He made faint protests that were full of the opposite: a clotted joy, a turgid ecstasy. He was bemused; his muse was being bad. But he couldn't either complain or rejoice completely, so he just surrendered to me, helpless. We stayed there a while, I getting lower and lower and he throwing his head back — or his head fell back — and he looked at the stars through half closed eyes then down at his muse and star half kneeling on the concrete at the side of the building. Then that dampness and odor of something plasticky and like mushrooms and up and we walked to the end of the long avenue block and around the corner and around the next corner back on the side street and to his little yellow building with a semi-peaked roof. And up the creaking linoleumed stairs and into his two rooms that smelled of dried things. And this display of mine had never been made before and was never again. It just came into my mind to do it and I did. It all came from my impatience with the walk by the recreation center, the visit to his workplace, the Gateway, after hours, the lingering together on high stools at the bar, the twiddling my thumbs waiting for the shy boy to call and finally calling myself.

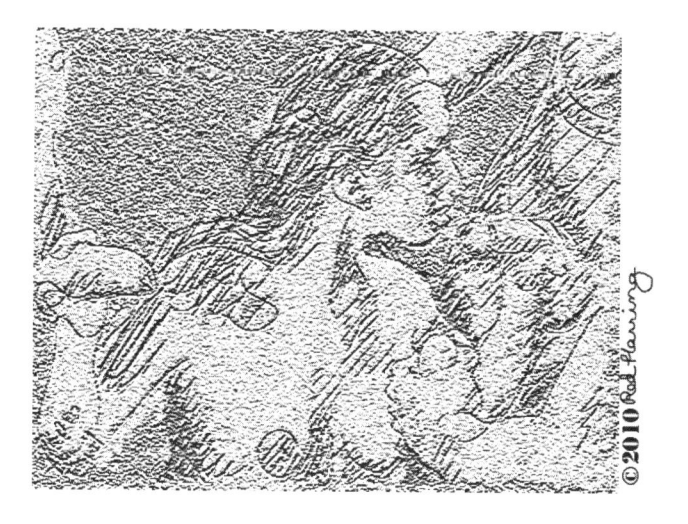

BEAUTY IS AS BEAUTY DOES
BART PLANTENGA

An ex-girl-friend-stripper-artist once told me that being beautiful — as painful as she found it to admit — was just as bad as being ugly, an Achilles heel, a burden that people hate you for. She may have called it "beauty persecution" or something like that.

Well, Emke saw it differently. Emke considered her considerable beauty to be like a lead guitar, the bumper on a '62 Cadillac, a backlit Ingres in the Louvres, a spring-loaded firearm…. Her beauty, simply put, made others nauseous. It had a destabilizing effect in crowds. Imagine Marilyn Monroe stepping off the Whirl-i-gig into Madison Square Garden during a cock fight. Everyone suddenly gets up off their haunches, standing erect as if saluting the flag, silent and humble for a few endless seconds as their cocks scurry about. Some people will never understand this almost vengefully ecstatic, life-fucking aspect of beauty.

Needless to say, it was great being seen with Emke; it was esteem by association as revenge for all the sins of those who did not take me seriously. And suddenly one day I'm walking around like Sly Stone or Grace Jones or somebody with a character-enhancing crick in his left knee.

I met Emke at a benefit for a battered women's shelter at CB's Gallery I'd been invited to perform at by Prudence P. — the stipulation being that I had to be cross-dressed to participate. Three hours of connived artfulness by PP and

VV, and I looked intriguingly like a young Joan Crawford. But I'm not the one to ask because I was high as the Acid Queen, having picked this auspicious evening with a city councilwoman, VV and Susan Sontag in the audience, nursing non-alcoholic drinks, with their six knees tightly cramped under a wobbly sliver of café table to test the psylocybin mushrooms that friends had been cultivating in their Brooklyn basement.

Evidence of their efficacy: I was queen with a boundless love for all mankind, warmly reading my short story about an aborted affair with Andy Warhol, well not with him, but with his wigs. An apprenticeship for which Warhol expressed his gratitude in his own affectless remunerative-affectionate way. I could *feel* the audience listening, grooving, repeating, masticating my every word like some gastronomic delicacy. People followed me into the bathroom to just gaze. One couple stood stiffly before me to declare: "You remind us of Rita Hayworth in *Gilda*."

"Yeah, a Rita a little melted around the edges."

People with names and affiliations shook my hand, squeezing it just ever so suggestively. You know, when someone grabs your hand with both their hands and doesn't let go? Did I really agree to work on the councilwoman's reelection campaign in the West Village?

Emke walked over to my table where I was sitting with PP who had come to NY to win the Marilyn Monroe Look-A-Like Contest sponsored by *Esquire* and L'Oreal. Was it the mushrooms or was I having my picture taken by a *Daily News* photographer flanked by — yes — *two* Marilyn Monroe look-a-likes? They gazed at and *into* each other like two women meeting in a strange psychic seam, at a crossroad where the personae they have assumed will either take hold or float away like a cool wraith-like breeze passing over us.

I wanted to pronounce the word *döppelganger* right, but when I did it sounded like the name of a utility infielder for the Milwaukee Brewers. And Emke and PP continued peering into one another's eyes and shaking hands as if their arms had become detached from their bodies.

"I have to meet you," Emke said in a warm, breathless whisper. She pressed a tightly folded wad of paper into my palm, "You're an impressive woman."

"So are you."

"I've been practicing longer'n you." She was gone. I stuffed the wad securely in my pocket and checked countless times on the way home to make sure I had not lost it.

I went to her place on East 20-whatever street, sniffed my underarms, took a deep breath before ringing her doorbell.

She greeted me in a low slung gown tied at the waist with a fancy sash "borrowed" from the Frick. She leaned mythically in her doorway as if there was a world of bedding and boudoir behind her. She stepped onto the welcome mat, closed the door behind her, fiddled with the doorknob behind her back. This did not bode well.

"I'm really, really, really sorry but this hand-puppet troupe from Berkeley breezed in a day earlier than expected. There's seven of them staying with me. It's like the Marx Brothers' stateroom scene but not as funny. They're stayin' a week; they've appealed to my weakness for good causes, which is to convince East Coasters to shed their leather shoes for shoes made of hemp."

"You can smoke'm after they wear out."

"Not that kinda hemp. They brought wine and they don't mind if you come in. We won't hang out with them. The tall guy with the dreads, he's my ex as in capital E, capital X. X right through his photo with a kitchen knife but that's long ago. He's better as a guy I just know."

"Really?"

"No, I'm making it up, he's going to decapitate you while you're making love to me."

After meeting the Punchin' Breaded Puppet Theatre, we retreated to her bed, in what the landlord listed as another room but was really just an oversized dresser drawer with a mattress stuffed into it, wedged under the staircase.

"My roomie's out of town — in detox, a kind of Betty Ford Clinic for underemployed genius post-punkers of a certain vintage."

Her silken bathrobe came undone as if by push button, will or magic. No amount of poetry, anatomy classes or pubescent studies of *Playboy* had properly prepared me for the perfection of her breasts. Awestruck is probably a good term here. We shared a bottle of wine, spending a long time trying to pronounce "beaujolais," repeating it until it took on a life of its own — Bo Joe Lay, Boo Shoe Lay, Bow Shjo Lay — until the giggles led to incursions of a most opportunistic kind, laughter as land mine removal, and the word "beaujolais" now meant just about anything to do with sex.

"I wondered about you and now the wonder is to be wonderfully consummated." And the way we slid together was so *glissando* that the fine lines between reverie and reality, between her quivering wishbone and my sinister prominence became a seamless weld of giggle and sigh, of heaving and delight. You must know this feeling. If you do not, you will just have to settle for religion or the big spiraling slide down at the pool.

"I'm really annoying when I come,[1] so, with respect for the present company, despite their didgeridoo music drowning us out, I cannot allow you to get me off here inside this…"

"Dresser drawer?'

"Le's go in the hallway. Discretion and all that..." A corridor of dog crap brown, mental institution green and jimmied open mailboxes. She shoved me under the staircase and yanked my pants down, spread some Chinese menus across the floor like autumn leaves so that her knees would not touch the truly gruesome fake-tile curling-cracking-pocked-with-cigarette-burns-melted-into-it linoleum.

Under the flickering hall light and in full sight of the front door, she sucked me off and at the moment of moanful crisis, she cocked my appendage, squeezing it and then cocked it forward and suddenly back to create a unique pump-action: My cock became a kind of firearm with the ejaculant hurled outward like a slow-motion Hollywood bullet hitting the wall with such force that I swear we could hear it as it dented the flaked-paint wall. My legs went gumby as we watched the sperm drool down the wall.

She held "me" firmly, bent over, gave it an Eskimo nose kiss before helping me back into my pants. "I'm intense, I don't stop at flesh till I get to the marrow. Now get outta here."

She passed by SS's studio to see where I "worked," dressed in a green fuzzy bathrobe — not much else, well, a halter, hotpants, heels — the 3 Hs. She wanted to hang — swoon — because, although beautiful, she was lonely, found NYC gals bitchy and was still clueless [at age 23!] about how to actually apply beauty to talent or talent to beauty.

The sickly light from the dangling fluorescent light fixtures hummed inside the powdery air, thread and tufts of fabric strewn about, columns wrapped in fabric, phone artistically melted into the shape of a steak, posters of basketball stars dressed in strange socks, no windows and a rack of CDs that bred pure contempt: Loggins & Messina, John Denver, Midnight Oil, Lionel Ritchie, Jew-2, an Israeli U-2 cover band.

"Ugh, these CDs are *definitely* an occupational hazard….
I bet you missed me — and my orifices."

"They DO function exceptionally well."

She sat down, "That's because they are so finely tai-
lored," on my lap, "to your wildest dreams."

"I just haven't found an on-off switch." She began writhing
on top of me as we wheeled around in the office chair.

"What's SS do anyhow?"

"Socks."

"He washes'm?"

"No, he designs'm."

"Tube socks must be the bane of his existence."

"I love a beautiful woman who uses 'bane' correctly." I
made Triumph TR6 engine noises.

"The real bane of his existence is the nagging feeling
that people will find out he's sham."

Her hand operated the stick shift as she made her own
vaginal Moulinex sounds. We twirled and zoomed across
the studio doing the office-chair waltz.

"Remember those socks with the different colored toes
like gloves for your feet, well, he invented those. He made a
fat million."

"That is creepy. Any chance anybody's comin' by?"

"Pro'ly."

"Let's go in there and see what's going on," she pointed
to the bathroom with its floor to ceiling mirrors, sock
images, an old *Laugh-In* "Sock it to me" poster, toilet paper
with his logo on it.

"Guy's creepy. Isn't he like half-Jewish or something?
Isn't a lightning-bolt SS logo asking for trouble?"

I took her from behind in the style of an old porn movie
and there was this electricity that shivered across her skin
as if her veins were electrified barbed wire. The hipbones

engage in a slithering, butter-churning movement, clavicle handholds for leverage, the febrile flexing of her buttocks, a place I didn't know even had muscles. And BOOM like that she becomes a craving werewolf with a Moulinex vagina running on 600 watts.

She pushed me to the concrete floor, buttons and pins sticking to my back. She sat on my face and holding my appendage for leverage, rocked so hard that her pubic hair chafed my face and it was finally my nose that sent her into the throes of orgasm. But orgasm, like cocaine addiction, demands more until the mind becomes a greedy suction device of unrequited need. And as my culmination arrived [67 minutes!] she squeezed my member, we stood up and then — yes, that pump action again — the sperm — WHOOOM! — shot a good ten feet onto the mouse pad. The glob glistened like a snail under moonlight.

"I'm a naughty meat puppet," she said as she manipulated my member, making the urethra mouth her words — yes — just like Shari Lewis used to with her Lambchop. "I am SO sorry."

"Insatiability is my Achilles heel. I'm *never* satisfied."

"I will always be ready to service you," I heard my urethra say. "You have the international human right to have your desires satisfied within a reasonable period of time."

I yanked up my pants and went to wipe up the sperm but she said: "Leave it, it'll mark our territory and prove that sex trumps senseless labor any day."

Fearing SS's return — he often worked evenings — we retreated, tumbled [stumbled?], north to Max Fish, me with the scent of pussy worn as aftershave and her breath smelling suspiciously of humid gonad and pheromone.

It was 10 PM — early in Fish time — a few stragglers escaping airco-less hovels. We sat at the bar balancing on wobbly [funhouse-purchased?] barstools. After only one Fuzzy Navel she was already teetering, admitting "I get drunk easy." We tried to behave, balancing on the stools, perusing the *New York Press.*

She whispered: "I'm gonna put the *Press* across your lap so's I can fish out yer dick cuz I just wanna play with it."

She surreptitiously fished "me" out. Reverting to her best Shari Lewis, she recited:

"'Oh mother, I have had such a fright! I saw a great creature strutting about on two legs. On his head was a red cap'…"

"Whazzat?"

"'All at once he stretched his loooong neck and opened his mouth so wiiiiide, and roared so loud, that I thought he was going to eat me up, and I ran home as fast as I could'…"

"Whazzat from?"

"My childhood. 'My dear child, the fierce thing you speak of would have done you no harm. It was a harmless cock' … Aesop, you sap!"

We embraced, her kneeling on the wobbly barstool. People from under ironic baseball caps yelling "WHOA!"

"I feel so close. Like we're co-conspirators." I felt a sudden tug and change in her demeanor. She whispered in my ear that she was watching some guy videotaping us in the mirror. Which only encouraged her to greater emboldenments. "This is as close to a movie career as I'm gonna get."

She faked spilling a drink, got a bead on the voyeur culprit[2] and smirked right into his camera as she dabbed my lap, exposing my half-erect member to the camera, twisting it so that the urethra could make a statement for the camera: "I am empowered to service her pursuit of happiness." Leaning down, she gave "me" an Eskimo kiss, then stood up, approached the camera to declare: "We are a perfect love team. Me with my perfect breasts, hungry pussy and attitude and him with his perfect dick." The boys in their strategically disheveled work shirts hunched in closer, clutching their pool cues.

She turned to the *bartendress*, an ethereal waif of terror, to declare: "He's got a perfect dick."

"So do I," she responded, as if nothing meant nothing and who cares.

Months later, I received a letter from friend Christine. In the envelope was a photo of the inside of Max Fish I'd instructed her to take as repayment for letting her crash on my couch. It showed the two barstools — one red, one green — me and Emke had commandeered that night.

I framed and hung this photo in my bathroom, which has allowed me to write this story and, whenever anyone asks, it allows me to climb into the cockpit to become a voyeur ravaging my own dream when for a short period of time ecstasy stopped all clocks, all aging processes, canceled all rental contracts, erased all memory, all the run-up beer tabs, something years of therapy could never hope to accomplish.

Notes

[1] P.J. Harvey plays a *castrati* in a Derek Jarmen film or the bleat of an injured mountain goat.

[2] Dan Queezie doing "field research" for his public access Channel 25 TV show, *Porn to Run*. Carol said she saw us on TV. Said she liked Emke's energy.

LAWRENCE FERLINGHETTI BOOK PARTY
AT GOTHAM BOOKMART
ERIK LA PRADE

he first book party at the new Gotham for Lawrence Ferlinghetti took place during early June 2005. In the process of ordering copies of his new book from the publisher, I began to collect every Ferlinghetti book I could find in the store, a vast number but nothing unique or rare. The invitations for this book party were printed and mailed out from Gotham. Then, Ferlinghetti's publisher, New Directions, also mailed out a set of invites. On top of this, an advertisement appeared in *The Village Voice* announcing Ferlinghetti's reading at Gotham. All of this publicity created a stampede of his fans that descended on the store that evening.

Whenever there was a book event, I'd usually leave work early to come home and walk and feed my dog, then I'd go back so I could stay to eight p.m. to cover it. My job was to circulate in the crowd and look out for shoplifters. On this particular day, I returned to work about five o'clock. When I got to the building, there were two police cars double parked outside the store, and AB was standing in the street. I walked over to him and he began to explain what happened.

It was Marie, the housekeeper's job to prepare food, snacks, etc., before an event. She would spend half a day in AB's kitchen, organizing trays of food. On this particular afternoon, it seems, Lois, a part-time bookkeeper, decided that she was also going to work in the kitchen to prepare some of the food. When Lois saw Marie putting pepper on the Munster cheese, a Romanian custom, she began to protest.

As a result, Marie physically pushed her out of the kitchen. Of course, Lois saw this as an assault and called the police. Why Lois didn't come to him to explain the problem seemed to confuse AB. The whole incident quickly blew over as the official book party was scheduled to begin at six p.m.

We made the mistake of letting people up to the third floor as soon as they arrived. By six thirty, it was jammed with freeloaders, Beat generation fans, academics and a large contingent of downtown poets and punks. The crowd on the first floor had to wait for the elevator as AB didn't want people walking up and down the stairwell. This created another problem as the elevator was slow and could only hold five people. AB took it upon himself to operate it, and that's where he stayed most of the evening, missing his own party.

Ferlinghetti sat at a large table and signed copies of all his books people stuck in front of him. By seven-thirty, every copy of *Coney Island of the Mind* was sold out. It was the book to get even more than the book Ferlinghetti was doing the signing for. Ferlinghetti played the old Beat, giving off the impression he was the spokesman for the whole Beat generation now that Ginsberg, Corso and Burroughs were dead. Whether he liked the role or not, he worked it well. He got up to read some poems around seven-forty-five and the crowd made room for him. By eight o'clock, the store began to thin out but there was still a mass of people hanging out.

By now, AB had stopped conducting traffic and stepped off the elevator to mingle: he and Ferlinghetti went into his office and as they sat there, they simply looked like two old book dealers.

There was a long black leather couch on the third floor of Gotham in the front, facing the windows. It was one of the most popular spots for employees to eat lunch, take a break, or just relax and read. Generally, AB was never on the third floor after twelve o'clock, so it was a safe area. There was a beautiful, Chinese lacquer table with a glass top situated in front of the couch and opposite this table was a cloth sofa, facing in. The whole front area was tastefully arranged with tables and deco-styled table lamps and two very large, antique, wooden bird cages with no birds in them.

But it was the leather couch that caught my imagination because it seemed comfortable and offered an ideal place to get laid. If you were lying down you couldn't be seen, since the couch faced the front windows. Anyone coming off the elevator would have to walk the whole length of the room to see if someone was indeed lying prone on the couch.

The late afternoon was probably the best time to have a tryst on this couch. But sometimes AB scheduled meetings with his lawyers on the third floor and then it was off limits to us peasants. Eventually, I did get laid on a black leather couch, similar to the one on the third floor of Gotham, but the event occurred in another apartment.

About a month after Kato Ghondi, the surrealist painter, died in September 2002, I got a phone call from a woman, named Denise, who was writing a biography on someone Ghondi had known; an art collector and dealer. She wanted to interview me regarding Ghondi's relationship with him. I said okay and met her for lunch the next day. I had some letters and knew the story of Ghondi's life as I had briefly worked for him; I knew of his relationship with this collector.

Denise had written some prestige books on people, generally filled with little-known facts about her subject's lives, private or public sexual preferences, formerly unknown lovers, bisexual encounters, literary successes and failures. Her last biography managed to piss off enough relatives and friends of her subject that the book wasn't reviewed in *The New York Times,* and as she told me, if you're not reviewed in *The Times Book Review,* your book doesn't exist.

Our interview went well and I was able to provide Denise with information from some of Ghondi's letters. About two weeks later, I found myself reading a four-hundred page manuscript of her book. I also began taking her on studio visits to meet New York artists she had never heard of. It was extra work for me but I didn't mind going out of my way as we'd become friends. She was meeting artists who were the real deal, picking their brains for information and ideas, all to write a better biography.

During the night of the Ferlinghetti book party at Gotham, Denise showed up about seven-thirty. She had just come from a party at her agent's office and the effect of two or three martinis showed. This was my first encounter with her drunk. While Denise was engaged in a conversation with some academic writer, I was busy looking out for shoplifters. At eight-thirty, the crowd began to thin out. Denise and I decided to leave. She was drunker after having two glasses of wine. We made our way to the first floor where a crowd was mulling about. During our exit, Denise continued talking with the same writer who followed us outside and lingered on the street with us. When I told him I was taking her home, he backed off and gave her his card. Then she kissed him goodnight. As we were walking away, I asked her if she knew him and she said no.

I wanted to get a taxi as it was raining mildly and in one hand I was juggling an umbrella and carrying a bag of books, while with my other hand, I was steadying Denise. But she didn't want to get a taxi, she wanted to walk; so we walked in the rain, heading west on Forty-Sixth Street. By the time we got to Sixth Avenue, Denise had fallen twice; once in the middle of the street and again at the corner of Sixth Avenue and Forty-Sixth Street. I now had to hold her up with my right hand. As I stood on the comer with her, we made eye contact and began to kiss.

We would walk a few feet and stop, either to kiss or because I had to pick her up from the sidewalk. She continued to refuse to let me get a cab. Somehow, after half an hour, we managed to get to the Howard Johnson's restaurant on Seventh Avenue and Forty-Eighth Street. I thought eating something might help sober her up. So we went in and I ordered two cheeseburger deluxe specials and two Bloody Marys. Denise was too drunk to eat anything but she drank her Bloody Mary. I paid for everything, got a doggy bag to add to the collection of things I was carrying and we went outside. By now, she was having trouble even standing up. I managed to hail a taxi, then we got into the cab and she passed out onto the back seat, lying across it. I squeezed in next to her and gave the driver her address.

When we reached her building, we went upstairs to her apartment. Inside, Denise slowly began to sober up, but her coordination was so bad she continued to fall down as she navigated the rooms. She sat in a chair and immediately fell out of it by leaning too far sideways. I decided to stay there until her boyfriend came home. It was eleven o'clock by now and I was wet and tired, yet I kept my vest and leather jacket on because I felt chilled.

I put her into her bed and she began to pass out, then

got up and went into the bathroom to take a piss. As she sat on the toilet, I stood outside the open bathroom door, wondering whether or not she would fall off the toilet seat. When she saw me standing outside the doorway, she mumbled that she knew what I was after. Then she wiped herself, stood up and sat on the edge of the bathtub. She immediately slipped into the tub and cracked the back of her head on the tiled wall behind her.

I pulled her up and put her back into bed. At this point, she invited me to lie down beside her, so I did. I mentioned that her boyfriend also slept in the bed, so she got up and ran into the living room, falling onto the black leather couch. I sat down on it beside her.

By now, Denise was more awake and we began to make out. She pulled on my leather jacket, asking me to take it off, but I refused. I was apprehensive about her boyfriend opening the door and finding us locked together.

After she insisted I have sex with her the third time, I decided, what the fuck. I pulled her red panties off, opened her legs, and performed cunnilingus for about two minutes. I thought she'd like it until she told me it wasn't working for her. She took out my cock and I began to enter her, and then stopped when I heard a noise in the hallway. I paused for about ten long seconds then went back to fucking. By now I was overheated and nervous and she was moaning in my ear, "O please, O please." I came quickly and as I lay on top of her, she now told me she loved me, repeatedly. I had lent her my set of the first thirty issues of *Evergreen Review* magazines a month earlier, and I kept reminding myself not to forget to take them with me before I left her apartment.

We stood up and as I put my pants on, Denise put her panties on and went into the kitchen and got a soda. I was hungry and began to eat my cold cheese burger deluxe with

French fries. I asked her what time her boyfriend was coming home and she said any minute. She began to clean the sink and refrigerator as I sat there eating her cheese burger deluxe too. Then, she poured herself a glass of white wine. I didn't feel any regrets about having just had sex with her. It had just worked out that way. Then she began to tell me how she could feel cum dripping down her leg and that she wanted to fuck again. I decided I'd better get out of there, got my things, kissed her good night and walked to the bus stop. Of course, on the bus I realized I'd forgotten my set of *Evergreen Reviews* with the laid-in Henry Miller autograph.

The next day was Saturday. I went to work and as soon as I got into Gotham, I called Denise and asked how she felt. She said she felt "great and had had a great time." I was relieved she felt so chipper. I thought about having her come to my apartment and fucking there under different circumstances.

The next time we met was a week later on my day off. She wanted to go to The Strand. I wasn't inclined to go to a bookstore on my day off but I met her anyway. After visiting The Strand, I said, "Let's get a beer," but she declined; there was a marked change in her personality: "agenbit of inwit" as James Joyce wrote. I realized we weren't going to fuck again. What brought this change about I didn't know and didn't ask. Maybe she'd told her boyfriend or her therapist, but she offered no explanation. I was disappointed. We parted and again I thought of my set of *Evergreen Reviews* and how to get them back.

I saw her two more times. The first was in September. She and her boyfriend had just returned from Mexico. I met them for dinner and she gave me a present. It was a cheaply published pamphlet, the kind tourists can buy anywhere. The pamphlet was titled, *How to Make Love to a Woman*. I assumed it was her idea of a joke but I wasn't amused. I didn't know whether or not she'd told her boyfriend we'd fucked. On my way home, I threw it away and decided to dump my relationship with her.

The second time I saw her was after another book signing party at Gotham. It was an academic affair; a book of memoirs on Edmund Wilson edited by Wilson's son, Ruel. The book didn't sell very well but the wine was paid for by the publisher. Denise was there with her boyfriend and by eight o'clock she was loaded.

We managed to make it to a small hamburger stand located in the lobby of the Parker Meridian hotel on Fifty-Seventh Street, a small, trendy dive that was generally crowded. After ordering, we had to wait as all the tables and booths were taken. Somehow, Denise zeroed in on two guys having a conversation as they finished their meal. She went over to them and asked if they were leaving soon. One of the guys told her they were. Five minutes later she went over to their booth and began badgering them for not leaving. They laughed at her and she began to yell. To say she was making a scene was an understatement. Our order hadn't arrived but I continued to wait with two other people, while Denise's boyfriend took her home. I was glad I wasn't taking her home again. She needed a caretaker. I sent her boyfriend an e-mail suggesting he get her into AA, but I never got an answer.

On October 6, 2005, I was unpacking and shelving books in AB's walk-in safe. I stood on the top step of a ladder and as I overextended my reach, the small aluminum ladder slipped out from under me. I fell about four feet onto a concrete floor. I tried to break my fall by using my right wrist — which I managed to fracture. Since AB was sitting at his desk, he immediately came into the safe and saw me getting up from the floor, saw the broken ladder, and asked if I was all right. Luckily, I had managed not to fall on any boxes or first editions.

I mention this incident because it took me a week to go to a sports medicine doctor, have my wrist x-rayed and get fitted for a brace, which I now had to wear. Workers' Compensation paid for all of it — I never took a day off from work. During this whole period, I didn't hear from Denise and she wasn't returning my phone calls. I finally reached her and told her I was coming over to get my set of *Evergreen Reviews.* She said she had company and was going out later, so I told her I'd come in the afternoon. She agreed to wait.

I arrived at four and met her and her girlfriend. They were both wearing short house dresses and seemed put out by my presence. Her girlfriend was an older woman, a poet, but someone I'd never read before. I sat in a chair, opposite her girlfriend. I had a direct view of her and noticed she wasn't wearing any underwear as she sat there with her legs slightly apart. I kept looking away, and then back again, stealing a glance at her snatch.

I couldn't tell if Denise was wearing underwear but she seemed in a slightly agitated state from afternoon drinking. They acted like schoolgirls. In fact, this woman was one of her oldest girlfriends; they had met at boarding school years ago.

I had a distinct impression they were also lovers, but whether that was me projecting my lesbian fantasies, I wasn't sure. I think I was hoping all three of use would crawl into bed that afternoon. I was tempted to tell the girlfriend that Denise and I had fucked on the leather couch she was sitting on. But I lost my nerve. I just wanted to get away from them.

I told Denise to give me my magazines and she collected them in a shopping bag. I sat there and counted them, then left. On the bus ride, I examined each issue and then discovered my laid-in Henry Miller signature was still where I'd left it.

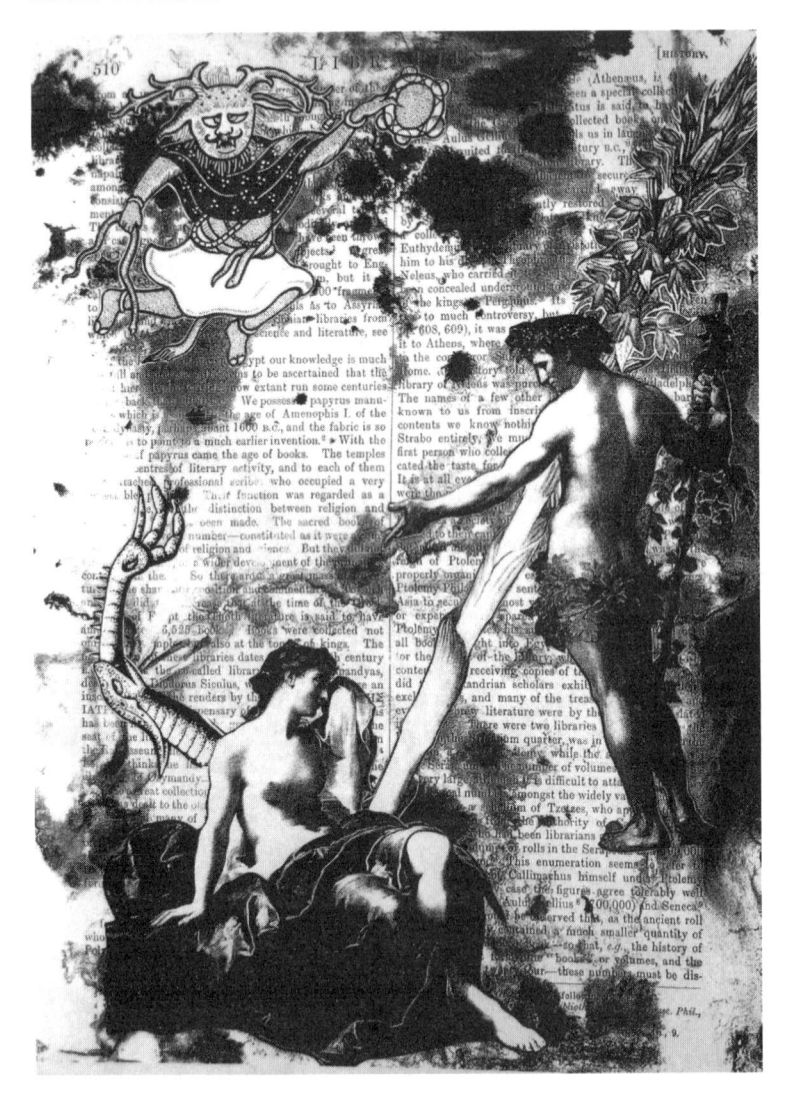

THE SUNDAY AFTER THANKSGIVING
ARTHUR KAYE

t was late afternoon, the Sunday after Thanksgiving, 1976. He couldn't remember exactly what he said, but it wasn't in anger he left, but in sadness and regret. He walked down to Riverside Park and then uptown for a long way, feeling empty. It was chilly and windy, and it wasn't too long before it began to get dark. He turned back towards Broadway and went into a pizzeria at W. 111th Street. He sat down with a hot slice. It wasn't good pizza. He looked up at a person who stopped at his table and was surprised to see Daniel Epstein, a stoned saxophonist — friend of some mutual friends.

"Man, you look like you want to go swimming in that pizza," Daniel said and then, uninvited, sat down in the seat opposite Josef with a slice and a soda.

"I'm okay," Josef said, resignation in his voice. Then, "Where's your sax? I don't think I've ever seen you without it."

"I'm cool," Dan smiled, spreading his hands, palms up. "I can't be playing all the time. Sometimes a man wants to lay it down, sometimes he picks it up, and sometimes he just needs a bite to eat. So what are you up to? I didn't know you hung around this part of town."

"I was just out for a walk. What's up with you? Still playing in that band?"

"Yeah, I'm in the band, but it isn't a great gig. I got a

new full-time job teaching. I dig passing it on to the kids."

Josef considered this. Daniel teaching made sense, so, good for him.

"You still see any of the other guys?" Josef asked.

"Some, the ones still in New York."

They both gnawed their way through their slices. Josef wasn't really in the mood for company. Walking away from Wendy still shook his world. It hadn't even been hours, yet here he was, sitting in a pizzeria acting as if everything was okay. Nothing was okay, the world was crumbling beneath his feet, a hurricane was rattling the windows of his mind. What was wrong with him? Why couldn't he win the heart of the woman he loved?

Daniel was finishing up and getting ready to go. It was too early to hit a bar and start drinking and too late to just hang around. Josef could see that Daniel was trying to figure out what he was going to do next.

"What's the matter?" Josef asked.

"Nothing much," Daniel responded. "I'm just feeling a little down. Girlfriend trouble, you know what I mean?"

"Tell me about it," Josef said. "What else is new?"

Daniel shrugged. "Lady I've been seeing, well, she wants to move in with me. I don't know if I'm ready."

"I hear you," Josef said.

They ended up on Riverside Drive, walking up to Grant's Tomb where they sat on the chilly steps tossing pebbles into the gravel, sharing a joint, quietly contemplating the puzzle of being in their mid-twenties and despairing over working things out, or not working things out, with their girlfriends.

Later on, sitting at the bar in the West End, they joked around for a while, then Daniel got up and parked himself in the phone booth. Josef watched him through the glass door, making up with his girlfriend. Daniel wouldn't sleep alone that night. The bartender filled Josef's mug again. A woman sat down on the stool next to him and asked him to pass the bowl of peanuts. Josef obliged, glancing at her. She was okay: brown curly hair, thin nose, thick lips, neither thin nor fat. He thought about chatting with her but what would he do if she responded? He wasn't in the mood to start something but he knew that getting laid would be a great way to start back on the road from heartbreak.

Daniel came back. He finished his beer, scooped up his change and put on his coat.

"I'm out of here," he said. "Laurie's willing to talk things over. I tell you, Joe, I may not be ready to live with her, but I want her."

Josef nodded. He understood. His situation was different and he knew there wasn't anything a phone call would do for him except make him sadder.

"Your friend's got girlfriend problems," the curly haired woman said, watching Daniel leave.

"Story of our lives," Josef replied without thinking.

"Tell me about it," she said. "Just as tough for us." She sipped her drink and popped some peanuts in her mouth. Josef saw that she had a nice face. "Sometimes it's easy, like when all a guy wants is sex."

"I think you're right," he said into his beer. "If all I wanted was sex, it would've been easy." He took a sip and turned toward the woman. "What's your story?"

"I got no story. I live in the neighborhood and I'd rather sit in the bar than have a drink at home alone."

"Do you have a boyfriend?" Josef didn't really care, but he'd rather she do the talking, so he kept asking questions.

"Nope, no boyfriend, no girlfriend and I don't want one." She ate a few more peanuts. "Relationships are problems. I'm better off by myself. No commitments, no fears, no angry accusations, no wondering if he loves me... nobody else's hair in the sink."

Josef nodded without conviction. I just walked out on the woman I love because I don't think she loves me, he thought. I'm not trying hard enough, but I guess you got to know when you can't win.

"Like I said, when all they want is sex, it's easy. But take a man home, cook him a meal, fuck him, let him sleep over and the next thing you know he wants to move in with you. I'm tired of men telling me they love me and then telling me how to live my life." She sounded a little pissed off.

"Somebody dump you?" Josef asked. He took a good look at her. It was hard to tell, the way she was sitting, but she might have a good body below that pretty face. Maybe... he let his imagination go for a moment.

"Not this week," she said. She watched him finish his beer. "I'm not looking for anything. I just don't want to drink alone. What's your story?"

Josef was trying to catch the bartender's eye. He wanted another beer.

"I'm just like you," he answered. "I got no story. I don't want a story. I don't need a story. What I need is another beer."

She shook her head. He liked the way her curls moved. "You're full of shit," she said, grinning. "You're down in the dumps and something's eating you up. You don't have to tell me anything, you don't know me, but you keep letting that eat you up and one day you'll wake up and you won't be there anymore."

Josef shrugged. What was the difference? He'd get women to make love to him. Like she said, that's easy. The hard part was getting a woman to love him. Wendy made love with him, then she'd fly. He walked out on her because he wanted more than she did. Would it all have worked out if all he wanted was to fuck her, from behind, in a chair, in bed with her on top, in the kitchen with her leaning over the table? He shook the vision of her ass, her breasts, her face, from his head. There was a pretty, curly-haired lady sitting next to him and everything she said made it sound like she'd fuck him if he asked her.

Yeah, he would go back to this lady's apartment, if she'd have him, but it was Wendy he'd be fucking. The mug in his hand was damp and cool. He took a long drink from it then put it down on the bar. It was nearly empty. The bartender reached for it, but Josef put his hand over it. No more for now, he decided. He was a pretty buzzed from the pot and the beer and if he drank any more he wouldn't be going anywhere but back to his own place, alone.

"So what's your problem?" she asked again.

Josef muttered one word, not loud but loud enough for her to hear him and hearing him, smile. "Love," he said.

"Have you eaten?" she asked softly.

"I had some pizza before," he said.

"Well, I haven't yet. Let's get out of here and get a bite to eat."

They walked downtown on Broadway. The neighborhood was seedy but he didn't notice, walking with his hands stuck in his pants pockets, gazing at the sidewalk. He was used to the junkies on the stoops, the dealers on the corner, the garbage cans lined up outside the walk-up tenements on the side streets.

At first neither of them said anything. The cold air felt good and it brought him back from the high he had felt in the bar. At W. 99th St. he glanced at her and wondered what her name was. She was wearing a peacoat buttoned to the neck with the collar turned up against the chill.

"My name's Josef," he said. "I'm sorry I'm such a bore."

She laughed. Her curls shook as she laughed. Josef liked that. She doesn't look anything like Wendy, he thought, and then he was momentarily shocked by a vision of Wendy's breasts.

"Nice to meet you, Josef," she said. "Shirley." She extended a mittened hand to him. He pulled his from his pocket and shook hands with her. "And you aren't any more boring than anyone else. You seem to have a lot on your mind."

"I guess so," he said. He wasn't ready to really open up, but here he was, at W. 98th St. and still going downtown. Much further and he'd be back in his neighborhood. "Is there someplace around here?"

"There's a diner on the next block," she said. In New York it seems there's always a diner on the next block. "We can go there."

"That'll work," he said. "I think I could use a cup of coffee."

"You need a lot more than a cup of coffee," she said. "I'm not sure what else. Maybe we can figure it out."

The diner was warm and smelled better than most. There was a hint of fresh baked bread under the aroma of hamburger and French fries. They sat in a booth by the window. Josef watched as she took off her coat and settled into her seat. He was wondering what a nice woman like her was doing with a bum like him, and what the hell was he doing there when all he wanted was to be a mile further downtown snuggling on the couch with Wendy, stroking her hair, maybe resting his head on her breasts. Shirley wasn't bad, in fact, she was definitely good looking, but she wasn't the one he wanted, not then, not yet.

The waiter took their orders and left them with cups of hot coffee steaming in front of them. Josef held his in both hands, hiding behind the steam. Shirley sipped hers, watching him. He could tell she was wondering. He was waiting for her to ask him something.

"So what happened?" she asked.

He almost laughed. It all seemed so predictable. He almost felt like crying. It was so weird. He could be with Wendy, but he was the one who walked out the door.

"I broke up with someone today," he said. His voice didn't seem to carry much emotion, or at least that's what he thought. "I told her I couldn't take it anymore and I left."

Shirley didn't say anything, just sipped her coffee and waited.

"It's weird," he continued, "I've never said goodbye to someone I didn't want to leave. I'm all broken up but I'm the guy who walked out the door. I ought to be relieved but instead I feel like I've been kicked in the stomach."

Shirley nodded.

"I guess there's a first time for everything," he sighed. "Love is so fucked up. You meet the person you want to spend the rest of your life with, she tells you she loves you, she wants you, but she's not ready to make a commitment, probably never will be, and what the hell is left? If I can't have her, I am out of there, but it sucks how much it hurts."

"You love her, she loves you, and you left?" Shirley wanted to be sure she had it right.

Josef looked at her. What nice eyes she has. I want her, I don't want her, he thought. I want Wendy but I can't deal with her anymore.

"Yeah, I guess so. I mean do we ever really know if we are loved? I mean, I know I was in love, but there wasn't a night when we were together I felt for sure that she loved me, and I still don't know. I just can't live like this, I want her and I want her to want me. I don't think she does, so I had to go. Feels shitty but I'll be okay. I'll get over it."

"What about her?" Shirley asked. "What did she say when you said it was over?"

"She said I was right to go," Josef sighed. And she was right, and Josef was right, and the sun rises on the right if you are facing north, and if you keep the river on your right you are always going to make it, and mom was right, if only I'd listened to her. Oh yeah, Josef's thoughts ran away from him, if everyone's so right, why the fuck am I feeling so goddamn fucking wrong?

"She said she loved me and I was breaking her heart but she couldn't move in with me, that she didn't know what she wanted, only knew what she couldn't do, and if I couldn't take it, then I was right to go. So I went. I walked out. I didn't slam the door, didn't tell her to go to hell, didn't make a scene, didn't yell or scream, just walked out the door, took the elevator to the lobby, walked out onto the street and kept walking, and here I am."

"Not with a bang, but a whimper," Shirley said.

"Not with a bang, but I feel pretty beat up." Josef looked at his coffee. "I think I want another beer."

"You're okay," Shirley said. "Have some of my fries." She pushed her plate across the table.

"Thanks for listening," he said. "I mean, I'll be okay, but it's nice to have a friendly face show some sympathy. But it must sort of stink for you to be spending your evening with a loser like me, listening to me beat my breast for the lost love of another woman."

Shirley laughed. "I'm not complaining."

"No, you're not, which is amazing. You're nice. You got me out of the bar before I got totally sloshed, and you're actually listening to me. You're okay."

He was not a one-night-stand sort of guy, but Shirley seemed a little different. Later that night, back at her apartment on W. 105th Street, lying naked in bed, listening to the steam pipes clattering, gazing at nothing while she rattled around the kitchen putting on some coffee, he felt rescued, knew that he'd feel better sooner rather than later, that Wendy would do what she had to do and so would he. Then Shirley was standing naked in the doorway, a true sister of mercy, her perky little breasts getting him aroused, the triangle of pubic hair an arrow pointing the way to sanctuary, a cigarette in the corner of her mouth.

He got up from the bed, put his hand on her breast, then took the cigarette out of her mouth and kissed her. She was smiling and he felt her hand on his cock. Yeah, he thought, it isn't Wendy but it's just what I need. They went to bed. Her cigarette burned down to the filter and Josef took another dose of the sex cure from Dr. Shirley.

Josef felt like he was dozing. The apartment was overheated and between that and the late hour, it wasn't surprising. Josef lay on his back. Forcing himself to not fall asleep, he was beginning to wonder how long he'd have to stay before he could politely leave. He wondered what Wendy was doing and with whom she was doing it. He remembered some of the good times and got choked up. He turned to look at Shirley. He was glad to have had a few hours with her, but he knew that was all he wanted, and he was pretty sure she felt the same way.

"What's up?" Josef asked. "You okay?"

"I'm fine," she said. "But I think it's time for you to head back to your own place."

"I was thinking the same thing," he said. "I didn't want to be rude. After all, we, um, we just…"

"And you were great," Shirley smiled at him as she slid out of bed, reaching for her robe that was thrown across a chair.

He didn't mind in the least being shown the front door. Downstairs, Josef stood on the stoop in front of the building. He looked up and down the street. It was deserted, and that was a good thing. It was a rough neighborhood. He walked up to Broadway, then decided to walk back to his place. He wasn't feeling much better but at least he wasn't horny. Shirley had been a nice interlude. He didn't say he was going to call and she didn't say she wanted him to. It was all so casual, an exchange that seemed of no consequence to either of them.

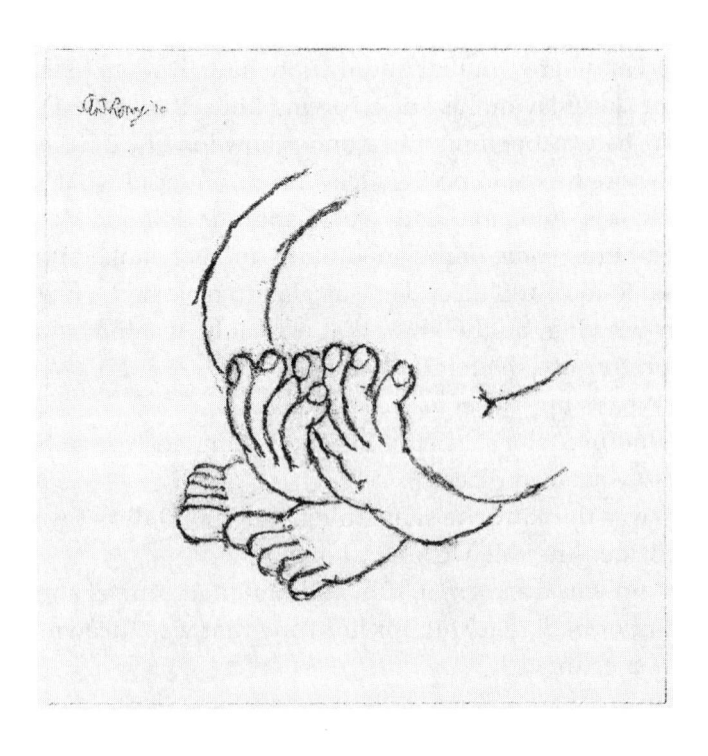

TIGHT WHITE LINEN SKIRT
MAUREEN KELLY NOLAN

He met me at Grand Central. We had e-mailed. Nothing spoken. Didn't know much about him. Didn't care.

I'd been waiting to be with him again. We had a brief encounter the year before, but I ran away in tears. I was not ready. I started watching him. I waited.

He sent me an e-mail. I had a picture of him that I put in my notebook. Cute picture. Cocky. I never spoke to him or if I did, I don't remember what was said. I was mute before him. The "will-someone-please-turn-off-the-talking-machine" Maureen was strangely silent. Words choked in my throat. The word "silent" was too loud.

I loved the way my small square hips fit into my white linen skirt as I clip-clopped across the beautiful stone tile of Grand Central Station in my toe-less Candies.

I liked the shadow he cast as he emerged from the platform, limbs akimbo, legs apace. A New York pace. It all happened in a New York minute.

I was nervous. "Let's go get a drink," he said. We cabbed it downtown.

We went to some bar that we'd never, either of us, think of going to unless we were looking to get laid. I was looking for it. I heard it. I felt it. Hoped my panties weren't too soaked.

I moved my knees a little closer on drink number two. I'd had enough. I only needed two drinks to make the decision to fuck him less of a "decision" and more of a consequence of "alcohol interference with ordinary sexual/bodily control."

So, one more drink for courage. One sip and I was transported to his apartment around the corner.

He didn't throw me against the wall and attack me like the year before. Not that I have anything against a sex attack, I was just afraid at the time. I was not afraid of sex with some guy I hardly knew. I was afraid of liking it. Too much.

One year later after watching him and not speaking, I met him at the train station on his schedule and ended up in his kitchen. He kissed me this time. It was an extraordinary kiss. I looked into a deep blue ocean and I steeled myself, "Am I ready for this? I have been single for so long.…" Happily single, I may add. I went for it. I closed my eyes and attacked him this time. I had that song played by Diana Krall in my head; "How deep is the ocean? How high is the sky?" I fell into the deep sea of his gaze as we mauled each other hungrily.

The kissing became frantic. We squirmed around in the kitchen — or I squirmed. He was making me squirm. He leaned me against the same wall as he had the year before, but this time, I threw my legs over his waist. We bounced around his little apartment and ended up on the floor as he took a minute to pull out the futon.

I needed a minute to catch my breath. So much for getting to know someone before you fuck. I was breaking the "rules." Look, I'm sorry. I was too afraid to talk to the guy because I liked him too much. I knew nothing about him. I liked him for no good reason. I had nothing to say. Afraid.

I was afraid he wouldn't really like me or love me, like I

wanted to love and be loved. I had reason to fear. I wanted him. This much I knew. I shut my eyes and went for it.

I played my favorite game of kissing the pink pony. I got him ready for me. I was delirious, my mind swimming as my full-swollen cum machine sucked the pink pony into me. All the way in. I went for a glorious ride.

I let him go before he came. He got me in the face! That was enough for another giggle. I was good. I was good three times over, not counting the orgasms in the cab, the bar, the kitchen, the wall, the desk, on the floor with his balls in my mouth…. I was good. I could breathe again.

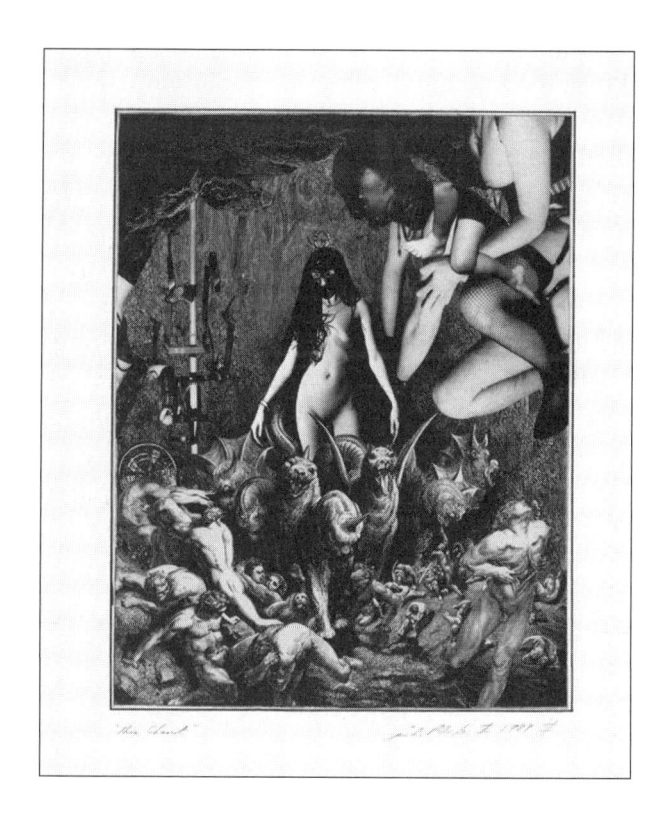

DICK
KATHE BURKHART

I couldn't breathe in Brooklyn. It was the kind of sweltering August night that drives people out of their apartments, in search of any diversion that includes air conditioning or water. It was one of those nights when I was burning up inside. I couldn't think straight, and I felt pissed off and potentially vicious — when you can't stop, and you just keep going. Maybe you don't know what I'm talking about.

I called The Safe to see if it was cool there, which it was, according to whoever had answered the phone. Then I put on my leather skirt and see through body stocking. I put a suit jacket on so the neighbors wouldn't see my tits. I tucked my black patent spikes in my purse and headed up Broadway towards the elevated train. The J took a long time to come, which it usually does if it isn't rush hour. It seemed like years before it came and started chunking and clunking west across the Williamsburg Bridge.

My nylon and leather stuck to me like bacteria to moisture — I was glued to my seat. I got off at Delancey and transferred to the F train, took it to Fourteenth Street, then walked west to Tenth Avenue.

The meat-packing district stank of dead carcasses as usual. When I finally went down the basement steps and entered The Safe I was relieved, like you are after you take a piss after riding home on the bus when you have to go wicked bad. By that time, I was a regular at The Safe. The bouncer usually waved me in for free. If I missed a few weeks, he'd always welcome me back.

I remember that summer, coming out, alone, as a dominant woman. Gay men and lesbians aren't the only ones who come out, you know. Het perverts do, too. I talked my girlfriends blue in the face before I actually made any moves. I did my research. Then I constructed it like a pilgrimage to Mecca, but closer, from the East River to the Hudson River.

Inside, the place was dead and it stayed that way. As usual, Dirty Foot was scooting around nearly nude in his filthy loincloth. Some said that in his straight life, he was a major executive, even an art collector. But there he was at The Safe on a sweltering Saturday night, an abject masochist chained to a cum-stained floor. I was bored to tears, sick to death of denying the desires of unattractive, seemingly subhuman foot slaves. I'd already given up on entertainment when I met Dick.

He was tall, long of lock and nose, and wide-eyed in a way that was both naive and jaded. He stared at me like an orphan at his long-lost mother. I recognized him immediately as the boy who'd knelt at my feet, rapt, in the back room just a little while ago, as I allowed some other slave the pleasure of licking the bottom of my spike heel.

Now, he persisted in striking up a conversation with me. He looked like a hippie. He was wearing a WFMU t-shirt, which I thought was okay, since I listened to that station, too. He told me his name was Dick, and offered to make a beer run. It was common slave etiquette.

The law kept sex clubs like The Safe from serving alcohol, because there was nudity, as if the moment a naked person had a drink all hell would break loose. So you had to bring your own bottle, or go to the deli for beers.

"What kind, Mistress?" he asked.

"I'd prefer a bottle of wine," I said, "but a couple Amstel Lights would be all right."

He nodded, yes-mistressing me, and went out. I yawned, and watched whatever pathetic scene going on before me. One man, wearing only athletic socks and shoes, masturbated his unusually large penis. Men look furtive when they jack off, I observed, especially in public. Sort of frantically pathetic. When Dick came back with the beers, we started to talk. He told me that he was straight, but he had strange tastes. He complained that he could never find straight women who didn't think he was weird.

"What do you mean?" I said. "You're submissive — right?"

"Oh, yes, I'm submissive," he assured me, eyeing my less than half full beer oddly. "Drink up. Would you like another beer?"

"Not right now," I said, not really getting it yet. "So — what are you into?"

"Well," he said bashfully, "I don't even know that many straight men who are into what I'm into... but...." He bowed his head and lowered his voice. "I'd really love to drink your piss." He looked up and smiled at me earnestly.

"Where?!" I asked. "In here?"

"Yeah," he said. "Go and get the key to the women's bathroom from the bartender when you're ready. There's a floor drain in there. People used to do it all the time in the old days, before AIDS. Just nod at me, and I'll meet you over there."

"Maybe," I said, "but I don't have to go right now."

"Don't worry," he said. "No rush. I can wait. You'll tell me when you're ready, won't you? *Please.* I really want to be your toilet."

His big brown puppy-dog eyes looked up at me hopefully. I stiffened, then felt wetness in my pants. That surprised me, but it was interesting, so I thought about it. I meditated on it some more. I wasn't convinced yet.

"Do you do this all the time?" I asked.

He nodded. "As much as I can," he answered.

"Aren't you worried about HIV?" I said. "I mean, when you drink it?"

"No," he replied. "That's what most people don't know. Urine is totally sterile when it comes out."

"You'd better be sure about that," I said.

He looked at the floor. "Oh, please, Mistress, *let me*," he begged. "Do you need another beer?"

I did. He opened one for me and I took a drink. Dick looked about seventeen, but he told me he was twenty-five. I didn't believe him. So he showed me his driver's license. He wasn't lying. It ruined my kidnapping fantasy that he wasn't as innocent as he looked. We talked some more. I found out that he lived in Greenpoint, just a few miles up the road from me. Said he was moving to San Francisco in a few weeks. The sexual subculture was supposed to be better there.

Finally, the beer went through me, and I had to piss. I let Dick follow me to the bathroom, where there was a line of dominant and submissive women of all shapes and sizes waiting. The women's bathroom was private, while the men's had no door and was open to plain view.

While we waited, I watched the action in the back room off to the side. The scent of musty, dried cum wafted through the stagnant air. S/M videos droned on. A portly Floor Mistress was tying up the genitals of a Hasidic Jew, complete with yarmulke, who was happily suspended from the ceiling. Nude or semi-nude men enthusiastically jacked off nearby.

At last it was our turn to go in the bathroom. I could smell that the floor drain had recently been used. How in the fuck was I supposed to piss standing up?

I soon figured out that I was supposed to squat on Dick, either on the toilet or the floor. I made Dick lie over the drain, but knowing there was a line outside waiting gave me performance anxiety. My bladder got shy and I couldn't piss one drop.

Failed perverts, we exited the bathroom. By that time, the club was thinning out. I was pretty drunk, and there was no place to go but home. He offered me a ride home in a cab with him. It was five o'clock in the morning, so I said ok.

Halfway across the bridge, he said, "Want to have another beer, and try again?"

"Sure," I said. So he had the driver go to the all night bodega under the train. I don't know why we decided to go to my place. How did I let that happen? Oh, well.

Dick sat cross-legged on the sofa in my apartment and rolled a joint.

"On the floor," I told Dick, "where slaves belong."

The puppy flopped down and paid attention to my feet. I got tired of him staring at me reverently while I was smoking pot. Maybe I was getting paranoid. So I blindfolded him with an old scarf I had. Then I tied him, face down, to a couple of pillars, and took his pants down.

I put a record on, Ministry or some kind of industrial dirge. Spanking music. Then I went to get my toys. He looked cute lying on my living room floor.

I came back and took down his shorts. I rubbed his ass, (nothing special), then spanked him with my hand. He wiggled around, moaning, and I could tell that his dick was getting hard. I didn't care. So I flipped him over, ready to gag him. But I stopped short when I saw the size of his cock. It was enormous. I hadn't counted on that.

I went to get some dental floss, and began his cock and ball bondage. Dick screamed for mercy, and was afraid I was going to beat him up badly, I could tell. He'd hinted at it before, something about sadistic women who just liked to beat young boys up. The more he talked about it, the more violent I felt, and the more I pushed his limits.

It's a good thing I'm not into blood. If I closed my eyes and spaced out for a minute, I could imagine that he was the last shitass I'd fallen for who'd fucked me over. When that happened, I'd forget who he was, zone out and pull the string around his nuts so hard he'd scream. Then I'd play with his hair, or cane him a little for his outburst, until he started whining again. I stopped for a minute, and petted his hair. Then I ripped his t-shirt off and pinched his nipples.

"You like that, don't you?" I said.

"Y…y…yes…," he moaned. That gave me the go-ahead to move on to clothespins. After playing with the dirty laundry for a while, he turned pale and started trembling. I knew I'd gone a little bit too far then.

So I stopped again. I noticed that it was getting light out. I cracked open another Amstel, and looked out the window absently. This was starting to get tedious.

"What would you like to do to me now?" Dick asked me.

"I don't know," I said, starting to feel tired.

"If I might make a suggestion," Dick offered, "I wish you'd put on your biggest strap-on and fuck my ass."

"Maybe I don't feel like it," I lied. (My harness was in my chest of drawers, but I'd used my dildo in a sculpture and didn't have a spare handy.) "Let me look at your cock. I might want to get fucked myself."

His eyes lit up like a Christmas tree.

"Oh, Mistress, I can't believe you'd let me! But aren't you going to allow me to be your toilet? Please," he begged, *"you promised."*

"Lean up against the couch, there, Dick," I said. "I have to examine your peter." He had a big mole on the side of it. "What's that?" I asked him.

"A mole, Mistress," he replied. "Does it bother you?"

"Not as long as you're sure that it's a mole and you wear a rubber," I said. It looked like a mole to me, but you never know.

"I don't have any rubbers on me," Dick said. "I usually need the Magnum size, but if you have a regular one, we could try it."

"All right, Dick," I said. "Get down and crawl over to my bedroom. Just follow my footsteps, but watch out for the pushpins on the floor." I punctuated the command with a crack of my riding crop.

Snap. He got down on his knees. Snap. He didn't know where the bed was, but he was a darn good doggie and followed his sense of sound and scent. I took off some of my clothes, just what's necessary for getting fucked. He didn't deserve the pleasure of seeing me naked. Piss he may get, the whole picture, fuck no.

"You may remove the blindfold," I told him. "Now get over here and service me."

"Will you mount me, Mistress?"

"Forget it, slave. Get on top of me and fuck me. Stop fooling around."

I shut my eyes. It was ok.

After I came, I pushed him off me. He was still looking at me in that doting way that was driving me up a wall. I might have been a piss novice that night, but I was still an accomplished control freak. As far as that went, I knew what I was doing. I knew that men who enjoyed water sports liked to come as they were getting peed on, or enjoying their beverage of choice. Dick sat up, and peeled his scumsack off.

"Don't even think of throwing that in the trash," I told him. "Take it into the bathroom and flush it down the toilet, like the toilet-slave you are."

"Yes, mistress," he said, getting up. I smiled, and let him go into the bathroom. I had to piss like a racehorse. I was now ready to assert my power by subverting his fantasy — since it was unlikely he'd come again so soon. I got up and went towards the bathroom.

"Dick," I said, "it's your lucky day! Still wanna be my toilet?" I smirked.

"Now?" he said. He looked puzzled. "But I don't have a hard-on anymore."

"I can see that, Stupid," I said. "Just lay down on the toilet and open your mouth."

"But I thought we weren't going to do this," he protested.

"Dick," I said sternly. "I thought this is what you really wanted. I just made you wait for it. Now shut up, and open up."

I straddled Dick, sitting squarely on his face, and making sure all my weight rested on him. It felt good. He started to lick my cunt. I slapped his head. "Who told you you could do that?"

"Mmmrbody," he whimpered from underneath my ass.

At which point I started to piss. I started sitting down, and then raised my ass up, directing the stream directly into his mouth. The sight of his grimacing, gulping mouth, with rivulets of urine running down his face, was turning me on more than I'd ever dreamed. It was one of those long pisses, the kind that go on dribbling for a minute or more.

Dick scooted around underneath me like a wiggle worm, making all kinds of noises. He appeared to be both enjoying himself immensely and behaving like an abject victim. When I finished, I got some toilet paper, wiped myself, and threw it on, rather than in, the toilet. Relieved, I went back to bed and looked at a magazine.

"May I use your shower, Mistress?" piped Dick from the peanut gallery.

"Yes," I answered. "But make sure that you clean up any mess that you've made first. The mop and bucket are in the broom closet."

I felt very tired, but contented. It was daylight outside again. I looked at a magazine for a while. Then I started to nod off. The last thing I heard was the sound of the shower going on.

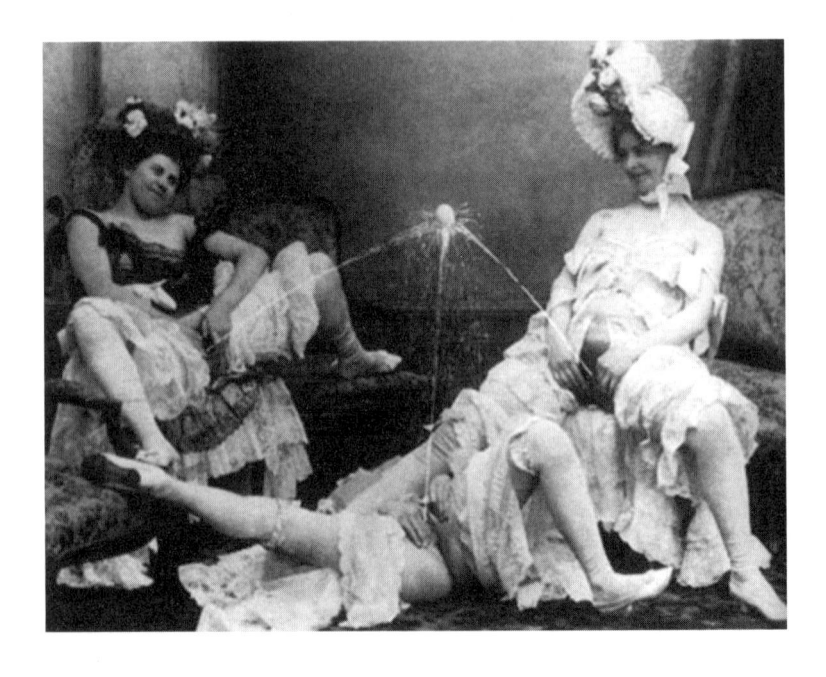

RAPPING, REDDENING AND 'RITHMETIC
THADDEUS RUTKOWSKI

The movie put her in the mood for discipline, though I didn't know that at the time. I thought the candy bar got her in trouble.

The picture was soft core — less than soft core, really. We saw one spank, one slap of a hand against a buttock. Continuous swatting did not occur. A grin, however, accompanied the one slap, and the camera had caught that grin, on the face of the woman getting smacked. But spanking wasn't the point of the movie. The point was that behaving hedonistically was more fun than earning a Ph.D. I couldn't argue with that. Still, the butt slap was what stuck in my mind.

After the movie, she said, "Today, I ate a candy bar."

"A whole candy bar?" I asked.

"Yes," she said.

"That's very bad," I said, "a very bad thing to do."

Sugar was hard on the teeth, and calories encouraged weight gain. The candy bar's nonorganic ingredients, its chemicals and additives, could not be good for the health. I would have to punish her for snacking.

I tried to speak softly, because that was the best way to proceed. Bluntness was not called for. Insistence was to be avoided. What I didn't want to do was to sound insensitive or impersonal. I didn't want to treat her like a masochistic mannequin. I wanted to compliment her, build her up, make her feel good about herself. So I said, "I'm going to have to spank you a little."

"What do you mean by 'a little?'" she asked.

"Just a few whacks with the horse paddle," I said.

"What am I," she asked, "chopped horsemeat? How about one smack, like in the movie?"

I didn't understand her response. After all, I'd always enjoyed spanking myself. Not my monkey, though I spanked that, too. I liked spanking whichever body parts I could reach with a handheld flogger. I remembered pleasant times, from when I was an adolescent, when I first went fetish crazy. The horse paddle had sentimental value for me.

I had acquired my first such implement at a harness shop. I grew up among plain folk, farmers mostly, and I bugged out when I saw that they used buggy whips, riding crops and horse paddles in their daily lives. In short order, I learned to whip myself into a lather. This froth extended to my monkey, which was always ready to get lathered up.

It took years of preparation before I graduated from spanking myself to spanking another person. I hung around birthday parties to get my fix and kicks. At some point during the festivities, the birthday person — usually a girl — would get spanked. In fact, some birthday girls wanted to be spanked. They were exhibitionists, in love with their own derrières. If I were lucky, everyone in attendance would get a turn at administering correction. That was how I lost my epidermal virginity. I stuck out my knee, bent the honoree over it, and whaled away.

Bachelorette parties were also good places to find some paddling. Unfortunately, due to my gender, I was never invited. The closest I got was one time on a city street, in a bar neighborhood, when I saw a group of women in formalwear approaching me. One of the women was wobbling on her heels. She was wearing a blindfold, her hands were behind her back, and her friends were holding her arms. When she passed, I saw that her hands were cuffed together. She was wearing police bracelets.

"This is humiliating," I heard her say.

"She's getting married," one of her friends explained.

I suspected that at that party, there would be some toplessness and picture-taking, followed by sharp teasing, simulated groveling and, most likely, real spanking. At least, this was what I heard happened at bachelorette parties.

But my days of random spanking opportunities were over. Now, I wanted to focus on paddling a target that was committed to me. My partner and I had been together long enough to communicate in a way that went beyond skin-deep.

Paddle in hand, I lowered my voice to a whisper and said, "Assume the position."

"What position?" she asked.

"The standard spanking position!" I exclaimed, not quite ejaculating.

She turned away from me and bent over. I knew this was not the only spanking position. There was the hands-and-knees-on-the-floor pose, reminiscent of a donkey before a cart. There was the basic over-the-knee position, favored by birthday celebrants. There was the handcuff predicament, preferred by ecstatic bachelorettes. And there was the spread-eagle exposure, practiced by recipients of the hardest-core inquisitions. But the basic toe-touch position was fine with me.

"Grab your ankles, please," I murmured.

She complied, and I de-pantsed her. I unhitched and pulled, until her outer waistband was at her knees. Then I grasped the inner elastic and peeled off the fabric, so that her gluteal nucleus was bare.

The act of de-pantsing triggered a wave of nostalgia. I remembered girls getting paddled when I was in junior high school. My biggest educational thrill — bigger, even, than acing a spelling bee or exhibiting in a science fair — was seeing girls' rumps roasted in class.

All of my teachers owned paddles; it was a school rule. Some of the pedant/disciplinarians just waved their whackers in warning. Others actually applied the hickory. It was boys, mostly, who felt the board. On rare occasion, though, girls also tasted the shellac.

Whenever a girl committed a school crime, such as note passing, gum chewing or public toenail clipping, she would be instructed to step to the front of the room. She would be told to face the blackboard, bend over and grab the backs of her knees with her hands.

She would gather her skirt — if she was wearing a skirt — as if for protection. But there was no way to prevent the slap of wood on bottom. As a topper, the girl would have to stand in a corner, nose to the juncture, ears to the plaster, and keep her hands away from her stinging keister.

In a way, I was now rewriting the curriculum. At the sight of the unprotected, heart-shaped target, my monkey, normally a slow learner, was ready to move to the head of the class. Or rather, the head of my monkey was ready to behave without class.

I started with the old horse paddle. I swung it like an angry jockey, first through the air, then in the direction of the untanned hide in front of me. When I heard the first whinny — a note of protest — I realized I would have to proceed differently.

I would have to start at the bottom and teach the three R's of spanking: rapping, reddening and 'rithmetic. These were the principles practiced in any European boarding school — I knew this from studying a wealth of material on corporal punishment on the Continent. I'd seen countless films — Swedish titles, mostly — with innumerable spankings in them.

The rapping and reddening would be easy, but the 'rithmetic wouldn't be for retards. This was the European way.

I set the horse paddle aside for later use. For the rapping, I began with a ruler. At the first thwack, my ambivalent apprentice said, "Ow!"

"You know," I said, "European women don't say 'Ow' when spanked. They say, 'Ai.'"

"Ai!" she shrieked as I swatted again.

But this wasn't a class in European women's studies. It was a lesson in the three R's of spanking. I proceeded with the ruler rapping, which led to a rosy glowing, then a deep reddening, accompanied by some crowing, as well as the jumping of my monkey. But when my whack-ee started bucking, I knew I would have to administer a stricter tanning. We would have to concentrate on 'rithmetic.

I switched from a ruler to a yardstick. "Do you know the proportion of a yardstick to a ruler?" I asked my unruly *compadre*.

"A yardstick is three times as long," she said.

"What does that mean?"

"You can deliver a harder smack with a shorter swing."

She had been studying her spankology. As a reward, I applied the wood.

"How many strokes should I give you for eating that candy bar?" I asked.

"Ten?" she suggested.

"That was a chocolate bar!" I reminded her. "Underpaid, nonunion workers harvested those chocolate nuts! Your consumption prolongs their poverty! That's worth ten squared."

I made her count, then, down from a hundred. To keep track, she sang a classic counting song, modified for a thrashing: "Ninety-nine bottles of spunk on the wall. Ninety-nine bottles of spunk. You take one down and squirt it around; ninety-eight bottles of spunk on the wall." And so on, with a percussive stroke and an "Ai!" at every change of verse.

My monkey danced the whole way through the aria. At times, though, my arm got tired, so I had to switch implements. I tried a hairbrush (it worked well both ways, bristles and backside, on her backside), a fly swatter (slapping with the flap was easier than swatting a fly), a wooden spoon (more fun than tossing a salad), a wire hanger (when straightened, the perfect shape for flailing), a fishing rod (had to cast about to find one), and a spatula (the flapjack flipper was springy and stingy). Then I went back to the trusty horse paddle. I put her through her paces as I worked on her haunches. The only thing I lacked was a meter stick, for the full European effect.

As she approached zero in her countdown song, I moved in to give her a monkey whipping. When excited, my monkey was a harsh master. He was King Dong. I held the creature by the tail and clubbed the butt before me. The monkey's head peppered the chocolate glutton's heinie, covered every inch of global territory, and came to rest at the gluteal entranceway. Then, like a primate possessed, my monkey dove right in.

When I heard my spank-ee reach zero, I let my chimp go ape.

MEHEC
JENNIFER BLOWDRYER

I used to call it the Mutual Exploitation Hack Erotica Cycle. MEHEC, if I was fond of acronyms. Which I'm not. MEHEC was what I called the sub world I stumbled into when I moved to New York City to go to the Columbia University's Writing Division on a slender fellowship. Thank you, Claire Woolrich, whoever you were, for the $2500.00 a semester. I didn't know anybody in New York, just a leather guy called Lou Rudolph who lived in Long Branch, New Jersey.

I seem to have at last turned into a kind of academic, in my own lifetime, because now I feel honor bound to explain what I mean not just by MEHEC but by Leather Guy. Oh, these heady days of being a forty-nine-year-old night person! There is so much to tell you! San Francisco, in the late 70s on up to the early 80s, was a gay Mecca. There were a few bars that were just for men who were fully into sado-masochism and what Bette Midler waggishly referred to as their 'accoutrements' — leather outfits, whips, masculine décor. Lou belonged to a gay biker club, the Rainbow Club, and wore an embroidered rainbow logo patch on the back of his denim cut off vest. This is what bikers call wearing your Colors, and it used to be enough to get you banned from certain bars. Yep, bikers were dangerous once.

I didn't know Lou well but he always was pretty friend-ly — his bar, The Anvil, was actually a collective, as it was so common to be a gay S&M club type that they had advanced to a profit sharing cooperative outlook. I doubt that, say, The Mineshaft was a collective. Really doubt it. I called Lou when I got to NYC, from my tiny dorm room on 125th Street at International House. That place was a rainbow situation, but not the open-minded kind. Students from all over the globe lived in a multi storied 1950s atmosphere of cheap rooms and a zesty cafeteria. Lou sent a copy of my first book, *Modern English: A Photo Illustrated Trendy Slang Dictionary* (Last Gasp, SF, 1984) and a cassette tape of my songs ("I Love My New Clothes,""Interpersonal Song,""I Wanna Kill My Roommate"), along to an apartment on Lexington Avenue and 27th Street, inhabited by porn star Annie Sprinkle and tattoo artist/bon vivant Spider Webb.

This phone call, and Lou's postal mailing of my materials, launched me into a world of MEHEC that I could still live in, if I was bored enough and hadn't come up with any other ideas in the intervening quarter of a century. To wit (sounds like a pompous academic phrase, something you'd say when you were furtively pissed off) — to wit, I have just been in two sex worker themed anthologies, *Working Sex* (Seal Press) and *Hos Hookers Pimps and Call Girls* (Soft Skull), and read twice for no remuneration at a gathering called Sex Worker Literati, all within the last year. I also read, confusingly, at the Hustler Bookstore in Hollywood, an event I took a public bus to and from. We all did well at that event, I feel, from adult star Sinnamon to a young lady who was emotionally raped as a call girl. You might call it Spoken Word. We got *Hustler* key chains as swag.

Back in 1985, we didn't hear the word sex work much. Hustling was what you did and hid. I was in a porn movie when I was nineteen due to financial desperation, and had tried to turn tricks unsuccessfully at a so called, because that's what they misleadingly called it, Swing Club. I was attending San Francisco State University at the time, and barely had $$ for the bus there and back. I'm pretty sure Nina Hartley, who is now a flagrantly public adult star, buck tooth and long in the tooth, was attending nursing classes at SF State and also working from the Swing Club, but that was way before she stood at Book Soup, after being in a group reading for *Ho, Hookers* etc with me and a cavalcade of other formerly and currently broke scrappers, and declared herself to be a Nurse who Healed through Porn Movie ensemble acting.

I hardly know how to act, now or then, and in '85 I freely admitted to Annie Sprinkle and the late erotica writer Marco Vassi that I'd slept around, been in an adult movie, and, lying helpfully, said I'd like to have sex with a game show host one day. I pouted and primped in photographs taken by Annie that subsequently appeared in *Velvet, Swank, Penthouse Forum* and *Adam,* prudishly refusing to take off my top.

When I figured out that Annie, Marco, Veronica Vera, and a handful of others were furiously documenting themselves and almost everybody who entered their apartments for pay in sex magazines, giving things an upbeat masturbatory slant, I decided that shame should not be part of the equation. Well, they never did seem ashamed, but remember, I was at Columbia University with Poets and Fiction Writers at the same time I was in *Velvet* and *Adam.* I never got invited to anybody's dinner parties, but attended a twenty-four-hour stripper contest in upstate NYC with Annie and Veronica, as well as an Adult Expo in Philadelphia.

That beat movement I read about in school was, similarly to the heterosexual biker coterie, not fun for the women, I concluded, but this weird stomping ground of commercial Smut consisted largely of flashy women makin' some change and photographing and writing fairly well, if in a surreal cloaked manner, so let's call it The High Heel School of Journalism. And we did. I ran many shows called Smut Fests, beginning in 1988, that mixed sex workers performing their own writing and movement to a clientele of thrilled intellectuals, perverts, scenesters, and tricks, and became for about fifteen years the person you saw doing that sex thing somewhere. Jennifer Blowdryer, hah. Now it's a good thing, something to work, but ladies and gentlemen, I only hustled for like a minute and I am so so tired of sharing about something that is no longer even taboo. Now that being an intellectual is possibly the most embarrassing thing an American can do, I shall take refuge in that.

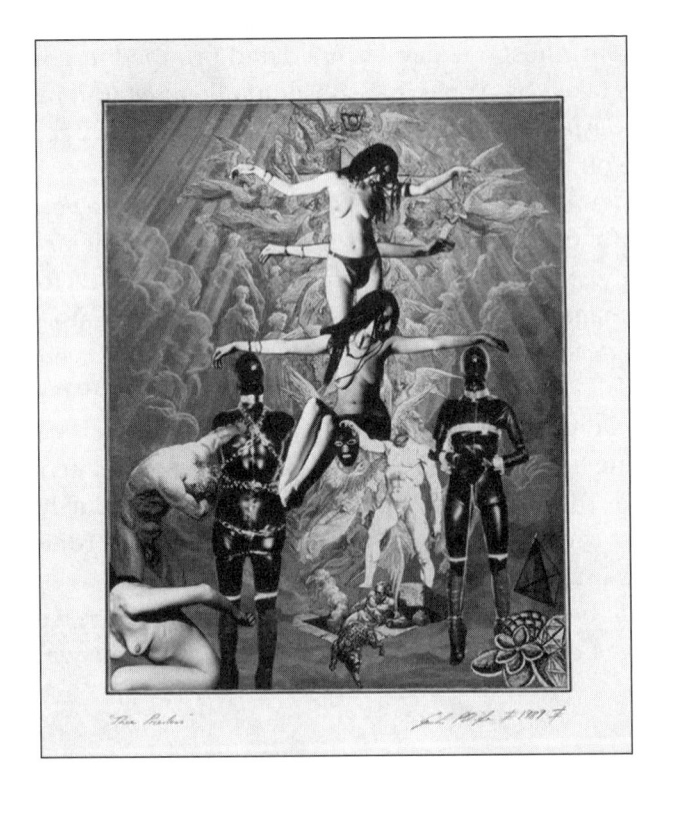

A BOOB STAMPING
ON A HUMAN FACE FOREVER
DAVE MANDL

I've been to topless bars on exactly three occasions, and each was worse than the one before. The first time was when I was a teenager, in the late seventies. A friend had the brilliant spur-of-the-moment idea to pop into a Times Square topless/bottomless joint one afternoon, after we'd seen a (non-porn) movie in the neighborhood. You'd think that a kid who'd only ever caught fleeting glimpses of naked breasts would have considered it heaven to be surrounded by four pairs of them, but no — the sad entertainment consisted of the minimum micro-movements possible by the obviously bored dancers; I was sold a beer of a highly suspect off-brand that I've never seen before or since, and charged $3.75 for it (an inconceivably high price at a time when $1.50 would have been considered robbery); and, though no one was pestering us, the place had a generally creepy vibe that made me want to down the can of piss I'd been served and get outta there as quickly as possible. My friend agreed, and we split.

My second topless jaunt was a few years later (by which time I'd seen a few bare breasts, thank you), and was even less pleasant. A bandmate of mine had been persuaded to hold his bachelor party at a downtown "gentlemen's club," and so I was obligated to go. Feeling uncomfortable being there at all, I retreated to a pinball machine, without a beer

(I'm not a big drinker now, and was even less of one then), and attempted to make the time pass more quickly by playing the silver ball. Since, in contrast with my Times Square adventure, this time it was late at night and the bar's festivities were in full swing, the place was being policed fairly closely by the management. One of them walked over and made it very plain to me that I was there to spend dollars on alcohol and not quarters on pinball; this wasn't really negotiable. I was a meek kid, but I didn't like being told what to spend my money on by gangsters, so I said goodnight without finishing my game and caught the next Q train home.

My third and worst experience was about ten years ago, at Billy's Topless on Sixth Avenue, a place that was known for employing non-traditional dancers, which mostly meant no silicone and a higher-than-usual percentage of artist and intellectual types. I was brought there, along with a handful of friends, by a female pal of ours with unimpeachable sexual politics and good intentions; once inside, the first thing I noticed was a bunch of women sitting right up front cheering the dancers on, in a sex-positive, You Go, Girl! kind of way, and showering them with applause and dollar bills. I hung back at the bar to shoot the shit with my friends. By then I'd learned the rules, and I ordered a beer practically before my second foot was in the door. But alas — I was unable to drink it quickly enough, and after gulping down most of it I paused for a few minutes with about a quarter of a glass left. This prompted the hostess to sidle over and sweetly ask me if I would like another drink. "In a minute, thanks," I replied. "I'm not finished with this one yet." Apparently satisfied with my answer, she walked away. But less than a minute later, one of the place's much more imposing male employees came over and asked me a little less sweetly if I were ready for another drink. There was still some beer left in my glass, but clearly it was too little — or there was some beers-per-minute rule that I had unknowingly violated — so I threw my hands up and said, "Why, yes, I'd love to have another one." Anyway, this would buy me some more time to catch up with the friends I hadn't seen in a while, and now I'd be sure to time my sips in such a way that I wasn't caught with an unacceptably small amount of beer in my glass.

But, unfortunately, pacing my drinking correctly was just one of the tests I was to be put through at Billy's. Another, as it turns out, was making sure I was standing in the right place. While talking to a friend in the large and amorphous group of us at the bar, I had unwittingly moved over to a spot on the floor that was supposed to be kept clear. One of Billy's bouncers walked over and brusquely told me I couldn't stand there. Where, exactly? And why? I wasn't sure, but it was clear that asking would be pointless, so I moved to a different spot a few inches over and resumed talking to my friends. The bouncer walked away, signaling that I was now in compliance. I continued drinking my beer at what felt like an acceptable speed, and monitoring the level in the glass to make sure I didn't violate *that* rule. But in the mild chaos of the evening — other friends who'd been invited, some of whom I hadn't seen in a long time, continued to trickle into the place, so I'd inevitably jump over to shake someone's hand — I strayed into the forbidden zone a couple more times. It was hard to know exactly where that was, and it seemed innocent enough, in a bar, to take a few steps over to greet this or that new arrival, but I was warned several more times, in an increasingly unfriendly way, to move the hell back.

This was now becoming embarrassing — I was losing a game that I didn't know the rules to, the ultimate penalty clear enough to this street-smart native New Yorker. My friends were chuckling good-naturedly if slightly nervously at my uncomfortable predicament, but I wasn't sure what to do, and I was getting mildly concerned. The place was packed at this point, and there were a lot of us crowded around the bar: Did I have to go stand in a distant corner somewhere, away from everyone else, and wait for a piece of floor in the safe zone to open up before I could come back? Was I required to sit by the stage and cheer on the dancers, whom I didn't feel that strongly about one way or another? My instincts told me that, at this point, the bouncers probably had me pegged for a troublemaker (and a light drinker), and were looking to bully me, so I started to think about heading out of there. The idea of getting the shit beat out of me for no reason at a bar I didn't even want to be in, and in front of fifteen of my friends, was not particularly appealing. The decision was made for me when I was confronted for the fourth time: "I fucking *told* you…" OK, time to go.

The next day, talking to one of the people who'd been at Billy's with me, I found out that on a previous trip there another friend had actually been ejected by the bar's security staff, and possibly roughed up, for reasons that no one exactly knew. The guy in question was a physically unimposing poet who would never hurt a soul. Had he stopped drinking for a minute to go to the men's room? Had he recklessly put his foot up on a stool? Regardless, it was clear to me that customers must have been at least threatened with violence at Billy's fairly regularly, for the mildest of "infractions." Why? People do terrible things every day and are successfully dealt with in various ways that don't involve being beaten up. Were the crimes perpetrated by Billy's clientele so much worse than fraud, kidnapping, arson, and grand larceny? More important, even if things rarely got to the point of physical violence, what does it mean for a business establishment—a place where people voluntary walk in and spend wads of money to have a good time — to be openly run like a jail or one of the ministries in *1984*? Was the average patron of these places — like a child of abusive parents who grows up under the assumption that regular beatings are just a normal part of life — cowed enough to think that this was a reasonable atmosphere to expect in a drinking establishment? Is this what bars in North Korea are like? And was this the only way to publicly fly your sex-radical flag in New York City in the late 1990s?

Which brings me to another question: Given the blatantly unliberatory atmosphere at Billy's, why should anyone go there for the purpose of cheering the dancers on? Because they're abused and exploited? If so, you've got your choice of much worse-off workers in neighborhood bodegas and garment-industry sweatshops to root for. Because they're *not* abused and exploited? Big deal! And with the dancers at Billy's providing a thin veneer of hipster sex-lib to a joint with such a strong stench of authoritarianism-cum-violence, who are you helping by cheering for them? It's all well and good for these women to engage in sex-positive work that they enjoy, escaping mind-numbing office drudgery in the process (the most likely, and most reasonable, explanation for the existence of the cheering section), but that positivity is more than outweighed by the almost sociopathic nature of the place. Compare the merely psychological warfare of, say, TV commercials aimed at four-year-old kids to a place of business where the threat of actual *physical injury* looms barely below the surface, to prevent the crime of nursing your beer a minute too long, or just to maintain some kind of arbitrary order. Being a dancer at such a gangsterish establishment certainly doesn't make you "complicit," any more than being the window washer at Bernie Madoff's office does, but it's a big leap from that to being at the vanguard of the sexual revolution.

Billy's closed its doors a few years ago, for reasons I was never curious enough to look into, and I'm not even sure what has replaced it. If there's any justice in the world, though, the spot is now occupied by a more customer-friendly and socially conscious business — say, a small camera-and-electronics shop catering to tourists.

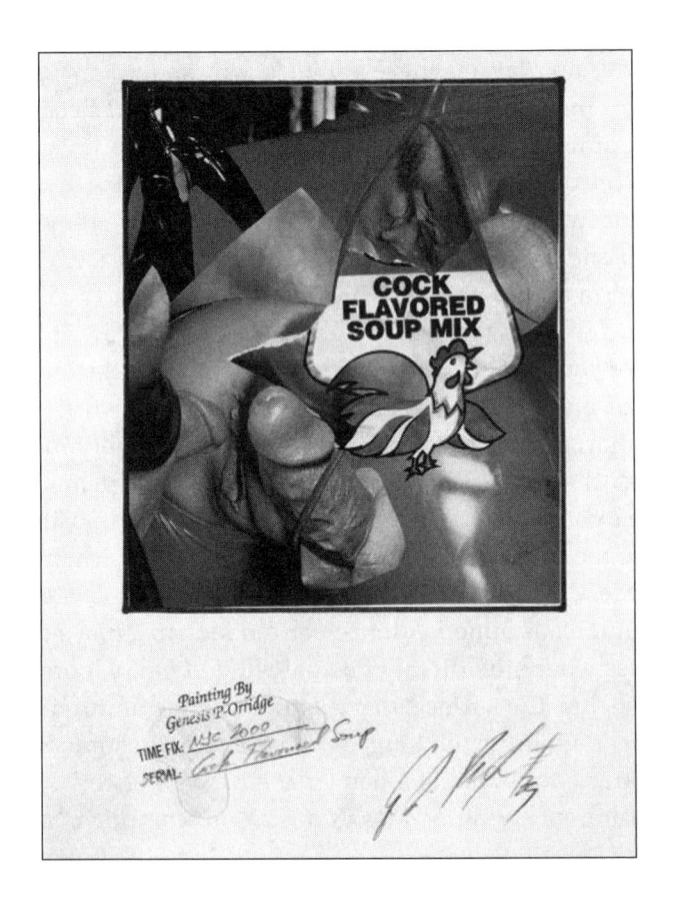

NIGHTS IN WHITE SATIN
MAX BLAGG

I t's reassuring to know that a great night out in Good Britain still seems to involve a lot of drinking and the subsequent random expulsion of chunks of half-digested food, just as it did when I was first initiated into the mysteries of Saturday night. Too bad the town square now is a no-go area after ten pm, as roving bands of teenage idiots perform their drunken rituals for CCTV, ready at any moment to thrash pensioner and policeman alike. A night out in New York seems much safer and simpler by comparison. Those of my friends who have somehow avoided hospital, incarceration and death, now enjoy a comfortable midlife, free of any real crisis beyond occasionally losing the key to the handcuffs.

But what do they do for pleasure on their nights out? I conducted a brief survey, not the Kinsey Report by any means, just a few fragments of the history of love in the 21st century. My friend S likes to meet new friends on Craigslist, where he has listed his age as 44, shaving a decade off his true birth date. His ad hints broadly at his domineering nature, and it garners a rapid response from a shower of submissives. He winnows this group down to a few likely candidates and finally makes a date with the one who claims to feel insecure at night unless she is handcuffed to her bed. They meet on a corner of the Bowery, now resplendent with new hotels, chic restaurants and lofts the size of department stores. Once they have both got over the shock of their actual appearance, as opposed to their online photographs, they wander along this latest Golden Mile of Manhattan.

S, who never plans on much financial expenditure, steers his companion into the lobby of one of the new hotels. It's quiet and plush — the tourists are still tottering around the cobblestones of the meat market 20 blocks away, from which the celebutards have long since fled. After a long, intimate chat on a luxurious sofa in the vestibule, the odd couple move discreetly to the public bathrooms one floor below that S has already scoped out on a previous visit. S invites his new friend, code name Jenny, into the handicapped toilet, which is almost as big as a hotel room and conveniently out of camera range. Once inside, he quickly handcuffs her to the steel rail conveniently located next to the toilet. S then threatens to abandon her there, as previously agreed in their email scenario.

This gets Jenny so excited that she pees her pants, which S carefully removes and places in a plastic bag. He then pats down the wet spots with baby powder and affixes two clothes pegs to her nipples, tweaking them like radio dials as she makes amends for her "accident" by performing enthusiastic fellatio.

Are you still with me, gentle reader? And where are all the other hotel guests during this time, the over-attentive staff, the physically-challenged visitors dying for a pee? Because they are below ground, and because the concierge and staff working the ground floor are quite intimidating in their crisp Jil Sander-style outfits, few people are aware of these luxurious subterranean facilities. S has the run of the place.

Giddy in her restraints, Jenny keeps her mouth full while S dials the simple pegs to various levels of pain and pleasure, careful never to exceed the volume. They both finally release their anxieties in the spacious cubicle. To Jenny's apparent dismay, S uncuffs the prisoner and, after unmercifully paddling her bare bum for two minutes, instructs her to depart, but not before they have made a date to meet in the men's room at Saks Fifth Avenue one week hence. Out into the night they go, Jenny still wearing the clothes pegs under her shirt. An excellent evening, S declares, and he still has an entire bag full of pegs, not to mention another pair of dewy panties for his growing collection. Just remember to leave them in the mailbox overnight, in case the wife makes a sweep of his pockets.

Just around the corner from this new hotel lives a painter of my acquaintance; we'll call him by his girly name, Betty. He has always loved boys and reefer and red wine, and continues to paint and party with a vigour and consistency that belie his advancing age. Although the years have been kind to him, he has grown somewhat wrinkly, so now he must adjust his sensual sights, find a new niche. With a little online research he discovers the "silver daddy" phenomenon, and becomes, on brief but magical evenings, the father he never was in life.

Apparently, there are innumerable young lads seeking a substitute for the daddy they never had or the real pop who beat them and buggered them black and blue. They want an Old to cuddle with, to reconstitute a past they never had, a twisted version of tender, loving parental care. Betty arranges to meet these likely lads at the Starbucks round the corner from his Bond Street loft, where he's lived since the early 1970s. Once again, the internet provides an unreliable stream of possible connections. Except, in this case, Betty doesn't have to lie about his age or post an ancient photograph. These boys are actually looking for old men.

Before committing to an evening of parental bonding, Betty sizes them up, and part of the thrill is the decision to take a chance that they will not rob and/or murder him if he takes them back to his elegant, art-filled loft. He's hoping for a nice cuddle and a cup of tea, but if they decide on a savage grudge pump with their daddy substitute, he's fine with that, too.

Quite often, the evening winds gently down with Betty dandling a boy on his lap, the lad all innocence again, stroking the older man's wrinkly head as he puffs on a joint. But parenthood has its price. A few days later he notices that small Ed Ruscha photograph has disappeared, purloined no doubt by the temporary son so recently lying around the loft in a loincloth.

There are those who pay, and those who don't yet have to buy their pound of flesh, who still get all they can eat for free. Men like Hyde (not his real name), a handsome, mustachioed hetero, single and solvent, who attracts women like filings to a magnet. And they are not backward in coming forward, some of them are even willing to bypass the dinner/nightcap routine, demanding that he jam them on the spot, in the nearest lay-by or public convenience, as if they can't wait long enough to get to his well-appointed bachelor pad. And yet Hyde brushes aside many of these eager beavers, preferring the calm and reverent treatment he receives at a select group of Asian massage parlours in New York's outer boroughs. Like a happy panda, he eats, shoots and leaves on a regular basis.

What is the operating frequency, how does one signal the desire for a little extra, a happy ending to a vigorous 40-minute massage? Hyde explains: "They usually ask what kind of massage you'd like, hard or soft, and you just tell them you want relaxing, very relaaaxing... ""Aaah, re-raxing," they say with a smile and reach for the string of artificial pearls. Their delicate hands become a blur and, after the joyous finale, there's an extra $30 in their tip cup.

And what am I doing with my nights out while all this scurrilous behavior is taking place? Some masochistic urge still draws me to poetry readings, and more often these days, as the Boomers go down, memorial readings for deceased artists and poets. What shams most of these events seem, teeming with tiny talents and massive egos. Poets consider them a great night out for several reasons: free food and wine, and one less voice to compete with in the shrunken universe of modern poetry. They are happy to sing the dead man's praises now, though they never did in life. They'll even condescend for one brief evening to read his work, rather than their own, in return for the public exposure. Or maybe just one of their own as well? It's short, only two pages. For some reason, the audience never rises up and pelts these blowhards with rocks and stones.

I keep going in spite or for spite, and every time it's less fun than being chained to a railing in a public toilet.

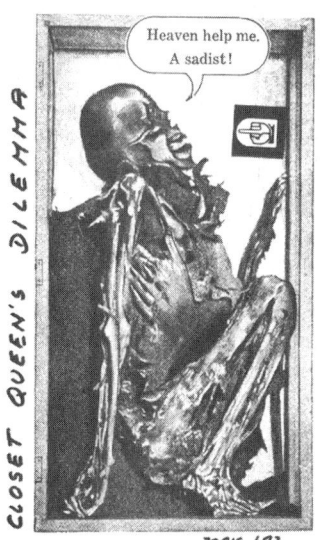

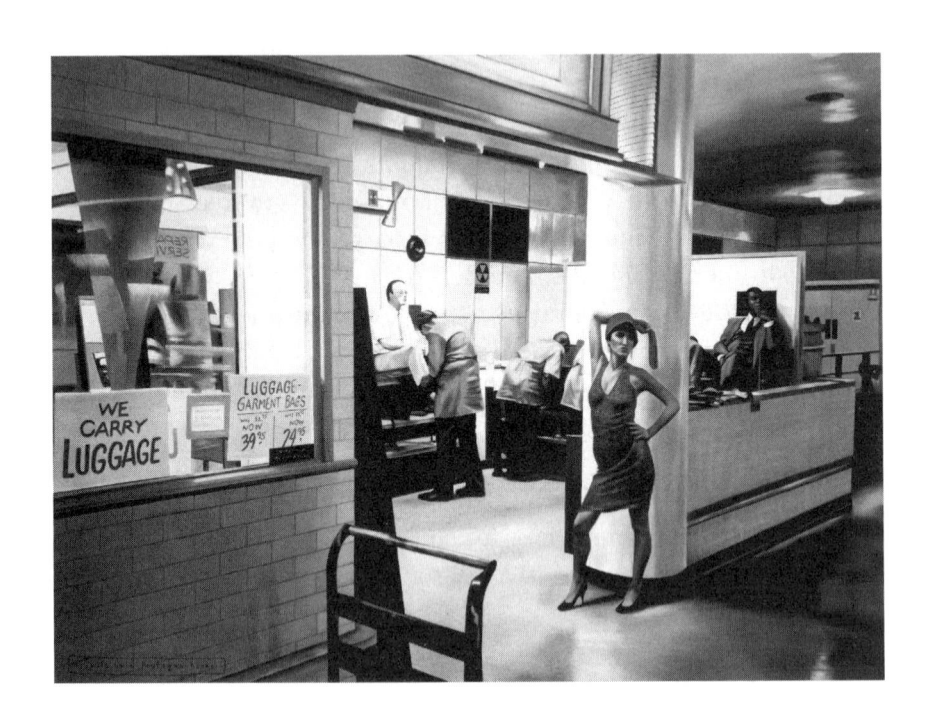

HOOKERS I HAVE KNOWN
CLAYTON PATTERSON

SEX — a word only thee letters long, yet one of the most powerful and content-filled letter combinations in the English language. These three letters can bring joy, intense expectations, companionship, friendship, and are often linked with love. For some creative types, sex is their muse, a mental aphrodisiac that inspires them to make movies, write poems and stories, take photographs, paint. It is a constant theme in entertainment.

These three letters also have a dark side and have been a driving force in the destruction of careers and marriages, tearing apart families, instigating murders, and are used to embezzle, intimidate, exploit, and blackmail individuals. This three-letter combination is connected to therapy, self-doubt, suicide, and addiction.

On the Lower East Side, for many — especially the young — sex is used, in some way, as a means of survival. It's a way to pay the rent.

In the late 70s and early 80s, I lived at 325 Broome Street, between the Bowery and Chrystie. From my second floor window I would look out and see the ladies of the night on a 24-7 hooker stroll — in this case, Black hookers. Other than buildings 325 and 330, the block was occupied by industrial and wholesale businesses, and void of much walking traffic. I never saw a cop.

I managed the building, and was not particularly bothered by this street action. For the most part it was on the other side of the street. When I went out I would greet them, and that was the extent of my interaction. They were too busy fishing to catch a John as they were driving by. The norm was to pick up the hooker, drive a block or two away and make a so-called date. If a date wanted more than a suck or a tug, there was a two-hour rent-a-room, hot-sheet hotel around the block on Delancey. We were cordial.

The front door to the building was set back about ten feet from the street, and a set of stairs led to a landing which was fairly dark, lit by a single Tungsten light bulb. It was like an urban cave, a perfect hideaway for the hookers. But since I was cool with them, they didn't cross the bounds of being neighborly — except one girl for whom being nasty was a way of life. She fought with the other girls and thought she owned the block. She did not last. Most of the girls would take their Johns off the block; she would service hers right there. Not smart!

In the middle of our front door at shoulder height was an unbreakable glass window. Because our alcove was accessible from the street, it was always a good idea to look out before exiting. One incident I saw when checking things out made me laugh out loud.

As I was approaching the door to step outside I could hear voices. When I looked out the window, there was Miss Nasty on her knees, facing the street, mouth in action on this redheaded twenty-something in a brown suit facing the door. I could have whammed the door open and scared the shit of both of them, but I stopped to overhear what this guy was saying. In his moments of moaning glory he said to her: "I can get you something really great." She stopped and said, "What, Quaaludes?" "No," he said, and a few seconds later he squeaked out the word "meditation" as his eyes rolled back and his bobby-pinned yarmulke bobbed.

I am not sure Miss Nasty was amused, but she did not bite his little precious, so I guess she was okay with it. It made my day, so I left them alone.

As mentioned, I was the building manager for the landlord. It was a good job for an artist. Normally I was the middleman — if someone needed a plumber, I would hook up what was needed. Being a hook-up guy is a skill that has helped me survive. There were times, like a sudden snowstorm, when there was no one to call and I would have to shovel the walk. But getting caught in the middle of a fight with the hookers and a tenant in the building was far worse than shoveling snow.

An idiot artist in the building lacked street smarts. He never realized that being friendly and respectful to the street people, especially those who earned their daily keep on your block by engaging in criminal activity, did not translate into friendship. He invited a couple of the hookers into his apartment and had them pose for a portfolio's worth of photographs. The next day, he got robbed of all his equipment. He called the cops and they picked up the girls. There was no proof, but the girls went through the system. Two nights later, the front door, intercom, doorknob and keyhole were attacked by a Montezuma's Revenge-type shit storm. The girls came back with a pile of human feces and, with their hands, did an abstract shit painting everywhere one would have to touch to get into the building. You could read in the strokes that hands and fingers had spread the shit. The pisser was that I got left with the midnight responsibility of cleaning up this stinky payback. Yes, payback can be a bitch, but it should not have been my bitch.

By 1983, Elsa and I had moved to 161 Essex Street, where we have remained. In the "good old days" these busy streets outside our homes always reminded me of rivers, and the sidewalks were the shores where the third world-looking strugglers hawked their illegal goods. The move from Broome to Essex meant we traded hookers for drug-dealers: again 24-7, again no cops, even though we were across the street from a well-maintained elementary school.

I made an ironic video of the school maintenance workers putting up a sign warning that it was a serious crime to deal drugs within 500 yards of the school. I guess none of the cops or drug dealers could read. Drug dealers surrounded the school, but they didn't bother the kids. The action was mostly with drive-bys.

The motor-driven boats would pull up to the shore and, with the motor still running, the captain or passenger would roll down the window and an exchange was made. Soon they would file their way back into line and follow the current off the block heading to some tributary. Who knows? Who cares?

Of course Essex Street was deeper in the jungle, which meant rubbing shoulders with dozens of shoreline dope peddlers and daily drug hunters. I never did what they did, but I was the curious, creative type. I realized that I had moved into their territory — they never came to mine — and I adapted to my new home, filled with curiosity. I wanted to integrate into this new landscape and find out more about these mysterious, sometimes mystical sellers and hunters of what? Ecstasy? Madness? Stupidity? Satan (as some would say)? I was not interested in experiencing what they did — I was interested in them.

Most were on the never-ending run to hunt down whatever fix was needed to feed their insatiable habit. I started photographing the street warriors in front of my front door and putting the photos in my storefront window, which meant that I could have an ongoing relationship with many of the people who occupied the street. But all my communications could be discretely handled on the street and not in my apartment, like the Broome Street knucklehead.

My explorations took me on many exotic journeys, which included danger and darkness and in-depth descriptions, unseen by me, but explained in graphic detail by the coke hunters. After they shot the coke, they would go into great detail about how their bodies were invaded by parasites, bugs; they had visions of both grandeur and hell. It was fascinating for sure, and who was I to question what insights this hyper-reality drug state yielded to them, or to question if the feelings taking over their bodies and their seeing microscopic invaders was real or not. It was not my place to question the authenticity of their realities; I was there to document their reality.

Once caught in the trap of addiction, with all that it takes to feed it, it is hard to have a job that will cover its cost, so prostitution becomes an option. I was documenting the street drug world and there was a natural overlap between drugs and prostitution, so my documentation included a number of the street strollers. I did not branch off into the other aspects of prostitution; only the one tied to drugs.

In the early 1980s, Richard Hambleton, with his Shadow Paintings, was one of the most recognized and respected of the emerging graffiti artists. He was famous before Keith Haring and Jean-Michel Basquiat. By the late 1980s, Richard was a desperate drug addict, still creating, but pushed to the fringes of the art world. When I met him, around 1989, he was living in a building at the corner of Houston and Orchard Street. The building was in legal limbo. Not quite a squat, it was caught between different landlords as it was being flipped during the middle period of the chaotic gentrification years. His apartment was a shooting gallery. Richard's art supported his habit. There was another constant — he always had some junkie prostitute living with him.

One day in the Orchard Street shooting gallery, when I was videotaping Richard's art and bedroom studio, I noticed a body sleeping on a couch. She woke up and I soon found out her name: Anne Hanavan.

The meeting from her point of view:

"At the time, I was living with the artist Richard Hambleton, with Steven, who used to run a magazine that folded, and with this crazy Canadian girl named Bonnie, who I never liked very much. She could usually be heard by our neighbors, and whoever was passing by the building, screaming about being dope sick and slamming doors. Bonnie believed that the louder she would yell the sooner one of us would shut her up with a bag of dope. It usually worked, but on more than one occasion the cops would show up, and at this point were on a first name basis with her. Actually, they knew all of our first names and we knew them by their last names. In any case we were all very familiar.

There was blood everywhere: on the walls, floors, ceilings, tables, chairs, counters, doorknobs, bedposts, sinks, showers, our shoes, the radio, Steven's TV, Bonnie's dog, Richard's bike, and the windows, too — you get the picture....

I woke up to a video camera aimed at my track marks, held by a huge man who looked like a Viking. I flipped. 'What the fuck is going on, Richard? Who the fuck is this?' Turns out the Viking was Clayton and Richard had invited him over to shoot the studio and I was indeed, at that moment, part of the studio. Clayton was completely calm and unaffected by the surroundings. I was intrigued. He smiled and introduced himself — he seemed nice enough. I soon learned that Clayton was genuinely fascinated by our lifestyle and had a connection to the subculture."

[From *Captured: A Film/Video History of the Lower East Side*, p. 532, Seven Stories Press, NYC.]

From this moment on we became friends. I was intrigued by her drug use. She was pale and thin, yet she always managed to retain her beauty. Anne had an innocent vibe and was always pleasant to deal with. Her hard lifestyle never made her hard. A drug addict, a carhop ghetto street prostitute, Anne was a little different than Richard when it came to her shooting up habits. She treated her body like a pincushion. She, like Richard, shot both heroin and coke. What was different about Anne was that she liked to pierce herself with the needle. Jam it into her leg. Draw a little blood, and pull the needle back out. Repeat this action, again and again, in and out, till her arms and legs were bleeding from these multiple punctures. As she pulled out the needles, she would wipe, with her bare hand, the droplet of blood left where the needle puncture was, leaving smears of blood covering her body. Eventually she would need to stroll, buy some more drugs, start the whole game over again. And again, and again. Out into the dark streets, into a car, the John not realizing she was covered in blood.

On the east side of Sara D. Roosevelt Park, particularly the stroll around Stanton, Forsyth, and Allen streets, the hookers were mostly white. During the 80s, when working this area, it was critical for the girls to be on point. This stroll was pure ghetto, and was as dangerous as being locked up in a large cell in the bowels of the New York City Tombs. Working this beat, a girl could get robbed, beaten, left for dead, or dead. This was one of the locations Joel Rifkin, the convicted prostitute serial killer, used to troll for some of his nine known victims.

There were tricks to survive working on the street. Anne Hanavan said she was sure Rifkin had approached her in his small pickup truck. She was about to get into this deadly creep's vehicle when she noticed there was no door handle on the passenger side. Desperate for a fix or not, her street smarts let her know that it looked like a trap and to move on.

I met Bonnie through Richard as well. Bonnie was the one prostitute who proved the rule: every group has a Miss Nasty. Bonnie was originally from Toronto, Canada, and she had the disposition of a bull getting speared by a matador: angry, nasty, bitter, and needy, always needy. Bonnie was ugly, not because of her looks, but because her disposition was foul and she did not take care of herself.

Bonnie was one of the people who shot coke and discovered that shooting coke allowed her to see the microscopic coke bugs inhabiting her flesh. With her sharp, long, dirty fingernails, she would pick and pick to get the bugs out from under the skin on her face. Soon her digging created large open sores. These sores on her cheeks could get to be the size of a silver dollar. Then she would dig deeper and pick at her wound some more. The tapes I made in the shooting gallery are not for public entertainment. My hope is that, someday, I will meet a medical professional or an addiction specialist who is interested in learning by observing behaviors related to coke addiction — to become enlightened about how shooting coke affects the human body.

Another street worker I became friends with goes by the name of Anntelope. She is a poet and a musician. Anntelope told me, when working a dangerous stroll, the first thing she did when getting into a vehicle was roll down her window. If anything weird happened, she'd distract the driver, grab the keys and throw them out the window. He had to go for the keys and she could run. When I met Anntelope, she was at the end game of her years on the stroll.

Mostly because of my relationship with Anntelope, I came to believe that shooting coke, with all its impurities and what it is cut with, wrecks havoc on the bones. Anntelope, by now in her late 40s, was suffering with severe neck and upper back pain. She could hardly hold her head up.

Anntelope was a proud woman. She asked me to accompany her to the hospital emergency room. The first emergency room we went to was at NYU and then we tried Bellevue. She could not tolerate the arrogant attitude of the doctors, and how they disrespected her as a person. I, too, was a little shocked at how rude and callous the doctors were. She found her way to Cabrini and eventually got better. As she recovered, she became more involved in making small paintings and writing poetry.

The story about how I first met Anntelope is amusing. At the time, I knew Linda Twigg, a short, good-looking blond. If you were her friend she could be one of the loveliest, sweetest, and most generous people you knew. She was a major pot dealer and not one to cross. Linda wanted me to record a situation she was involved in. She would not explain what she needed recorded, just that she had to have a record of the evening's events. I went along with it. Accompanying Linda was a stocky, tough-looking butch; I assumed, a friend of hers. The pace was fast, conversation was terse. We got to the location on First Avenue and Sixth Street.

Anntelope rolled up on her bicycle. She had the skinny build of a person who had shot drugs for years. She was about 5′ 9″ tall, in her mid-40s. She was still pretty in an older woman way, and you knew she had been a real good looker. Her demeanor was serious but pleasant. In a past life, a few years before, Anntelope had also been a big time pot dealer. They both worked for this guy Bruno, and Anntelope was Linda's bodyguard. Anntelope may have had the junkie look; however, in order to survive for so many years on the street, she had become a formidable street fighter.

It turned out that a fellow dealer who lived in the hood had ripped Linda off. It was a mistake. Linda wanted to send this woman a message — you fuck with me and you will pay a price. The thief's building had a glass front door. Linda impatiently and steadily started ringing the woman's bell, and then began pushing all the bells. The woman answered the intercom. "Get down here." Soon the woman, followed by her boyfriend, showed up. The woman opened the door to talk. Anntelope was the first one in. Linda, soon after, took over this opening, spit in the woman's face, and started to punch her. Anntelope, a container of mace in her hand, stepped between the two, and gave the woman a warning to clear up her debt. Soon the problem was rectified and the woman moved.

I was angry with Linda because she compromised my value system by suckering me into her plot. I do not document or participate in crime. I do not want this kind of information to be a part of my archives. While it is true that using drugs is against the law, I thought of what I was doing as recording addictive behaviors. Besides, until the mid-90s, the section of the LES where I lived — between Houston and Delancey — was a full-on drug using and dealing zone.

Soho was known for its art galleries. We had drugs.

Linda saw herself as a Gangster Bitch. Through some Italian friends she expanded her business from dealing pot to selling gambling supplies. She was given the rare and unusual contract of gold-stamping clay chips for high-end casinos. Later she had a much younger, good-looking boyfriend. The problem was that he was too young, too naïve, too stupid, and too infatuated with the mythology of what he imagined a gangster was supposed to be. He shot a cop, thus ending one life and ruining his own. Linda died of a heroin overdose.

But, through this nightmare, I got to be friends with Anntelope. In my archives are a number of videos of Anntelope reading her stories and poems, and explaining the meanings of her delicate watercolor paintings. In a film and video history, it is not unusual to highlight an actor. Since she is a featured in my archives, I wanted to give her the opportunity to give the world more insight into her character. She wrote an article about the life of a street prostitute for *Captured*. Her chapter is called "Whoremoans," by Anne Lombardo Ardolino. An excerpt:

"That's when I received a really good lesson about just how raw things can get out there in the 'sportin' jungle.' Because I was left speechless while 'Li'l Bit' ducked between two parked cars, raised her skirt, then squatted and spread her legs, and since she had no panties on, what she did next was wide open to my view and let me say, it was rank to witness as with no apology. She reached up into her hairy, steaming vagina with what appeared to be all four fingers, stirred them around, then popped them out abruptly. With that there came a rush of cum, leaving her hand shiny with the goo, and I was aghast as she flung it, I mean she just let it sling off her person and go flying, finally landing on the window of somebody's car, after which it hung there in sticky strands, just a-swayin' in the breeze.

As she was doing this, 'Li'l Bit' was busy cursing the chap in the automobile, saying quite loudly for all to hear, "WOULD YOU BELIEVE THAT LOW-CLASS MOTHERFUCKER? WOULD YOU BELIEVE HE CAME OUT HERE FOR A FUCKING DATE AND DIDN'T EVEN BRING A PIECE OF FUCKING TOILET PAPER?"

Wiping her hands on the inside of her skirt, she lowered it back down, smoothed it out, then ran her filthy fingers through her greasy hair, preparing to go back to work, but not before she asked me if I had a cigarette, which I handed her quite gingerly, trying not to touch any part of her person. While she was walking away, I heard her saying to no one in particular "I HAD TO GET HERE FAST BEFORE IT DRIPPED DOWN MY LEG."

Over the years I have met and befriended many individuals who worked in or were connected to the sex world. Recently I met Zoe Hansen and Gerry Visco, both ex-working girls. In the past, Zoe was a drug addict. She survived to tell her fascinating war stories. And Gerry was never intrigued by or curious about drugs. She worked the high end of the escort business.

What surprised me about all these women, including Bonnie? First, they were all very intelligent women. Anne Hanavan, once she recovered and got sober and before gentrification killed her business, ran her own very chic and profitable boutique. During working hours you would find her at her clothing stores. After work she built a solid reputation as an avant-garde filmmaker and became the President of the Board of Directors of the Filmmaker Co-op. Recently she married a businessman with movie star looks. Zoe is working hard at expanding the audience for her writing. She married a well-known rock-n-roll legend and has a young son. Gerry works at an Ivy League university and has acquired several degrees. She, like many of the girls, is very active, leading a full and productive life. All these women have had their writing published. Bonnie reads all the time, but sadly stayed curbside. I'm not sure if she is alive or dead.

Another surprise for me is that except for Bonnie and the war stories, none are of these woman are bitter about their life choices. Anntelope saw her profession as a service to mankind, a way to relieve some of the pain these men were suffering from. It was the guys who had the mental issues, not her. Zoe and Anne come across as perfectly adjusted, normal women.

I'm not sure why, but I never documented the sex world. I never engaged in their activities. I appreciate intimacy. This world is void of intimacy. For those who use it, I say — good. Better a momentary, impersonal engagement with a prostitute than a serious relationship outside of marriage or a partnership. Spitzer was a good governor and, assuming he had a solid family life and loved his wife, who cares if he visited a prostitute? Better that than having a girlfriend.

But there is no question that knowing these women has enriched my life and broadened my understanding of humanity.

(Thanks to Monica Uszerowicz
for her editorial assistance)

FUCKING PIG!
ANNE HANAVAN

Fucking pig! So gross. Trying to get over on a street ho who is charging twenty dollars to suck a dick. Pathetic. You would be surprised on how many of this type I came across. Funny thing was I thought so little of myself I just accepted the unacceptable. The number of rapes and robberies I endured by tricks over the years were countless. I never once reported an abusive trick to the cops. I just chalked it all up as part of the game — shoved the feelings deep down under bundles and bundles of dope and kept on moving.

The cops I dealt with were not like the ones you might see on a "Law and Order" episode. No way were they going to waste any manpower on tracking down the dumb fuck who raped me in a stairwell on Fourteenth and Second after I willingly lead the motherfucker into the building. Granted the encounter was to be conducted as a business transaction, not as me being forced to have sex with him while he held a knife to my side the entire time he fucked me from behind while pushing my face down against the filthy staircase. I can still taste the filth in my mouth whenever I think of that day.

Or do you really think a cop is going to give a shit about some guy who punched me in the face and demanded his money back because he couldn't come? I don't think any of the cops I ran into could have cared less. The lowest of the low were the cowards who pretended to be undercover cops threatening to bust you if you didn't give them a blow job. This happened to me every now and again. Sometimes I submitted and sometimes I called them on their bluff. If they looked like they might get violent, I would usually submit.

This one fat fuck picked me up in his disheveled black Buick Skylark. It was a fucking joke. I don't know who looked worse, the car or the pathetic loser at the wheel. The car was so jacked up the owner probably had to bribe the inspector who issued the registration sticker to keep it on the road. It was rusted out with worn tires and the front bumper was literally being held up on one side by a wire cord. The moron behind the wheel had a mop of scraggly blond ringlets sitting on top of a swollen, oil-slicked head. Pinkish pockmarks peppered his cheeks. He looked like the type of guy who'd have a film of sweat on his brow in the middle of a snowstorm. Totally pathetic. He circled the stroll three times. But when he pulled over, I jumped right in. I was only focused on the dope I could buy with the measly twenty bucks I was hoping to get.

"Goin out?" I asked.

"You know it," he answered.

"Cool. What are ya interested in?"

"Whatever you got."

"I got a lot... depends on what you want." I knew this guy was going to be difficult. Sometimes tricks and hookers play a semantics game. No one wants to be the first to really flat out say what they want. Everyone is afraid the other might be law enforcement. With this guy I sized him up and determined he was too fat and stupid to be a cop.

"Depends on what it's gonna run me."

I figured he could barely afford a replacement bulb for the hunk of junk he was riding in. So I gave in.

"Blow job, twenty. Straight, thirty. Half-and-half, forty, unless we hit the hotel. That's extra."

"Sounds fair."

As we drive to this little side street down by the Con Ed building over at the end of Fourteenth Street he makes stupid chitchat. Where am I from? Why did I move to NYC in the first place? Does my family know where I am? All the wrong shit to ask a hooker who works the streets. Be smart enough to keep it light. Current events, weather. Stay away from personal questions. I hate this guy.

We pull over, he shuts the car off and the bullshit starts.

"Listen sweetheart." Sweetheart? This guy is a complete idiot. "I'm a cop," he says.

"You're a cop?!" I know this pathetic loser was in no way a cop. This man could not even hope to be a security guard.

"Yes, I am a cop. We can do this two ways. I can take you in to the station or we can work something out between the two of us."

At this point I am trying not to laugh in his face but at the same time I am so enraged that I am so fucking far away from the stroll and will, of course, have to walk all the way back to Eleventh and Second to catch a real trick. I cannot believe my fucking luck. I knew I should have never jumped in this hoopty piece of shit car.

"Work something out? Work it out h-how?" I ask in a slightly exaggerated fearful tone.

"I think you know how," he says, as he glances down at the crotch of the old pair of ill-fitting jeans he most likely picked up at Sears and Roebuck. Oh my god, he is totally serious. Mind you, I am a tall gal but in my days as junky whore I weighed in at 105 if I was lucky. This guy is HUGE in every way. His head is huge, his hands are huge and it looks as if he has a huge basketball stuck under his frayed green sweatshirt but I still don't get the violent vibe from him. "Look, you got two choices here." He is starting to raise his voice now. "You give me head or I take you to jail. I am serious."

I stare into his face then slowly lower my eyes to the fly of his Sears specials, count to three in my head, then slowly lift my gaze to his and say, "You know what? I'll take jail. Yep...I will definitely take jail."

"Don't fuck around with me girl. I am serious!" He's yelling now. I had no idea his face could get any redder than it had been but it is quickly turning fuchsia. "I will take your ass in!"

"Take it in. I am not sucking your dick. I want to go to jail. Ya know what? I am fucking exhausted. Jail would do me good right about now. I got no fucking home. I'm fucking starving. If you lock me up, I got a place to get some sleep and get me something to eat — before ya know it, I'm out."

"I am starting the car and taking you to jail. We can do this another way," he says, trying to reason with me.

"I am stickin' with jail."

As he turns the ignition key all you can hear is a loud clicking clanking sound... errr err errrr err... his car won't fucking start. He's staring at the steering wheel with such intensity as if he's trying to will it to start but it just keeps making this horrible noise every time he turns the key.

"How do you expect to take me to jail?" I yell. He looks over at me not saying a word. I start to crack up. "You better call your partner, Mr. Police Man, if your radio still works! Where are you hiding it? Under your shirt?" I yell as I unlock the luckily manual lock on the door and jump out. "Where's your back-up now?" I scream as I slam the door. As I start to run down the street I turn and yell, "You ain't no fucking cop, but you sure are a fucking PIG!"

BROTHEL WORK
L.Z. HANSEN

I climbed the stairs in five inch platform shoes, with Bill's cocktail in hand. I had difficulty walking on shag carpet in high heels and I twisted my ankle grabbing the shaky wooden banister to steady myself. I would need to get used to these heels again.

I expected to see a little old man sitting in his underwear behind the door, thankful that any pretty young female was going to have sex with him. I felt the nerves spark in my stomach. My mouth went dry, but there was no time to have performance anxiety.

I took a deep breath and closed my eyes momentarily. Here goes… I changed into my alter personality Lizzy. I put my hand on the doorknob, looked skyward, made a sign of the cross in my mind and turned it. I opened the door to my first trick in four years.

"Nice to meet you," I said with a fixed smile, walking confidently over to the man sitting on the bed. I held out the glass, which he took, not saying a word. He took a large swallow.

My first thought: Rude. OK, I can handle rude. If the price is right.

"So how are you today, Bill?" I asked, standing in the shadows. It was as though a pre-recorded tape was playing and all the right words were coming out of my mouth without any thought from me.

Only a small pink bulb shone from an ugly old lamp in the corner of this deep blue room. I viewed my surroundings. The four corners appeared dark and endless.

Allowing my eyes to adjust to the shadows, I focused properly on Bill. To my surprise, he was in his mid-twenties, handsome, with a mop of dark messy hair, and a muscular torso. But I couldn't fully see his face as he was hunched over staring into his half full drink.

"Is the drink OK?" I asked cheerfully. I was beginning to feel a bit uncomfortable. This man clearly was not a talker or in any hurry to have sex. Both not necessarily bad things. I was on the clock and his time was my money.

Bill smiled and stood up. I stiffened at his movement. He walked over to me and looked into my eyes. He just stared and smiled to himself.

OK… I've met many tricks like this. He's playing a mind game, right? He's one of those guys who wants to mess with a girl's head. I took a deep breath.

Money! I suddenly thought: I gotta get my money. Then he can mind fuck to his little heart's desire.

I looked over to the table, maybe he'd left it somewhere. Nothing! Only the basket with lotion, Lysol, and rubbing alcohol. All right, I will let him unwind for the next two minutes, and then I would have to ask for my money. He gulped the rest of his vodka cranberry down in one mouthful and wiped his mouth. He appeared preoccupied, nervous.

OK that's it. Now I must collect my money.

"Err, um, Bill… I have to ask you to…." He silenced me by putting his fingers to my lips, pulling his wallet from his back pocket. He took two one hundred dollar bills out, and tossed them on the bedside table.

Good. Thank you very much. Now we have that taken care of. I didn't care for him shushing me. In fact, this whole silence thing was beginning to piss me off.

Bill then reached out and touched my arm softly, caressing my skin. I got goose bumps and shuddered. He held my neck, to kiss me. I don't like to kiss clients. I felt his lips cold from the cocktail. He smelled like baby powder, sweet. His body felt firm, young. He held me. I felt his hard cock against my thigh.

He pulled the top of my dress down and kissed my breasts. The stubble on his chin brushed my skin — it felt arousing, my nipples reacted. I tried hard to stay focused, to be professional.

He moved me carefully to the bed and sat me down. This was feeling all too much like a real date. I went to the button on his jeans. I must gain some control. I kept saying over and over in my head: Control. He moved my hand away and unbuttoned the jeans himself and pulled them off. We lay back, he moved on top of me.

Do I tell him now it's going to be an extra hundred for him to give me oral…? I had forgotten so much… I was getting turned on, but work is work, and nothing's for free. He went down, kissing me lightly all the way. By the time I felt hot breath on my clit, my professional instincts were disappearing. I was impressed at this young man's ability to completely disarm me. He was winning. I wasn't in control, and for that moment I didn't care. I wanted him to fuck me… but… I still wanted my extra money!

I felt as though I'd been under a spell. How did he make me respond like that? I never got so turned on while working, before. It wasn't as though I was hungry for sex — I had great sex at home, regularly, well maybe not as often lately.

I reached over to the table and with one smooth movement I grabbed the red Trojan I had placed there. I ripped it open with my teeth, and moved out from under Bill's body. I put the condom in my mouth, making sure it was the right way, the round rim between my teeth and inside my lips. I pushed him gently back and rolled the condom onto him with my mouth. A well practiced trick I learnt from one of the older women I'd worked with a few years ago. I lowered myself onto hard cock. He stroked my hair looking deep into my eyes with such love, it made me uncomfortable. My leg muscles had stayed surprisingly strong. He could get a good visual from this position, and relax while I did the work and gained control. He stared at my tight stomach muscles, my breasts bouncing as I played with myself, while I slid up and down his cock. He stared at my face, kept looking into my eyes. Why was he doing that? It was irritating. He was becoming too personal — making this session too much like real sex. It wasn't supposed to be like this. I swiveled around with him still inside of me, so he could grab my buttocks. I continued riding up and down on his dick. Now I could tell he was having trouble holding on, his breathing was getting heavier, and his fingers dug into my ass cheeks.

"I love you, Sarah, I love you...." He murmured so quietly no one was meant to hear. Sarah. Who's that? I looked straight ahead and counted in my head.... Five... Four... Three... Two... One... B...I...N...G...O! Done! I heard a 'cha-ching' in my head. Every time I made a man come it was two hundred bucks in my pocket.

I carefully got up so as not to pull the condom off, and grabbed some tissues and handed them to him.

Bill patted the sheet and reached out, as though he wanted to hold me. Sensing this, I resisted and sat on the edge of the bed. I never liked to lie or cuddle with clients. He took my hand and spoke for the first time.

"What's your name?" he asked. "You're lovely."

"Thank you, and it's Lizzy." I gave him my professional Lizzy smile.

"No, your real name." Oh no, not this line. It annoyed me that he assumed Lizzy was not my real name.

"That's it — Lizzy," I said.

"Lizzy. Very beautiful. So is that short for Elizabeth?" he asked, brushing hair from my face. I swung my head so the hair fell back down again. His gaze was a little too close for me to feel comfortable.

"No, just Lizzy, plain old Lizzy." I said, leaning back a few inches. This might be a long hour. I looked at the buzzer on the wall that would sound when our time was up.

"Lizzy," Bill said, "I have to tell you something. Since I feel we have a connection. Do you feel the connection?" I looked at his pretty boy face, dark almond eyes, long lashes, small straight nose, really quite a good-looking man. If I met this man out in the real world, I might date him... maybe.

"Do you have brothers and sisters?" he asked. It seemed like a harmless question.

"Yes." That's all I was going to give him, for now, till I knew where he was going with this. "Do you?" I asked.

"I do, yes, I have a sister."

Bill searched my face again. I felt like a prostitute bug under a microscope. There are so many strange men who I had come across while working as a sex worker; who knows what's behind this man's thoughts? I didn't care at this point, I wanted to complete the hour successfully and get paid.

"Sit." Bill patted the bed again. I obeyed.

"I think we have something, I think you're special." He was serious.

Sure we do, as long as you're paying me, we got something, all right. I smiled and took his words as pleasant compliments.

"Would you think it strange if I told you… I've been having sex with my sister?" Bill looked at me solemnly, yet visibly nervous, waiting for my reaction.

My gaze shot back to him upon hearing the words "sex" and "my sister." Was he joking? Is he serious? I don't like jokes.

"Really, wow, your sister…." My mind raced as I thought hard about this one. Incest repulsed me. Actually it frightened me beyond belief. Isn't that what separates us from cats and dogs? The ability to not fuck everything that runs across our path?

What type of shit has he been through? What sort of childhood had this man had? I felt a mixture of pity — and disgust that I just had sex with this guy. Although it was just work sex, and not real sex….

"You and your sister, really… wow! Um… err. Where does she live?" A strange and irrelevant thing to say when someone has just confessed to screwing his sister. But, I was at a loss for anything constructive, it was just the first thing that came to mind.

"She moved to Philadelphia recently. The reason I wanted to see you is well…. Nina told me about you, and what you look like, she knows I like long dark hair and bangs, fair skin… the way she…my sister looks…" He drifted off into a dreamy far away look, "and… well you actually look very much like her."

Now this was getting weird.

"Oh no, I can't look that much like her…." I was getting curious.

"Really, you do! Actually it blew me away when you walked into the room. That's why I didn't talk much, I was in such shock — it was as though she was here, you were her. We've been having a sexual relationship since we were children. She was thirteen. I, sixteen. I love her so much. I was her first… I… umm, took her virginity. I want to marry her. I just can't be with anyone else. I've never had a relationship with anyone but her." Bill lowered his head and looked so torn inside, so confused, so broken-hearted. I felt sorry for him. I wanted to put my arms around him and tell him it was going to be all right, that he'd fall in love with another woman — someone he could have an honest healthy relationship with, and not to worry. But I didn't.

I sat and listened, transitioning into psychiatrist whore. I was also wondering if this was an incest fantasy, and his telling me was part of the turn-on. That was certainly possible. But he seemed too sincere and emotional for it to be a fantasy.

"She's getting engaged to some asshole — she doesn't want me any more. I can't believe it. She's throwing our whole life away. I love her so much. I can't live without her. My therapist told me to come to a professional, you know, like yourself, to try and develop feelings for another woman. Do you think it will work? Do you think maybe you'd want to go out with me?"

Bill was now staring at me with urgency — he really seemed to want to know if I would date him, which I definitely wouldn't.

"Oh Bill, well, you see, it's like this. If I saw you outside, it would ruin what we have in here, all of what we have." I swept my hand around the dark dusty room, and found my statement a little amusing….

"I understand, you can't see me outside of here. But I can come see you again here, right?" He waited for my response.

"Oh, of course — I will look forward to our next meeting." He seemed very pleased with the prospect of our next visit and smiled an honest wide happy grin that looked so sincere it made me feel touched that I had meant something to this man, that our future sessions were that important.

Bill got up just as the buzzer on the wall finally sounded.

I had made good money, and Bill seemed happy. A win-win situation.

Bill got back into his tight blue jeans, and black long-sleeved shirt. I thought I'd met all kinds in my life. But a sister-fucker? This was a first! At least he wasn't a mother-fucker, or brother-fucker.

We walked down to the first floor. When we reached the living room, Bill pulled his wallet from his back pocket. I assumed he was about to hand me a tip. I stood on the landing saying how nice it was to meet him, and I reassured him that I hoped to see him again, soon. I looked at his wallet as he pulled a small photo with worn edges and handed it to me. I took it and gasped at what I saw.

"Oh my god!" I exclaimed. She really did look like me, it was uncanny.

"I told you," he said, smiling. Staring at me again. Pleased that I had such a strong reaction.

It was just a weird coincidence, wasn't it? The eyes and nose were the same, even the shape of the face, but her's was longer and she had a fragile look.

"OK, then… have a great day," I said, with a professional smile pleasantly fixed on my face.

"Nice to meet you," Bill responded. He leaned in, kissed me softly on the cheek, and slipped a hundred dollar bill into my hand. Which made me perk up, and hug him.

"See you very soon," he said, with a lingering look.

I waved and watched Bill disappear down the stairs and out of sight.

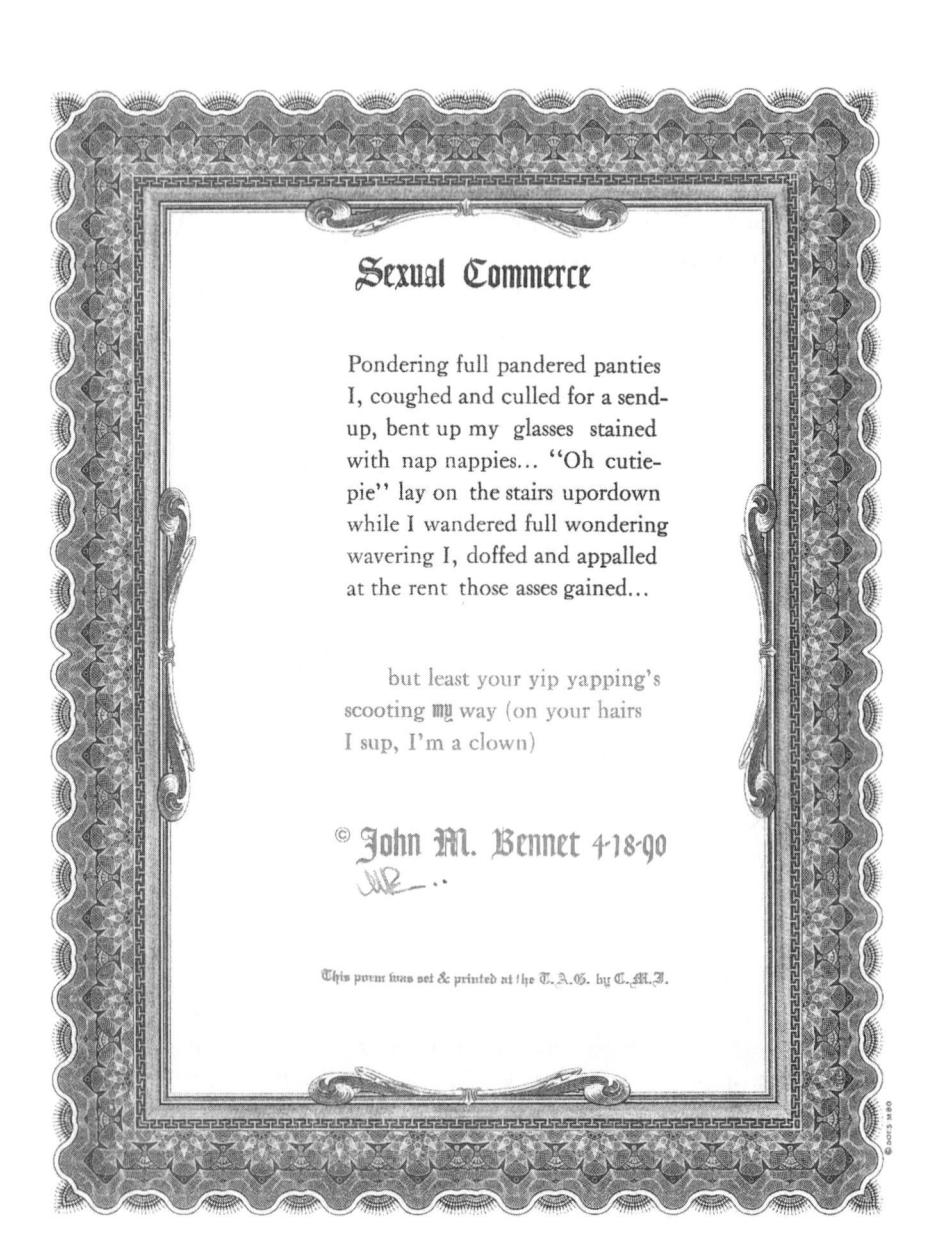

Sexual Commerce

Pondering full pandered panties
I, coughed and culled for a send-
up, bent up my glasses stained
with nap nappies... "Oh cutie-
pie" lay on the stairs upordown
while I wandered full wondering
wavering I, doffed and appalled
at the rent those asses gained...

   but least your yip yapping's
scooting my way (on your hairs
I sup, I'm a clown)

© John M. Bennet 4-18-90

FROM IN THE LAND OF ADULTS
MATTHEW FLAMM

A fringed Pretty Baby lamp atop a small dresser threw a soft halo across the room, turning the water-damaged walls into ruined frescos. Aside from a *Penthouse* pinup hanging opposite the bed the only other brothel touch was an elaborate headboard, its curlicues of fake wood filled in with tinted mirrors.

College Girl was spreading out fresh white sheets. I had considered telling her not to bother, but I'd already upset her routine by refusing to shower, insisting I had showered an hour ago.

A wave of her hand indicated the bed was free. Dropping onto the mattress edge, I bounced up and down until a look from her made me stop.

"Where do you go to school?" My voice sounded shaky. What a ridiculous question, too. But she could have taken it as a joke.

"You don't want to undress?" Jade asked.

"That's okay." I leaned back carefully against the bumpy headboard, shoes staying clear of the sheet. "I just want to talk."

Slipping off her clothes, she tossed them onto the dresser and lay down on her side, one thigh over the other. I helped myself to a glance, not sure it was right to feast. Silver rings pierced the nipples of floppy ghost-white breasts, while below her waist the thin green snake coiled

111

once, then tapered away towards her crotch. Contrary to what had been promised in the living room, the creature did not have two heads.

Propping her chin on her hand she stared at me. I forced a smile. Without smiling back, she danced her fingers lightly up my thigh.

"You can't talk with your clothes off?" Away from the others she spoke more forcefully, though still in a spacey I'm elsewhere voice. Maybe Sarah Lawrence.

"I'm trying to be good."

"Then why are you here?" A neutral question, as if the subject didn't involve her.

"Seriously — research. Also, it's a long story, but my girlfriend says I'm too pure." The two watery scotches had made me chummy.

"Then she'd want you to take your clothes off."

"Probably not."

"Should I tempt you?" Her fingers played spider for a few more steps.

Showing no strain, I managed to say, "Talking is tempting enough."

She nodded, but not like she agreed.

"What's it like when Zack makes the delivery? Does he ever…? You know…" Was that being creepily personal? It was hard to know if anything was personal here.

Jade chewed her lip. "Are you a cop?"

"Hell no."

"Cops don't take their clothes off."

"Cops don't deal herb."

"Maybe it's oregano." She yawned, folded her free arm across her breasts, and pulled up her knee so that her thigh blocked the view beneath her waist. Like a lot of heavy women, she looked better naked.

"I'm not a cop. And I'll pay you anyway."

"Pay me for what?" she asked.

"For talking. What's it like when Zack makes the delivery? Is it different from when I did?"

"Who's Zack?"

After a few seconds of silence, I felt around in my jacket pockets and brought out yesterday's perfectly rolled half-smoked reefer and a book of matches.

"Tell me if this is oregano."

Holding the joint with both hands, she took a shallow puff, well aware of how strong it was. I did the same and told her to keep it.

"You could still be a cop," she said blandly, putting out the joint with moistened fingers and reaching over to set it on the dresser.

Quickly and methodically I removed my clothes, just as I would at the doctor's, and climbed back in under the top sheet, which Jade held aloft for me. It must embarrass some guys to be seen naked. Propping a pillow against the headboard I returned to the position of a moment ago. I would never talk of this evening to Carla and never think about it, so it would be as if it never happened.

Like bubbles popping in champagne, a light tickling sensation traveled over my skin — the super-weed kicking in.

"I'm writing an article about Zack. 'The World of a Dealer.' Don't ask how I ended up subbing for him. Any gangsters ever show up here? You know he works with gangsters?"

Ignoring my jabber, Jade stretched out her legs and pulled back her arm, revealing patchworks of tiny veins in nearly translucent breasts. Further down, the tail of the snake didn't just fade away, but continued in a sinuous line to a cropped covering of rust colored hair.

"See that?" She swiveled her hips to provide a better view. The snake did have two heads after all. "You see where the tongue goes?" Like a spit of flame it lunged toward the winking pink flesh.

"Very nice." My voice reached the room swaddled in cotton. She put out her hand, palm up.

"Right," I said, and felt around on the dresser for my bloated wallet.

"You know it's four hundred for the hour."

A little more — a little — than I'd expected! And who asked for a whole hour? But it didn't seem appropriate to haggle.

"Plus tip."

A tip for talking? Good luck, sister. I counted out the bills twice. Hopping to the floor, Jade flicked the money into the dresser's top drawer and pulled out a foil packet and tube of KY. The place changed, becoming a cramped and squalid maid's room, as if it hadn't been that all along.

Cargo in hand, Jade clambered languidly back to bed.

"Anything special Zack does as a dealer?" I could still leave, once we'd finished talking.

"I'm really tempting you?" Reaching beneath the sheet, Jade ran her fingers lightly up my thigh, but this time didn't stop. "There we go," she said. "You still want to talk?"

Her nipples were the flesh color of childhood crayons. Carla's were café au lait.

"I do." I stared at a ruined wall, wondering if the Carla thought would pass. Nothing would take place with her in the room.

"I think you'd rather fuck me."

It wasn't too late to get dressed, except that whatever went on would all be over in a little while, so what, really, was the difference?

"Yes or no?"

As from a distance, I heard my answer: It would be better if you didn't.

But whose fault was it if my conscience whispered? Not a soul in the world would listen to a voice like that.

I nodded, and a wave of sadness washed over me, the undertow dragging me away. And then a louder, stronger voice burst out: "Yes."

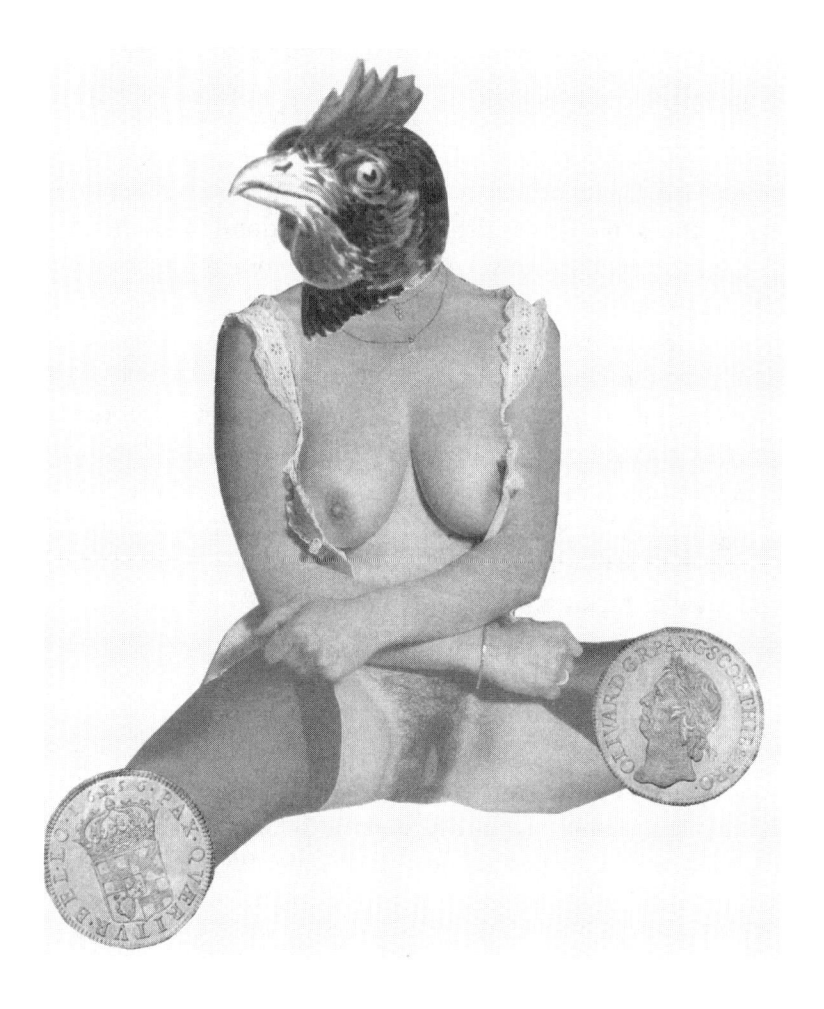

GIVING THANKS
JORDAN ZINOVICH

The erection stood up pink in the palm of Sophia's hand. It wasn't particularly large; a nice size, really, the size that wouldn't hurt her if he asked to stick it in her ass. It was even kind of pretty. She squeezed a cool dollop of KY jelly out on the head and rested her index finger on top of it. "This is the first time I've done this," she said, making a fist and spreading the goo down the shaft in one quick stroke.

She felt the man pulse and heard him groan. "The first time you've fucked for money?" he rasped.

"Of course not," she said, stroking hard for a few more strokes, making him groan again. "I'm a prostitute. But this is the first time I've ever put jelly on under a condom."

"I need it," he sighed. "Otherwise the latex rubs me raw."

"I don't know," she said. "Are you certain it won't slip off while we're fucking?"

"It won't," he said. "It just makes it move a little more freely. Trust me on this."

Sophia glanced down at his face. It was quite a pleasant face; the kind of face that normally told the truth. His eyes were closed, but just a minute earlier they'd been open unable to pull away from her and she'd known from his look that he'd knocked on her window because she was black. She glanced into the mirror beside the bed. She was definitely black; ebony black, so black that her nipples were the only darker possible shade of black: roughened velvet extensions of her breasts. Everything about her was black: hair, eyes, skin only her teeth, her nails, the palms of her hands and soles of her feet, and the bright pink slash of her cunt weren't black. She smiled, letting the black light in the room turn her teeth blue. Then she looked back to the pale erection, warm now, and throbbing under her hand. She stopped stroking and carefully rubbed the excess gel into his thigh before reaching for a condom.

"All right," she said, unrolling the latex sheath down the shaft. "I'll try it. But I'm going to feel to make certain it stays in place."

She bent over and took the pretty penis in her mouth, closing her lips around the head to work its sensitive ridge. The man groaned again, completely her captive now. In a few minutes, when he was near, she'd straddle him and take it up inside her. But she was going to try to be careful, not take him too far along so he'd come too quickly. She wanted to enjoy this first-time experience.

As she felt his hips rise toward her mouth Sophia thought again of the Sudan. The girls she'd grown up with, the ones who hadn't fled with her, would be excised by now. They'd have been slashed and sewn up, and were probably unable to even pee easily. And, if they'd survived the operation, for the rest of their lives they wouldn't feel anything but pain when they had sex, torn open and re-sewn each time they had a baby.

Life in the West isn't so bad, she decided, slipping her mouth past the glans and as far down the shaft as it would go. Just four days of this each week and I can pay my rent and go to school. Perhaps I won't work so hard tonight. I'll let this one stay with me a little longer than usual, just to celebrate a bit.

A CURE FOR HUNGER
AMY OUZOONIAN

His head rose from her saliva-slobbered vagina. She let out a yawn and her legs snapped shut like a beaver trap.

"Well it's not the first time I've been disappointed," she said in a nearly consolatory tone.

"You mean I didn't do anything for you?" The man's cheek was resting uncomfortably on her outer thigh. She didn't respond. He propped himself up and stood, waiting for her to say something. Nothing. He turned to his glass and carried it to a window that looked out at a bridge that had been around since before he was born.

"I didn't do anything?"

He was trying to sound sympathetic but the words fell flat, doused in whiskey, opium and were, for the most part, unconvincing.

A roach or a waterbug scaled the bed's headboard. The woman shifted closer to it and smacked it with her bare hand.

"Do anything? No, it didn't."

"Do you want me to tie you up?"

"No rope."

"Got any food around here?"

"Jar of sauerkraut, can of anchovies and there might be a tomato in the fridge," she answered without moving.

"I could go out to the marina and catch some fish," he said.

"We could sell the boat," she answered.

"We're not selling the boat."

"You're not selling the boat. I'm getting my nails done." She sat on the edge of the bed and filed her left hand.

"Why do you need your nails done? We don't have money for that."

"Marla's doing them for free."

"Marla's a whore — she doesn't do anything for free."

"Why don't you fuck your little dingy and leave me alone."

She walked to the bathroom and slammed the door. A chunk of ceiling fell beside his feet.

He thought about the woman he saw at the Gem Marina yesterday. His boss' niece. What a fine piece of ass she was. She was dressed in black tight pants, black lacey spandex shirt and had a snake tattoo winding up her arm. She noticed him and smiled and laughed with her red lips parted so he could see her stained two front teeth. Her hair was an oil slick pulled back tight in a ponytail, away from her colorless cheeks and stone eyes.

She was beautiful and hard, like how Stella was when he met her. Now, ten years later, Stella was just hard.

"You still here?" she yelled from the bathroom.

"Yeah."

"Well make some dinner will ya? I'm hungry."

He went to the kitchen, got a bowl from the cupboard, cleaned out the webs and chased a spider away with a dishrag and opened the refrigerator. The sauerkraut wasn't expired but the tomato was growing white and green hair. There was a can of beans, a half can of anchovies and a carrot. He opened the can of beans, tossed that in, then mixed the jar of sauerkraut and cut the carrot up and tossed that in too. He hated anchovies, so left that out.

Within minutes all ingredients were mixed and dinner

was ready. He dished out the contents into two smaller bowls. He found a packet of saltines with two crackers and garnished the bowls with a cracker each and some pepper.

"Presentation counts for something," he said to himself.

As he entered the room she was applying lipstick, using the turned-off TV as a mirror.

"Dinner is served." He placed the bowls on the bed that now served as their kitchen table.

"How long have we been in this dump?" Stella asked him as she sat beside dinner.

"Three months." He answered between mouthfuls.

"This is disgusting." She poked her fork in the concoction to see if it moved.

"Cures hunger," he said, nearly finished with his portion and now eyeing hers.

"Hunger's such a catholic reaction to absence," she spoke to the frosty glass window, worn by salty air and dirt.

"What's religion got to do with being hungry?" he asked.

"Not catholic with a capital "C," I mean catholic with a little "c," you idiot!" She knocked the bowl on the floor and stood with her back to the door, waiting for something like a punch or a tackle to the ground.

"Why'd you do that?"

"Because I knew you wanted to eat it."

"Thanks."

"Clean it up. I'm going out."

On his knees, he used his hands to scoop the bean, carrot and sauerkraut mush off the wood floor and dumped it in the bowl. She watched him briefly, half in delight and half in disgust.

"I'm leaving." She grabbed her bag and shut the door behind her.

He stood at the window, facing away from the figure who

trudged through the field of high grass and up the long dirt road that became asphalt and then dipped beneath a bridge and at some point would erode into water, sand and sea.

"I love you," he whispered to the bed, and then with eyes shut he repeated it to her dinner. He could not manage to sit or sleep or think of anything, hunger, to eat, to drink. His thoughts were a flipbook; a fish out of water, longing for atmosphere undiscovered.

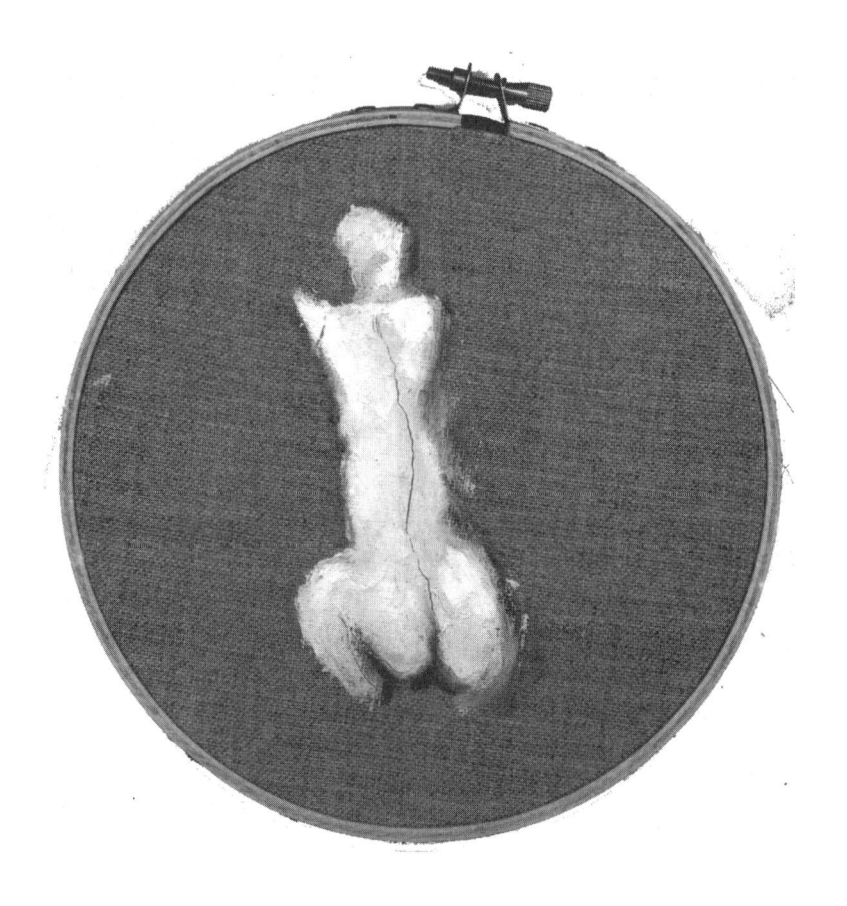

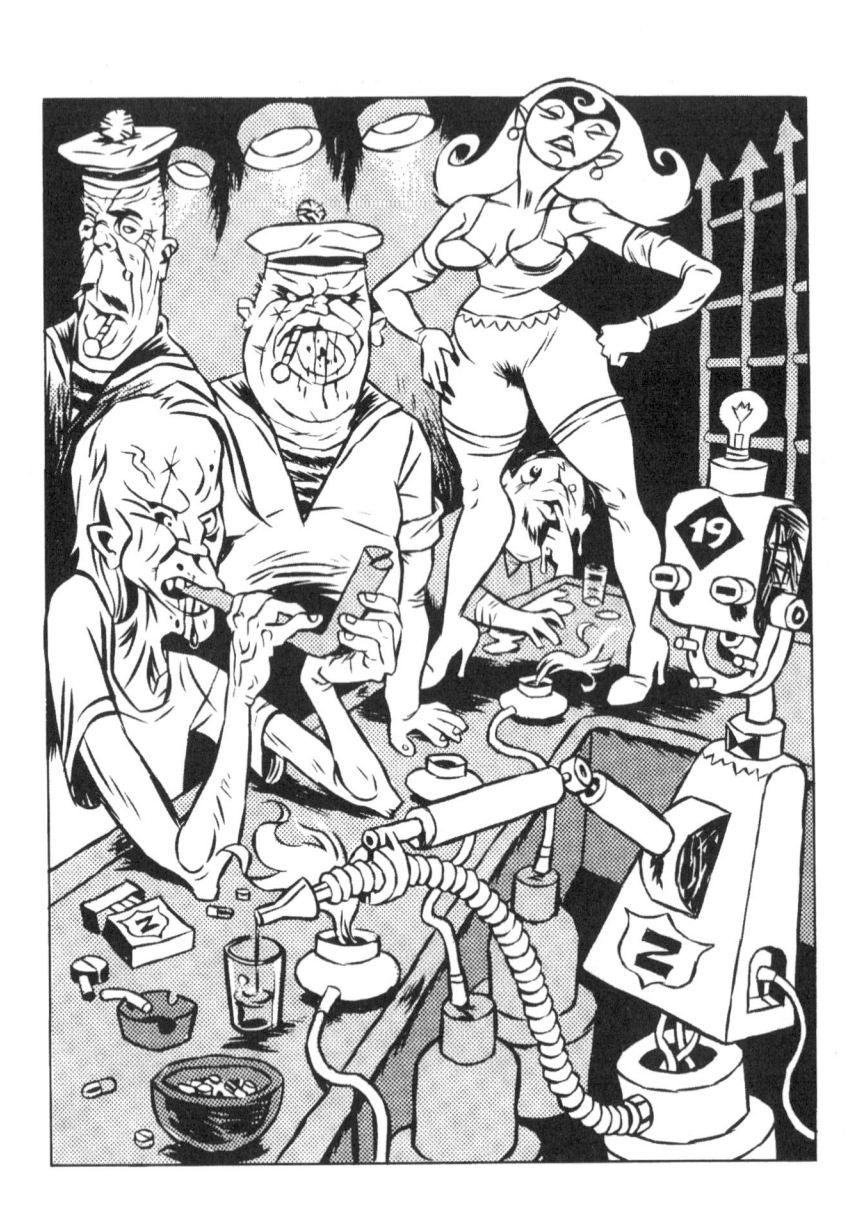

BACKWARDS THE DROWNED GO DREAMING
CARL WATSON

Being on the road caused me to miss most of the major social and so-called youth movements of my day, preoccupied as I was. As compensation the 'Skid Row' world was about to provide me with my own alternative 'Summer of Love.' But it would be depressants: alcohol, barbiturates and heroin, which would fuel my mini-revolution, and not the hallucinogenics and good vibes of the free love generation. No tie dye. No beads. No Woodstock Nation. I wanted to forget about Tanya, and the 'Little Death' was one way of doing it.

I met Patsy Little Death at the bar. That wasn't her name. I never knew her name. I don't know if she had one. Patsy Barfly maybe. I walked in the bar because I heard a song on the jukebox. "Summertime and the living is easy." It's interesting how banal the pivots of our lives can be.

I ordered the shot-and-a-beer special because it was still happy hour. I was minding my business, watching a television show about insects taking over the world. A couple of red ants were killing some black ants, when this pale, baked redhead in blue jeans walked in and grabbed the elbow of my black jacket. "Doesn't all that killing depress you?"

This didn't seem like a pick-up line so I said, "What?"

"Never mind. Listen, could you give me a hand a second? I got a problem."

Apparently one of her friends was getting beat up by one of her other friends and she didn't know how to interfere without showing favoritism. She needed some passer-by with no personal interest. I was that passer-by, even though I was sitting perfectly still. "Of course, I mean you don't have to, if you're not feeling up to it. But I really would appreciate it." she said, unsubtly brushing my leg. My sense of 'duty' was fueled by the vague promise of 'intimacy' on down the line.

The fight was half a block away. We broke it up simply by screaming at the same decibel level as the participants. Then we went to Patsy's place where, as she had hinted, I was to do as I pleased. I guess that was my reward. I doubt if it was hers. She went about the task mechanically, then offered me her back. I let some time pass just to be polite — at least five minutes before leaving. She thumbed a magazine while I pulled on my pants. She started cooking a fix while I laced my shoes. She lit a cigarette with great intent as the door closed behind me.

I did see her again though. In the same bar on a different day. I said hello. "Do I know you?" she replied with little conviction.

"No," I said, somewhat relieved, but also embarrassed because she probably thought I was trying to pick her up. But then I doubt it. She was listening to the men in the Seven Seas. Seemed like weeks had passed. Days at least. And they were still talking. They had circumstances, facts, figures. It was so many millimeters. It was German, no Japanese. Probably cost so many dollars once. And the kid was a loose canon. But the gun was also to blame. Apparently it was one of those guns that did things on its own. The people who held it often had no responsibility for their actions. It robbed people. Made men treat their women mean. Just having it on the table could cause a fight. A gun, a girl — little things, big events.

I thought back to the previous night. Perhaps my presence may have been what stopped an act of violence. It was arrogant to think so. But it turns out that Toby, the guy with the gun, was the husband of the woman who had been in the fight. He was recently out of jail and pissed. She'd been the one fucking the guy up in the park. Toby had gone up there to scare her. Or threaten her. Or him. Or so he claimed. The guy happened to be Patsy's ex-boyfriend. This was no secret. And now it was quite possible he knew that I had screwed Patsy too, even if it didn't mean anything. The net was tightening. My neck seemed to be in the way. Everything's connected they say. The universe is a seamless web. Or maybe just a seamy web.

When we'd had enough to drink we went out and yelled at some people. It was like starting the relationship all over — no baggage. We were young, dumb, belligerent and dumped on. Owed and angry. We went to her place again. She got high straight away, not bothering to wait this time. She knew there was nothing to wait for. Certainly not desire. In fact, I don't think we even wanted to do it, just following a script, some scenario written in some time immemorial by some lonely scribe — an act of joy rendered as an act of attrition. Millions of men and women in bars across the country are forced to end their evenings with sexual intercourse, no matter how useless and empty they know it's going to be. They see the little bead of a human skull in the clown gallery in the back of their minds and they have to shoot at it with something. Knock one down and prolong your life for a second, or a day, or a year. It's a carnival game. The ancient gene engineers and the modern dramatists had got together on it. There was nothing anyone could do.

"Are you done?" she asked.

She went to the bathroom. I stared out the window. A man standing under a streetlamp, smoking hard, stared back. Smoke hovered around his head like a cloud. I heard the toilet flush. "There go my children," I thought. A tear came to my eye as a tugboat cruised up the Willamette River, crossing under the Burnside Bridge.

Then the door opened. "There you go again. Stop feeling sorry for yourself," Patsy said, and with that, she walked back to the mattress and passed out. I gazed lovingly at the passed-out woman, and thought how delicate and vulnerable she must have been, once. Then I poked around some more: a cat-o-nine-tails hanging on the wall, medieval headgear. She made me feel like a kid. Down the dark hallway of her building I thought I heard a bottle break. I heard a muffled argument in another room. It was starting to rain. I felt a slow dull rhythm building up in my brain. I went to the bathroom too. There was a picture of a little boy stuck in the mirror frame. A little boy on a truck-tire swing. No doubt Patsy Little-Death stared at this picture every day with a touch of remorse.

My summer of love continued. I was shooting pool with this Japanese guy named Akira Hiro. We were headed from one bar to the next when this chick grabbed my arm outside the Silver Moon on 19th. I called her a chick, but she was probably 35 years old. We went back to her apartment.

"What's your name, Baby," she said.

"Frank."

She said hers was Sherri, Sherri White Flower. Something like that. Her boyfriend worked nights.

"Boyfriend?"

"Yes… oh, but it's okay, he's at work. If he comes home early though, he'll kill us for sure."

"Yeah?"

"Yeah, probably. But I don't think he will." She laughed.

"What? Kill us?"

"No. Come home early." She chuckled sardonically to herself. But the strain split me in two. I became two people — one watching the door and windows, the other watching her. I also watched my self make a bad decision. I felt light and heavy. Totally alive and dead at the same time. Only women and fear can do this to me. And certain chemicals.

Sherri released the snap on her bra, as she continued her intimidation. Apparently, Sammy, her boyfriend, had been in jail on and off for years on battery and manslaughter charges and he was a jealous man, etc., etc., etc. Once Sammy had found her screwing a friend of his. He beat the guy so bad he was in the hospital for a week. And that was a friend.

"C'mon, we better hurry." She was ready. I balked. "Nervous?" she said, watching the clock and scratching her thigh.

"Why should I be?" I lied.

"Well then let's get it on, Daddy. We ain't got all night."

I found it interesting that she would use the word 'daddy,' when she had called me 'baby' a few minutes earlier. I began to think her plan was simply to poison the womb of her enemy — her husband. She'd get pregnant. He would kill me. End up in jail where she could taunt him daily with a white man's child. It was a savage plan, and a bad movie plot. But this was the real world and it probably would happen. Or, he would kill her. I wouldn't say anything. I might not even know. There would be a mention in the paper. Actually, I would be a major suspect. I hadn't thought of that. But whatever she wanted, she was out of luck. The giant picture of Tanya floating in front of my face was choking the blood flow to my loins.

Tanya had said after all, "I just don't want to know about it." But she would know about this if it made the papers after the murder. But maybe I wanted her to know. Maybe I was getting back at Tanya for her infidelities with Reggie and Fat Mike. Much of the sex drive is based on revenge they say. You not only gain power over the person you screw but power over those who know about it. Of course, they must actually know. You could hope they divine it. Or you could brag about it. You could try reverse psychology — say nothing. Be subtle, subtlety being really just a way of screaming at certain people. Or you could act suspiciously. But in cases of revenge sex, suspicion doesn't always cut it. Tanya wouldn't know unless I told her. But she could suspect, and that might drive her crazy. A sort of delicious persecution. But then I knew she knew already. She was in the room, watching me in the mirror. "You're not hurting me you know. I'm in jail," she said. "So I hope this is fun for you."

I didn't know if it was fun. I guessed it probably wasn't. But then why go on with it? I looked at the woman below me on the bed. All that was lacking was the frame of reference. Maybe Walker was right. Maybe we were all gravitating toward some iconographic degree zero, based in self disgust. Sherri seemed nonplused, if a little miffed by my remoteness. I hadn't even realized that we had started, that I was already doing her. Suddenly, the baby started crying. Sherri unplugged and left the bed to check on it. I, in my isolation, was sure, for a second, that I heard a key slide in the lock. But just for a second. She came out with the kid at her breast. The kid's name was Billy.

"You better go now," she said, "I'm sorry." But I was already on my way out. I had just seen what I swore was a man's shadow outside the window.

A week later I saw Sherri again. She was crawling up the

chest of a 300-pound, seven-foot three-inch one-eyed thug with a buck knife on his concha-studded belt and a tattoo that read 'San Quentin '72.' We exchanged a few words, during which I noticed outside a tall grim figure standing under a street lamp on 19th, smoking a cigarette. It was the same damn guy, waiting for me to join him. I ordered another beer. Somebody put a quarter in the jukebox.

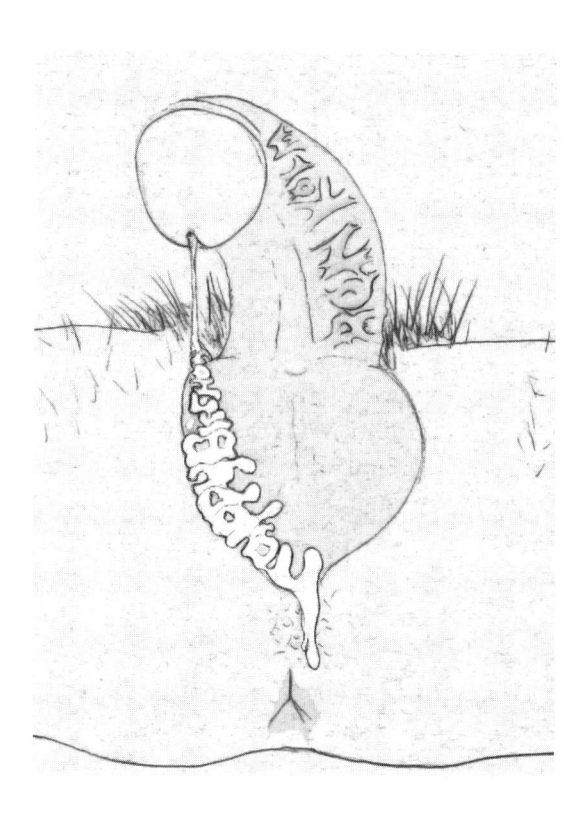

MAUPIN ROW
RON KOLM

We were totally unprepared for the winter of 1968; it was bleak and cold, and it seemed to last forever. My wife and I were from the North — Reading, Pennsylvania — and we had joined a government program to help organize the dispossessed so they could eventually help themselves. This program was called VISTA, which stands for Volunteers In Service To America. What it really was was my ticket out of Vietnam — if I volunteered to help the poor, then I wouldn't get drafted — it was called "alternative service."

The folks we were supposed to be helping were Southerners. Poor Southerner whites. Rednecks. After training in Atlanta, we got sent to Tennessee, to the tri-cities area on the Tennessee/Virginia border — the three cities were Bristol, Kingsport and Johnson City. We ended up in a hollow just outside the Johnson City city limits. The locals had named this particular hollow "Maupin Row," and it was a sad collection of dilapidated wooden shanties lining several narrow dirt roads, which were clustered around a polluted creek.

If you were driving on the city road that circled Maupin Row you couldn't actually see it — you had to turn off the main drag and cut through a sort of high hedgerow — the "community," such as it was, then opened out below you.

We lived in the same type of housing as the people we'd been sent to help — basically a two-room shack with a tiny kitchen hanging off the back. We also had an outhouse. Maupin Row was zoned outside the city limits so it had no sewage system and no garbage pick-up — the people who lived there only got cold running water, and the city was going to keep it that way if they could. Putting in sewers and picking up trash cost money and as the poor weren't able to pay any taxes, they simply weren't worth wasting time on.

Our neighbors were actually very nice to us. Mrs. Jones, who lived with her family on the dirt road that intersected with ours, tried to show us how to bank a coal fire so it would last through the night. The secret was to surround the heart of the fire with enough combustible material to provide fuel for it, but not enough to smother the life out of it. A coal fire banked correctly would smolder slowly, lasting almost until dawn. The only drawbacks were the inevitable fumes, but the shack we lived in was so drafty that that problem was moot.

I never did get the hang of it. Once winter settled in, we had to punt; we drove to the local discount store and bought an electric blanket and a large electric heater; we figured that this would be enough to make one room livable; the bedroom. The rest of our tiny home we abandoned to the cold — and it was so cold in the living room that we could put the milk and soda on the floor below the window, where they kept just fine. Meats, and any other frozen goods, were stashed on the windowsill, where they stayed frozen. I guess I should mention that we didn't have a refrigerator — the house didn't come with one, and we didn't have enough money to buy one, so we ate most of our meals in fast food joints.

They got to know us pretty well in the local McDonald's.

The bitter cold made sex difficult, almost impossible. Moving around under the electric blanket created a storm of static electricity that snapped and crackled and gave us a continuous series of painful shocks — it was like trying to couple on a bed of hot coals. If we threw the cover off, we froze our asses, and if we made it to any kind of climax, the wet cum would almost short the damn thing out. We ended up huddling together under the toasty blanket and watching a lot of late night television — Johnny Carson became our best friend.

We finally came up with an ingenious solution to solve our sexual woes; we'd hop into our half-ton pickup truck, drive to the East Tennessee State University parking lot, and fuck in the cab while keeping the engine running and the heater on. We'd usually keep the radio on, too.

Of course, this solution had its drawbacks. Because we were never sure if some sort of security would eventually show up and chase us off, we had to work quickly. Foreplay was minimal — a little making out, and that was about it. My wife would then kind of sit on my lap, where I'd be hoist her up and down on my trusty dick, gripping her by the hips, groaning in the throes of ecstasy, and she'd end up hitting her head on the window, or on the roof of the truck cab, with each thrust, shouting out more in pain than pleasure.

On good nights, when we weren't fighting and had time to plan ahead, my wife would wear a dress that buttoned up the front and dispense with undergarments altogether. Sometimes she'd really get into it and wear a garter belt and silk stockings; she knew that turned me on. Unfortunately, whenever she wore them they usually got runs and were ruined.

"Shit, Ronnie," she'd say, "I'm gonna have to throw this pair out, too! Take it easy! This fucking truck fucking thing is really pissing me off! Maybe we should just stop having sex 'til spring...."

When it snowed, she'd wear high leather boots, and she'd be stomping all over my feet when she did finally get off — the puddles of melted snow on the floor of the truck cab would squish and splash, and splatter the truck's interior in interesting ways.

One time, after we started humping, things devolved into a huge fight. She was pissed off that I hadn't brushed my teeth before we left the house, and the fact that I probably hadn't bathed in awhile didn't help; the smell in the truck was pretty ripe. The only time we could take a bath was when we visited with the other VISTA volunteers, which wasn't that often — most of them lived in Kingsport, a long drive in the snow. They had been assigned to help a more urban population; mostly folks who lived in projects. So those volunteers had been placed in regular homes with bathrooms and refrigerators. Whenever we did drive up to Kingsport, it was a real treat to get cleaned up and become almost normal again.

Anyway, after we screamed at each other for awhile, she jumped out of the truck half-naked, but with her boots still on, and ran off into the snowy night. I zipped up, and charged out after her. I was slipping and sliding on the ice covered asphalt, but I finally caught up with her and we tumbled down onto the ground together. I picked her up and we made our way back to the warmth of the truck. I was scared; this was something new. Our fights had never gone this far before. I clung to her tightly; she was shaking from the cold, and I turned the dashboard heater up as high as it would go.

OR WHEREVER YOUR FINAL DESTINATION MAY BE
DENISE DUHAMEL

The spring before my husband left me, I sat next to a flirt on the plane. He was a businessman, kind of cute, with curly black hair. I did my best to flirt back. I was so unused to aggressive men that, though I was flattered, I cringed when he lifted his eyebrow.

"Your voice is so sexy," he said.

"What?"

"I mean, you end each sentence by lowering your voice."

I realized I was not being myself — I usually ended each sentence in a question. People pointed it out all the time.

I didn't say anything because I was self-conscious.

I was coming home from a poetry conference in Arizona. I was sitting on the left side of the plane — there were only two seats in our row.

"So when did you get divorced?" he asked.

"I'm happily married," I lied.

"Sure you are," he said.

"I am." My voice was suddenly squeaky and high.

"You compartmentalize," he said.

He hadn't seemed interested when I told him I was a poet. He told me that in his job he had to know how to sum up people. He drew squares on his Jet Blue napkin. "Here is your brain, here is your heart, and here is your sex drive." The last was the biggest square.

I felt myself get wet, which hadn't happened in a very long time. I thought I never would again because of my age.

"You're a jerk," I said.

"Whatever." He leaned over to me and whispered, "But I'd still like to take you to my hotel and fuck you."

I wanted to take his hand and put it between my legs. I wished I were wearing a skirt instead of jeans.

"I'm going to ask to be moved to a different seat," I snapped.

"No, you're not."

I tried to look as much like a stone as possible. I kept my eyes in my lap, wishing I had a book or magazine. We sat in silence for a long time until I finally fished out my headphones and clumsily plugged them into the armrest between us so I could watch the TV. I stared at CNN and soon I heard the flirt snoring.

I turned to him in his window seat. He was more ugly than I originally thought. His shirt was polyester, not cotton. Probably middle management. I was middle age. This was my future, I thought, if I left my husband. I didn't know then that my husband had plans of his own.

The flight attendant came by to pick up our cups. I shoved the flirt's napkin, his sloppily drawn squares, into the trash bag she held out.

The stranger didn't wake up until touchdown when a young woman's voice on the speaker wished us a safe trip in Fort Lauderdale or wherever our final destinations may be. The man gave me a big smile, as though we had spent the night together and he didn't regret it. His teeth were straight and white — he was the kind of man who, as a kid, wore braces.

I was the first to hop up and get my luggage down from the overhead bin.

As my sleeves pulled, I felt my shirt rise. I wondered if the flirt could see a strip of my belly skin. For a second, I imagined his fingers reaching for my button, my zipper. He said something like I had one last chance. I said something like I had to get home to my husband. Then, without looking back, I pushed my way down the aisle — the metaphor not lost on me. The steward blessed each of us, *thank you and have a good evening.* I bolted to the taxi stand like a late bride.

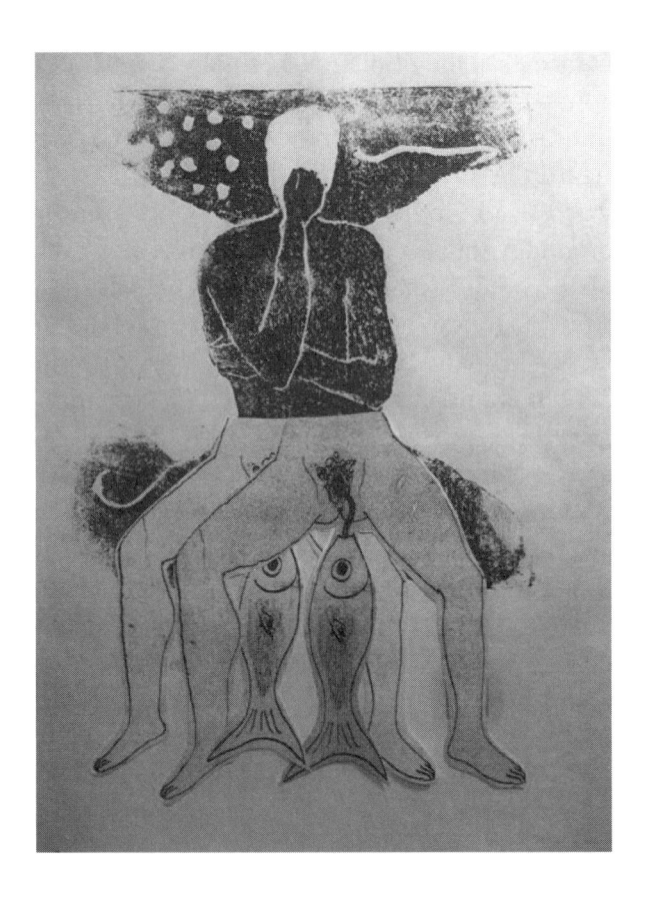

BAKING STRANGE STORIES OF THE WHITE GIRL SHUFFLE AND HER SWIM WITH THE SWANS

DOROTHY FRIEDMAN

Life is made up of expenses, expensive splashes of
       ectoplasm,
of organisms and experts with expensive tickets to
       fancy evenings
in which you wear just white satin gloves.

In orgasm after orgasm, in dream after dream that invokes
a woman's life after dinner: after the husbands and dishes
have been put away, and you browse through the family album,
as you brood about the afterlife of husbands and dishes,
dishes and husbands whose names you can't pronounce,
like Adolphus and Principus and Heathcliff.

After the dishes and husbands have been put away and you
still tawny in the nipples run out to the beach, eager
to see and be seen, sun and shells browse your flesh
and you are ready for show time, as you bake strange stories
of the white girl shuffle and the strange swim with the swans.

MEG
LYNN CRAWFORD

cannot say *Anna Karenina* is my favorite book but it is one I pick up and flip through often. For the descriptions (cold winters, rich food, riding boots, puffing engines, chirping birds, Turkish towels. Tea, gazebos, fields, satin dresses, trembling train platforms. Anna's different red bags and purses).

And lines like this one from Anna, "I so wish you would all love me as I love you."

And descriptions of Vronsky losing touch after he falls in love with Anna, perceiving people as objects; beds, trees, lampposts.

But I also return to this book for its irritating opening sentence: 'All happy families are alike; each unhappy family is unhappy in its own way.' Irritating because that sentence is filled with the importance of TRUTH while it is and is not true. Can you follow the logic and say: All happy people are alike, each unhappy person is unhappy in his or her own way?

Happy People.

Not self realized people who, like Job, survive, even grow from, loss, punishment, degradation.

But: men and women who effortlessly enjoy good fortune. Who have a spring in their step; whistle in the shower; are liked by neighbors, children, spouses, strangers, co-workers; make new friends but keep the old. Can you say those people are all alike?

I hope for happiness — try, even, to have faith it exists. But believe it is unhappiness that ignites existence or, in any case, breeds stories. And if I know one thing it is this: people need stories. Even the ones who say they do not.

Some look to literature for their stories. But even those who do not, even those who read for detail, rhythm, visuals, reshuffled tropes, are plot dependent. What is gossip but a series of stories; what are politics, what is religion, what is self-esteem? And what, in fact, is love?

Everything I have just said is grossly simplified and arguably untrue. Still, I have spent so much of my medium length, medium quality life not saying things because I think of all the exceptions, all the points that could contradict, even detonate, my own. I'll now try to do something different with my broad, if arrogant, inaccurate, statement. Generalization, pushing something forth, brings on anxiety. Yet, I remind myself, sweeping statements did not worry Tolstoy. So maybe I should try not to let them worry me.

Here is a truth: I recently learned my husband is having an affair.

My first response, rather than ask him who, why, say that I am crushed or even just break down and cry is to tell him he must move out of our house at once. Hoping, wishing, he will say, NO. Or, PLEASE LET ME STAY. Hoping to hear him describe, haltingly, the love — cavernous, frightening — he has for me. To hear him admit that he is self-destructive. Deeply so. And to tell me I must understand his affair under the umbrella of that self destruction. Hoping he will say behavior that seems cruel, coarse, is, in fact, a frightened shout for love. Or at least I hope he will tell me he screwed up, perhaps because of a mid-life crises.

But rather than do any of those things, he becomes stone cold. All that comes out of his mouth are concerns about property and statements that completely miss the point: "Listen, I never did anything with her inside our apartment, or even the restaurant."

This all takes place just when we move out of our apartment, temporarily, during an extensive renovation — making two medium sized apartments into one large one. The plan is to stay at my aunt's, who is abroad indefinitely. Her apartment is just a few blocks from ours and our restaurant. Or maybe now I should say, the restaurant.

When I learn about Dino's affair, I send our daughter Althea to Dino's sister, Georgia. My sister in law does not take her brother's side. I stay at my aunt's, hoping Dino will visit. It is where I am now.

What a picture; me, sprawled on a leather lounge chair in my aunt's complexly decorated dressing room. There is a large mirror in front of me. Looking in it I appear to be resting. But I am not resting. I am distraught, agitated, spinning out of control. I look away from the mirror, to the wall facing the street. It has a large window, covered by heavy, closed drapes. A narrow ribbon of light breaks through a small gap between the two bunches of material. I do not want to open up the drapes and let all that is outside in. I am just barely able to handle looking at the little strip of light.

My aunt's apartment is never boring. It features a rich collection of chairs, sofas, carpets, tables, paintings. She encourages me to wear anything in her wardrobe, which is an instructive exercise in restrained chic. I learn so much from examining, trying on, wearing, her high necked coats, sleeveless ribbed tunics with uneven hems, leggings, lace tops, capes, ballet flats, shoe boots.

Now, I am in one of her dressing gowns, a deep pocketed, silky, leopard patterned wrap that hits just below my knees. On my feet, her embroidered mule slippers, velvet, black, covered in tiny gold tulips. This attire gives me a feeling of living some grand, impressive life; definitely not mine. I fall asleep, looking at the wall, the drapes, the thin strip of light.

Dream: Dinner, in a castle, overlooking a sparkling lake, in a mountainous European country. Twenty guests occupy a long, wide, glass legged, glass topped table. The table is so wide that it is impossible to converse across it. Little microphones are set at each place setting. Next to each microphone is a number; one through twenty. If you want to speak to a guest you press his or her assigned number.

A vague, bloated figure presides over the dinner but it is never clear who this is, or where he or she is positioned.

Communication goes smoothly: #thirteen pushes #seven, #twelve pushes #one. Now, recounting the dream, I picture potential interference problems. What if more than one person or even every person wants to speak with #thirteen? This does not happen in my dream. But maybe this is the same thing as other things that do not happen in dreams: drinking, cooking, kissing, eating, instrument playing.

The dinner is packed with tall handsome men, apparently interested in me. I decide: enjoy the attention, do not: worry, be skeptical, question their sincerity.

A series of platters line the table's center; oysters, duck, asparagus, pomegranates, champagne, whip cream. No one eats or drinks. It all stays put: one sexy, varied still-life.

A band plays. Guests dance. I wear a billowy blue-chiffon floor-length dress with a wide sash, a dress unlike anything owned by me or by my aunt. She favors, and has taught me to favor, straight, form fitting dresses in blacks, browns, maroons. My hair is piled up high on my head. I wear heavily jeweled, dangly earrings, am concerned their weight might over stretch out my pierced earlobes. One of the taller men takes my hand, leads me onto the dance floor. We move; his hands grip my waist. "Inside decoration, inside decoration," he whispers in my ear, "inside, inside, inside decoration."

Guests at the table tap their glasses with forks and knives, signaling we should kiss. Just as our lips touch, the tapping grows unbearably loud. Tap tap tap. Tap tap tap. Tap tap tap. The elegant ball room becomes a drafty school lunch hall. Tap tap tap, the lunch hall patrol raps on the table, tells us to stop food fighting....

Tap tap tap, tap tap tap.

My eyes open to the sliver of sun shining through my aunt's heavily brocaded drapes. I regret waking up. My dream, even the part in the school lunch hall, is much nicer than this real world.

I finger the cigarette lighter in the robe's pocket, wish I smoked, think, why can't I start. Tap tap tap. Someone knocks. My husband! I jump up, tell myself: slow down. I pinch my cheeks. Breathe. Tighten the belt, loosen the neck of the dressing gown. Glide to the door. I stand there, hand on the knob, pull in my stomach, push out my chest, open it.

It is not my husband. It is my aunt's partner, Kitty, long blond hair, creamy fleece shawl, shimmering silver tank, slim dark pants, asking do I plan to move over to the bed she turned down for me in the bedroom or stay here in this dressing room on the lounging chair. Also, am I hungry because she is making a beet and carrot soup.

Here is what I honestly feel to be true but hope to be false. My husband loves me but does not LOVE me and is relieved to now have to end our marriage. Somewhere deep in my gut I understand this. Understand that it is futile to hope for, to fantasize about, him coming here to confess great love, beg for forgiveness, admit shame, guilt, but my thoughts still scamper in that direction. I, overcome with heavy helplessness, stand and stare at Kitty, not answering her questions about rooms and food. She kisses my fore-head, hands me a glass of sherry, a ceramic plate with a beautifully cut, fanned-out pear, says, "Drink, nibble. I am going to finish the soup."

I take the plate, the glass, and return to the lounge chair. See myself in that mirror: a disheveled woman, worn out, perhaps from living for so long in denial.

I turn away from the mirror, to the other wall, the one opposite the drapery. There are several book cases. I take a sip of sherry, walk over to them. On top of the case is a Bible. I open it to this passage: 'If a man is lazy, the rafters sag; if his hands are idle, the house leaks.'

I know this phrase, heard it paraphrased: idle hands are the devil's worktool.

I am troubled by such infatuation with busy-ness. Does work make you free? If you spend all of your time being busy, then when do you have time to reflect, contemplate, imagine, sort out?

Still, there is something to be said for productivity to lift one out of moping, brooding periods of self disgust.

I stare at my aunt's other books; novels, fairy tales, his-tories, including a volume about Henry VIII and his six wives. A small pile of blank notebooks sits next to it. I pick one up. Inside its front cover is a pen. Without thinking too hard I start scribbling, making up a story about Dino and his woman, his new woman — who happens, like him, to be a chef, a gifted chef. I decide; my portrait will make her out to be fantastic, witchy, wily, spellbinding, modeled after Henry's second wife Anne Boleyn; tiny waist, delicate skin, sharp teeth, six-fingered, left hand. No one can blame a man, king like Henry or a simple chef like my Dino, seduced by an enchantress. The seduction just cannot be seen, in that case, as their responsibility.

THE LOVER
LAWRENCE SWAN

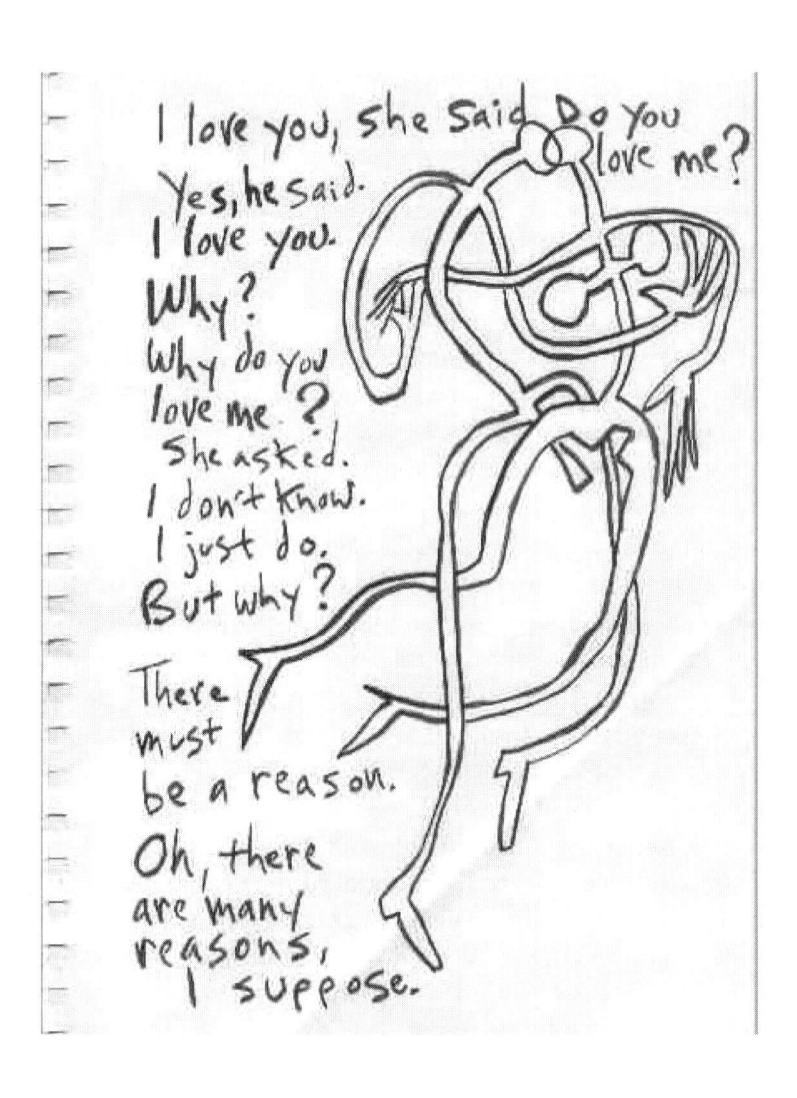

I love you, she said. Do you love me?
Yes, he said.
I love you.
Why?
Why do you love me? She asked.
I don't know.
I just do.
But why?

There must be a reason.

Oh, there are many reasons, I suppose.

Tell me one. What do you love most about me?

I guess what I most love about you is your love for me.

Your love for me often seems to surpass even my own love for myself, which is great. Your love is worthy of my self love and that is why I love it and it is what I really love about you.

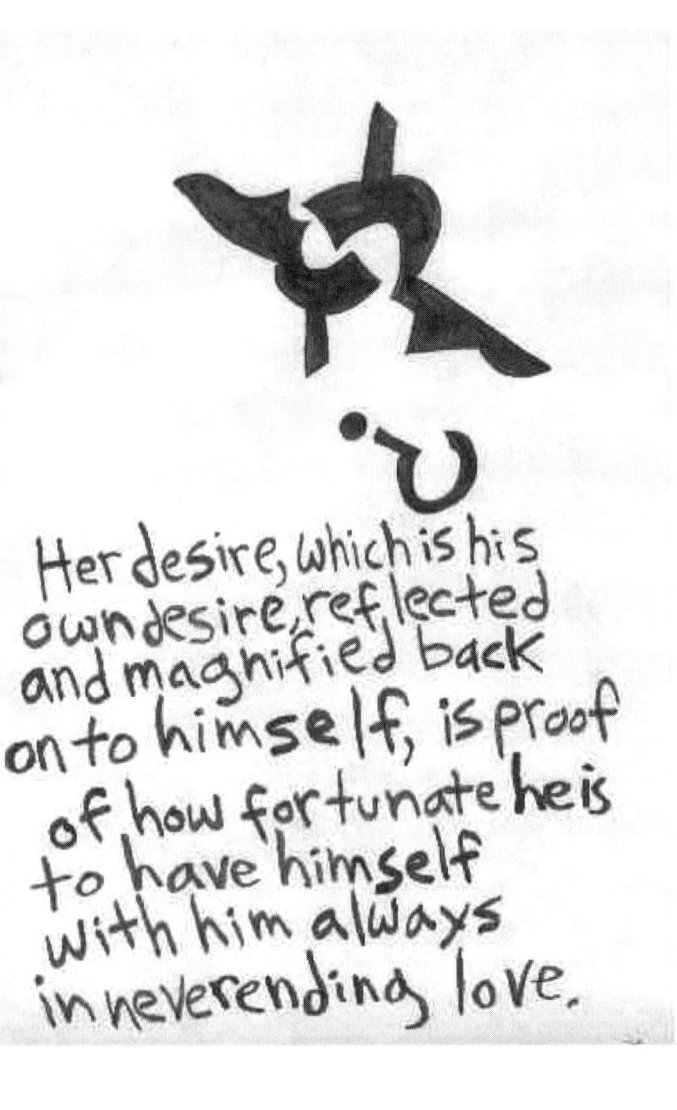

Her desire, which is his
own desire, reflected
and magnified back
on to himself, is proof
of how fortunate he is
to have himself
with him always
in neverending love.

LONGING LASTS LONGER
PENNY ARCADE

I awake at 4:30 AM and go outside. There is a burning behind my eyes. I think, "Those must be tears." But they don't flow. They're hard, frozen, behind my eyes. I only cry when I am with you. Outside, sitting on a low wall, I pinch myself. I think, "Maybe it's a bad dream."

You wake up and I am lying there, back in bed, staring at the tree outside the window.

The cypress tree that makes our bedroom look like it is in Tuscany. I am sad, sad beyond belief, and you too are sad. Two days before you said, "I don't want to be married anymore. I want to be self-contained. I want our relationship to change."

When I am sure you are asleep, my face in the pillow, I sob myself to sleep. Then night after night I wake up suddenly, at 3 AM, 2:30 AM, 4 AM. You are deeply sleeping. I leave our bed, so I won't wake you, leave you sleeping, leave the house and I walk the empty streets, smoking cigarettes, me and the other homeless people, all of us outside, trying to find a place out of the wind. I do that night after night for ten nights. Me and the moon and the near empty streets. I know how to do this. I am practiced at being homeless. I walk the places where the ragged people go, the street whores and hustlers, pimps and drug dealers, the schizophrenics, psychotics and borderlines and me. All of us wandering that other city, the city of night, the barely lit streets of LA, all of us stumbling around in the dark.

You didn't do that to me, that is what I do to myself.

Yes, it is sad. A vacuum. Emptiness. A terrible surprise, where there was so much warmth and love and sanctuary.

I wonder if it is my Saturn square Venus. My astrologer said, "You have that Saturn square Venus, it has been there all your life, you must be used to it by now." Saturn, the difficult lessons of life. Venus, love, a square, an obstacle. "Oh," I said, "you mean when the man who deeply loves me wakes up one day and doesn't want to be with me anymore? Oh that? No, I am not used to that yet. I don't think I will ever get used to that."

No working out issues, no discussion, no counseling, just change to what you want now.

At breakfast, your fist is balled on the table. I am making you angry as I lay out my thoughts. I ask, "Couldn't you have done this by phone? Did I have to come half way around the world to hear this?"

"No," you reply, "I have too much respect for you."

Somewhere during this breakfast I start to see clearly the anger you are holding towards me.

I believe my outburst at the beach last August was fueled by what I had been taking in psychically, by my feelings being controlled. I tell you, "I was expressing some of your suppressed anger." This is not received well. You do not remember your anger at your family, only at me. Perhaps that anger got pulled away from them into me.

It is easier to end a marriage than to end your relationship to your family.

But marriage as such means little to you. You are your father's son, your brother's brother. Slowly you begin; you talk of your long unhappiness with me.

There is only me and your unhappiness…our great love

gets acknowledged in passing but your unhappiness has center stage.

"I have been unhappy for a long time," you say.

You put in ten years. It is enough. You are by nature a loner, with tremendous social skills.

I am a loner too with my own set of social skills, the kind that go over really great with other loners.

"This is all about me," you say, "very little of it is about you. I can never last more than seven years with anyone."

When I mention things that make me angry, your teeth set on edge. You do not want to be challenged at all.

I bring up the links between what happened during our argument at the beach the August before and what you call having 'snapped' and you look at me incredulously. But I see you are finding holes in your own story of our ending and this too makes you angry.

"Maybe I will stay somewhere else," I say, half hoping you insist I stay home.

"Whatever you want," you reply soothingly.

"Maybe I could get a place on the other side of town," I add.

Silence. Then, "I don't think that's a good idea."

"Because you want autonomy?" I ask, using a word you have used.

"Yes," you reply, "that is what autonomy is."

"No," I think, "that is what privacy is," but I don't say it.

Later, by the car you say, "Perhaps this is the road back for us."

I speak with Hilary, who you have told about your issues. She is a good listener.

She asks, "Has he drawn a line in the sand? I thought he was saying you and he had stuff to work on."

After all what can I do? I can't beg. It would do no good.

Maybe you have been able to just forget our love. It is a relic now, a souvenir from another time. You are ready for the new. The new you and the new life that waits unknown.

I am falling inside myself. You are still my love, I can't change that fast. Even with my resentments, my thoughts of what it would like to be with other men, live other lives; you are still real for me.

"Look, there is your age," you said. "You are still young now. This is a good time to do this. I didn't think this was an issue ten years ago, but ten years from now you will be 68 and I will be 57 — it will be an issue then."

How can this be? This road I cannot follow you down? This road you don't want me to follow you down, this road you wish to walk alone.

Fifteen years before in Sydney, as I wandered the streets of Kings Cross, one night at 3 AM, walking the streets alone, walking off another failed love affair, a homeless man read my palm. He looked deep in my eyes and said, "It is really too bad that you have given up on love." And in that moment I realized for the first time in my life that I had. And he said, "There is a lot of love in the world for you, it's just, well, excuse me for saying it, but it is just that you have been so damn unlucky."

Before I returned to you, on my trip, in Palermo, in Fuerteventura, Gerona, in Marrakesh, I started to feel bereft, like I was all alone in the world. And I felt poor, terribly poor and I wondered where this emotional poverty was coming from. I scrambled to think of ways I could earn money, reinvent myself, go back to answering phones in a whorehouse, too old to whore, menopause would make that impossible. Perhaps across the distance, I now believe, I felt your thoughts. You packing me out of your life, dismantling our relationship, our family, our love.

"Last night I was heartsick," you said, "or maybe it was a stomach ache."

On the phone Steve said, "I never saw it coming. I thought you two would be together forever." Yeah, me too.

I have a hint of what you look forward to in your autonomy. Being able to hide your bad feelings from prying eyes, leave after you fuck. Take nice lunches, breakfasts, dinners, and short trips. You are a good date. That is how I felt when you picked me up at the airport that morning, like I was on a great date. Everything, even opening my car door for me.

"Oh," I thought, "he wants to make things better with me." When you told me about the spa we were going to on our trip, I looked for a romantic hotel that was not too expensive. An hour later, after you told me you wanted to end the marriage, I looked for a cheap motel. Why waste money? But in the end we didn't go. Too much crying, both of us, all through the night, we were exhausted.

Steve said, "The last day I saw you, you said, 'I loved my trip. I feel satisfied. I am ready to be at home with him for the winter.'" Steve had smiled, "I never heard you say you were satisfied before."

And I had crowed, "I'm satisfied!"

I, too, felt like you in Palermo, when I called you from the pay phone jetlagged, forgetting momentarily that it was our ninth anniversary. I, too, was disconnected, but I found my way back to you. I planned a little surprise for you for when I returned to celebrate our anniversary: Malibu, the motel there. But you, too, had a surprise for me.

There are no shortcuts through peoples' personalities.

You are leaving me how I found you, alone and isolated. Somehow, something in me unlocked the secret heart of you and you let me in past your sensors. I walked this whole way with you over rocky terrain; desert, perilous, and now you are dropping me here. You are leaving me how you found me, alone and broken.

And you are going on alone. Your smooth demeanor has returned, within which you hide your nervous and conflicted self, blanketed from the world.

"I feel like a heel telling you this," you said.

You made this decision all alone.

I felt so angry when you went weeks without resolving your feelings after our argument at the beach in August. For weeks and weeks before I left for Europe, I suffered and was angry. But even that anger I slowly gave up as I traveled and felt my freedom and understood that home was where you were.

I am like you. I have the same crazy need to see myself in bold relief.

In these past few years I have lost my mother, my health, so many friends and an entire way of life. And now to lose the love of my life, it seems too much.

"I realize I have laid a lot on you," you tell me at breakfast. "I am willing to feel your anger. I know I deserve that."

"You don't deserve my anger," I tell you. My anger is under so much sorrow like jagged rocks under a rushing stream. I am having trouble fording the sadness that wells up unexpectedly. I am, after all, an ad libber, filled with one-liners. Your face draws me in as it always has and I want to be under your chin, in my place there.

Yes, I am older than you. Yes, menopause has been a drag for us both. But how I longed to love you. You have no idea. And I was afraid, very afraid, that I would not emerge from it to love you again as we had in the past. Our past. Our romance. How many ever find a romance like ours?

"You carried me for a long time," you said.

Yes, but all I carried was your will to live, to be in the world, not your immense talent, not your lovely mind, not your deep integrity.

"I can't become who I feel strong enough to become in our unit," you said. "I have to sacrifice us for me."

I fell. Toppling from a high place. From that high place I saw great beauty in the valley below, not such a long way off. We were growing together and had been growing together for so many years. The sense of peace I had in our love. The shelter of your mind, your arms, your embrace, your support.

Yes, I wanted other things to happen between us. I thought for sure if we saw a therapist together and were quiet as each of us spoke, we would see what the other was, what the other wanted and needed and it would be easy to get there together as we have gotten everywhere else together in the past.

"I don't need to do anything legal right away," you said.

Right away? But 'eventually' hung in the air.

I find I can't be kind to myself. I can't be angry with you.

I see your problems, your issues, I know you deep, deep within me. Yes, I had shouted at the beach "I hate you! I hate your mother! Your family!" Meaning I hate the stuckness.

I heard something snap in you when I said it.

"I didn't know those words were going to come out of my mouth," you told me at breakfast. "I didn't know I was going to say I want to end our marriage."

You say you didn't know but when you speak, I hear the script you have written for yourself and it has an ending.

I am an improviser and I go along and speak, then think. I have no ending in my piece.

"Many people will be shocked," you said.

Yes, many people will be shocked, beginning with me.

Where is your shock?

I often saw your passion for me behind the rocks of your anger like a sea held back by a rocky promenade.

What are you doing? Why are you throwing me away?

Are you going to give your self to someone else?

Are you forsaking me?

I better look up the meaning of that word.

Forsake:

1. To quit or leave entirely; abandon; desert, to give up or renounce, to deny, reject, foreswear, relinquish, forego. To leave altogether; abandon, decline, refuse, to deny. To give up something formerly held dear.

I think I am simply addicted to the chemicals that form in my body from my constant longing for you. Longing lasts longer, longer than anything else. Now that I think of it, I used to lose you all the time. In supermarkets and parking lots and galleries and museums, airports and nightclubs. It always felt like I would never find you again, never see you again. Maybe I have always known that eventually you would leave.

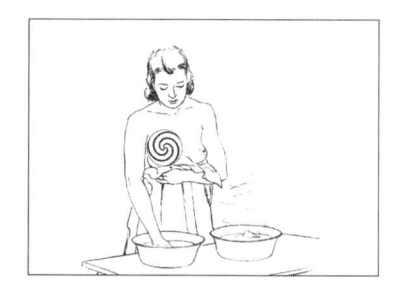 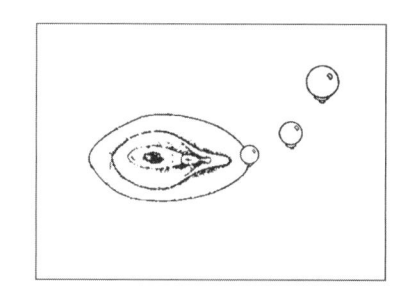

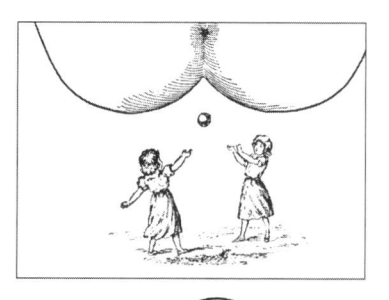 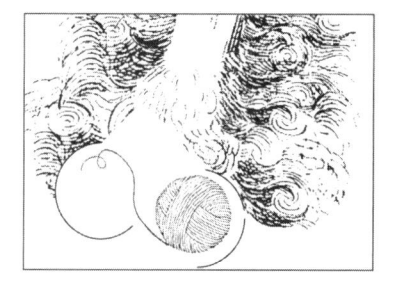

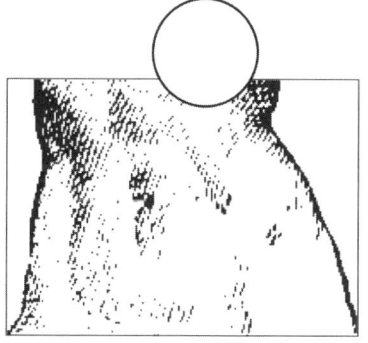 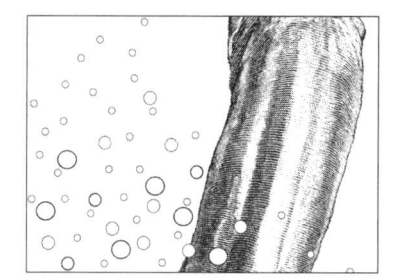

"Your words were sweeter than syrup, " she paraphrased Plutarch, "but war was in your heart".
"A fizzy beverage, rather," he suggested.

M. Kasper

RUN-IN
TSAURAH LITZKY

My ex-husband grew up on a farm. Once he bragged to me he learned to do it so good from watching the animals. When the hog mounted the sow, he said, the hog was an unstoppable force. "But I'm not a pig," I protested. "Yes, you are," he told me. "You are a pig for me."

It was true. All day when he was at work, I hungered for his cock, at night I feasted on it. With my mouth and with my sex, I swallowed it up again and again. After we split, I did not want his cock meat or any other part of him; or so I told myself. Still, five years later, I find myself dreaming that he is moving inside me, then in the morning I wake with my hands between my legs.

When I ran into him last Friday on Broadway in front of Dean and Deluca's, he didn't look like a farm boy. I hadn't seen him since he moved back to Canada. He was wearing a black leather jacket that had to be expensive and black velvet slacks. I wondered if he was dealing drugs again, but I wasn't going to ask.

His first question to me was, "Are you still with Paul?"

I told him, "Yes, of course," lying like Pinocchio, and then I quickly changed the subject.

"What brings you down here?" I asked.

"I have a show coming up at Castelli's," he answered. I wondered if he was making the show up to impress me, but I didn't ask that either. I was distracted because my nipples had suddenly hardened into sharp little spikes. He still had that effect on me.

"You and Paul happy?" he asked.

"Ecstatic," I answered. I didn't tell him how I had taught Paul to replicate all his farm-boy moves. Then my ex went on, "I heard your novel was published. Am I in it?"

I answered him, "Absolutely not. It's a fantasy, a total fantasy." The truth was he was on every page.

"Listen," he said, "If you're not in a hurry, let's have a drink, for old time's sake. We could go to Dante's. Is Larry still working there?"

"No thanks," I answered. "Why should I have a drink with you? Anyhow Larry's been gone for ages." I started to walk away. He came after me. "Come on. What are you frightened of?" he asked. I was walking a shaky tightrope suspended over a bottomless pit. I fell.

"Okay," I said.

Dante's was packed, three deep at the bar. Many of the patrons were already looped, talking loudly, wild eyed. "We are the Evil Empire, we are the evil empire," bellowed a bald fat guy wearing dark glasses. The crowd was all around us and he seemed to be yelling right in my ear.

"Yeah, sure," the man standing next to him said. "Three thousand soldiers dead in Iraq, three thousand and counting." He was an old gent with bushy white hair.

The bald guy pushed his face into his neighbor's face. "It's your fault, you dickhead. All you do is read old Robert Heinlein books. When did you last see the inside of a voting booth? Now we got a fascist country," he hissed.

His friend shot back, "It's always been a fascist country, that's why I read sci-fi."

The young guy behind him, his arm around a pretty red-headed girl, cut in.

"You both stink. Your generation blew it. You sucked your flower power up your nose. You jumped ship after Watergate. Now that maniac is in his second term. Next, he'll outlaw thinking."

They turned on him. "Who asked you?" the old guy shouted. "Stick your head in the toilet," yelled his friend.

The kid snapped back at him. "Going to make me?" he said, raising his arm, his hand curled into a fist. His girl-friend pulled his hand down. "Cut it out, Roger," she said. "Don't even go there. Everyone's nuts."

"You're so right, young lady," said the bartender, break-ing it up. "Let me buy drinks all around."

"You yanks are still fucked up," said my ex, as he pulled me down the bar.

"More then ever," I told him.

We pushed our way to the back of the room where we found a narrow place to stand by the long counter opposite the bathroom. He went back to the bar, scored us beers and brought them back.

"To old times," he said.

"I don't want to drink to that," I told him, 'but the future is too dismal to drink to." We stood silently facing each other, our eyes locked. The crowd pressed in on us, forcing me so close to him our bodies were touching. His jacket was open and my tits brushed against his chest. My nipples were still hard, so hard I wondered if he could feel them through the fabric of his shirt. My body always speaks true, that's how it betrays me.

We started to drink our beers, still looking at each other. A big brunette came out of the bathroom, wearing a low-cut red scoop neck sweater. The tops of her fleshy white knockers were visible down to the rosy nipple. He did not even glance at her titties; he was looking so intently at me, his mouth open slightly. I could see his thick pink tongue glistening, the same tongue that had licked my every inch, even between my toes, even my back hole.

I could not resist the dark force of desire growing within me. I reached my hand out, grabbed the waistband of his pants and just pulled him behind me the few steps right into the bathroom. I turned and locked the door. The small bathroom was designed for one person at a time with only a commode and a sink. I stood in front of the sink, took off my coat and dropped it on the floor. I bent over, hiked my skirt up in the back. It was he who pulled my tights and panties down to my knees.

"Bend over, bend over more," he said. I grabbed the sink for balance, bent over more and shut my eyes. I heard the sound of a zipper opening, then his hands were on my bottom, cradling, stoking, showing me he remembered ass play always drove me wild. Then one hand moved down and around, until his fingers found my clit and circled it, first stroking it, and then twisting it until I was crazy with wanting him. His other hand went to my nether lips, pulling them wide. I curled my hips up, offering myself to him and then he was inside; it was a perfect fit, like always, the hog and the pig.

Little oinker that I am, I started to squeal and came immediately.

"Can I let go inside you?" he asked. "I don't have a condom." Neither did I. I felt like saying go ahead, so much did I want his white fire inside me. Then he said, "No, I better pull out, we have to protect Paul." Good old Paul, I thought.

I felt the hog twitch and swell deep in my belly; maybe he was going to come inside me anyway. He was grunting hard, "uhh, uhh, uhh," but he slid out just in time and shot all over my ass. He rubbed it in with his big hands. I had forgotten how much I loved to have his hands on me.

I stood, pulled up my panties and tights. I opened my eyes and looked at myself in the mirror. My hair was standing up all over my head as if I had been electrocuted.

There was a loud pounding on the door. "What are you doing in there?" a shrill voice called out. "No getting stoned in the bathroom."

I put my coat back on and he zipped up. When we went out, the three women standing in line looked at us furiously.

Our beer mugs, now nearly empty, were still on the counter.

"Let me get us another," he said.

"No," I told him, "I better get home."

"Home," he echoed in a bitter tone, "home."

"Well, uh, good luck with your show," I said. I turned quickly. I couldn't bear to look at him, and made my way through the crowd and out the door.

EX-MARRIAGE
INGRID HUGHES

My husband — I haven't learned to call him
my former husband, but I correct myself —
has made more progress
putting our marriage behind
him than I have. He calls the bed
where we slept and made love,
where I nursed our children,
where we squabbled and dreamed ourselves
from youth to middle age,
our ex-bed.

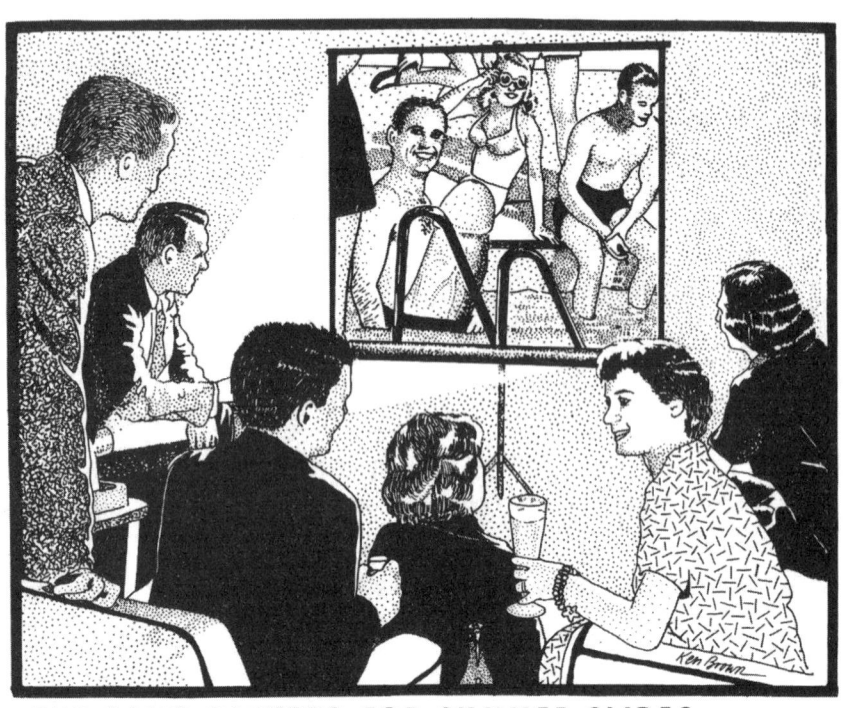

THE GANG GATHERS FOR SUMMER SLIDES

MYSTERIES OF MARRIAGE
ROBERT HERSHON

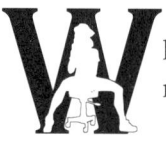ho knows the secrets of someone else's
marriage, she said

We had dinner with them twice a week
for 23 years and now we've heard
(nobody called, we just heard) that she's living
with her aroma therapist and he has a thing for
teenage boys
    Specifically, it's redheaded teenage
boys having sex with fox terriers in
restaurant basements while he, dressed in a sailor suit,
watches from a dark corner
This would make casual sex very hard to come by,
I would think, but maybe it's more of a scene
than I know

We promised ourselves (because who else cared
to know what we thought) that we would not take sides,
that we would stay friends with both of them,
that we would alternate Chinese dinners with
him and vegetarian dinners with her and be nicer
than hell to their new partners, but in fact
we haven't heard a word from either of them
I thought I saw her crouch
behind a mailbox when she saw us coming,
holding hands and skipping as we often do
Everyone thinks we're so goddamn happy

HERE I AM, RUBBING
BARBARA ROSENTHAL

Here I am,
Rubbing myself off to sleep again.
Expectations of a better evening come to this.
Congratulations for
Waiting so patiently for no-show lover.
Give myself a great big hand.
At least with two hands, I do not have to sleep alone.

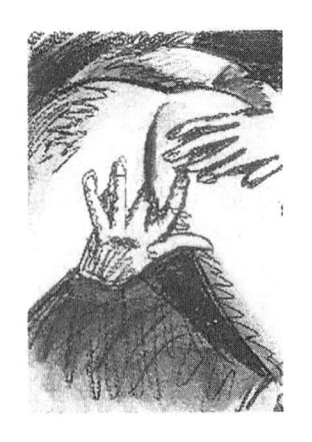

RUG BURN
FRAN GORDON

I had my first orgasm with the shortstop. I wasn't auto-sexual and didn't have any of the usual experiences; say, a hand-held shower head (too environmentally waste-ful), or the less-than-usual first experience of my ex-husband: an electrical belt meant to take pounds from the thighs and hips of his abundant mother; a device which was not entirely useless when used on a boy facing the "wrong" way.

Clothed, I came first with the shortstop, in the family room, on the rug. It was late, my parents were asleep in the dark white colonial; we had to be very quiet. I rolled on the rug, loving the plush spring of it. We started out just kissing, two virgins, the shortstop and me. Side by side. Then, with his hands on my bottom, he swirled our bodies, until he lay on his back, my body spread on his, and as we kept kissing, he began to hold his breath; and though he didn't thrust, the static pressure of his cock caused a surge, then sparks, as it were, between my blue-jean-clad legs. The jeans were the first pair I'd bought myself; tight, short-waisted for my long torso, they cupped my ass and cut almost painfully into my crotch, enhancing and, at times, distracting from the exquisite feelings beneath.

I'd read about sex, but experienced only inklings from the page. Knew of contact, and had also read of culmina-tion, but didn't get the relation. And so I didn't know what drove me, and expected nothing, no better pleasures than those I endured, no destination to end the slow, hard rub, not knowing a grind might hurry the process, not knowing there was a process, or goal, my electric flesh kept going, toward what I knew not. There was, for me, instead of anticipation, a superconducting perpetual loop. The shortstop kissed me harder, I squirmed and he began to breathe. My cheeks were slick with his sweat. "Am I too heavy?" I panted softly in his ear.

"No. No. *Oh no*...." His entire body seized up, rigid.

I compensated, scraped my jeans against his; the discomfort, exquisite, escalated. I was sweating now, crushing his hardness — could that happen? I wondered, then became still; his hands moved my hips, rocking them. His chest, broad for a boy of sixteen, heaved. I — led only by a complete lack of control, well, with one exception, volume — said, "*Shhhh.*" We musn't wake the parents. And so in the moment, there was just us, quiet, and an ingenious indecency that god willing, would persist. Then, oh then, I felt a great opening, and in an instant I knew what the Sydney Sheldon novel I stole from sis was talking about. I convulsed into exquisite shudders that shocked the whole of me into blessed loss of thought. Silence did have a place. The shortstop groaned, and as I covered his mouth, I felt his cock jerk beneath me, a tickle. Or via Sheldon, "an explosion that became a delirious ecstasy an unbelievable shattering journey an arriving and departure an ending and a beginning." The shortstop's jeans turned a darker blue beneath mine. I saw on his face the unlikely union of pleasure and pain. My physical intelligence had surpassed my erotic education.

Recently, a friend who was speaking about masturbation mentioned with awe that his male friend had experienced "the big O" first through sex. And so I told him, sans details, of my first orgasm. "Romantic, oh wow that's so romantic," he said with admiration. Romance, I thought, *the fiction that owes no allegiance to the god of things as they are.*

***

Sex is natural, but not if it's done right. I tried chocolate sauce first. The shortstop lying on his couch, who lay waiting for a mouth, freaked at a stickiness not his own. I wasn't sure then I'd like toppings. (I don't.) But there would be no way of knowing, with him.

All this would change with the Bedouin. He would indulge me. Tame me.

Before him, after the shortstop, I licked off champagne, and once, at the urging of short-lived lover who lasted too long for my liking, cocaine.

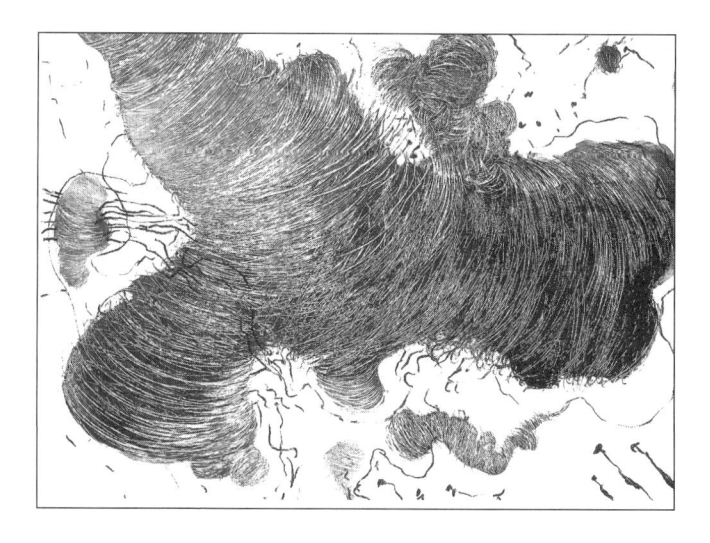

SEPTUAGENARIAN IN LOVE
Tune: A Teenager in Love (Dion & The Belmonts)

Ooh ooh wo-ooh wo
Ooo ooh wo'ooh wo

Each time we have some sex
It almost breaks my balls
Cause I am so afraid
We will not come at all

Each night I ask the stars up above
Why must I be a septuagenarian in love?

One day I feel so horny
Next night I feel so blah
Guess we'll have to take the whoopie
Whoopie with the BAH!

Each night I ask the moon up above
Why must I be a septuagenarian in love?

I try to fuck you
Every body and you
I'll be the hardup one
If you all think I'm thru
Well if you want to make me cry
That won't be so hard to do
If you should say 'FUCK OFF!!' today
I would still whack off to you

Each night I ask Venus up above
Why must I be a Septuagenarian in love?

I'd love to fuck you
Everybody plus you
I'll be the lonely one
If you say we're thru
Well if you want to make me cry
That won't be so hard to do
If you should shout "FUCK OFF-GO WAY!"
I will still whack off to you

Each night I ask the Satellite above
Why must I be a Septuagenarian in love
Why must I be an alta kaka in love
Why must I be a septuagenarian in love
Why must I...(spoke): Ya know I think I'd rather be a
teenager in love
(mumble & Then I could make a whole set of new &
exciting mistakes...

Major physical sex changes, as indicated by the numbers in illustration above: In the male, the pituitary gland becomes less active, (1); a gain in weight takes place, particularly at abdomen, as a result of decreasing male hormone, (2); there is likelihood of prostate gland enlargement, (3); there is a decrease in sex hormone produced by testes, less frequent and less vigorous erections, and testicles become smaller and less firm, (4). ● In the female, the pituitary gland becomes less active, (1); there is recession of mammary tissue and breasts become less firm, (2); ovaries cease functioning and menstruation ceases, (3); the womb becomes smaller, (4); the vaginal lining becomes thinner and the labial folds smaller and thinner, (5).

TULI KUPFERBERG

HOT
ROBERTA ALLEN

He wants me to look hot. So I look hot. As hot as a sixty year-old woman can look on Halloween without a bra. I'm jiggling under a shiny black teddy, trimmed with lace. Until I tried on the teddy in the thrift shop, I felt like those old women with long flapping breasts in ethnographic films, sitting in grass huts, kneading something dough-like.

In my short butt-hugging, stomach-crunching black skirt — another thrift store bargain — I feel squirmy, worm-like, narrow enough to inch through tight spaces like the thought, 'Why am I doing this?' which sneaks through my self-admiration.

I had trouble pulling up the black tights so there wouldn't be space between the crotch of my tights and that of my panties which someone might see when I sit. On my feet, black boots with heels, of course. Pointy-toed would've been better than round-toed but the thrift store didn't have my size.

I always scoffed at Halloween, even at ten, trick-or-treating with kids on 63rd Drive in Queens. Once a voice said *Nobody's home!* when we knocked. But this Halloween is different. Up here, they make a fuss, squeeze every ounce of fun they can out of it. I'm all for fun. At least, I'm trying to be though I'm not sure about my date. He was dead serious when he told me to look hot. He called me three times in two days to discuss my costume.

"How about a bikini?" he asked.

"I don't have one. How about my Chinese bathrobe?"

"What would you be in a Chinese bathrobe?"

"What would I be in a bikini?"

"Hot! You'd be hot. Is the Chinese bathrobe hot?"

"No. Not really. I have a sarong from Bali."

"Is it hot?"

I picture myself in Bali, sarong tied at the waist, tee-shirt on top, rubber sandals on my feet. "No."

"Don't you have something low-cut? Something sexy? Something tight?"

It's a big deal party he's taking me to.

When he picks me up on Halloween night and takes off his coat, he's wearing a Japanese robe with Japanese letters on the back, over a tee-shirt and exercise pants. I wonder who or what he's supposed to be. But I don't ask. I figure he was too involved in my outfit to give much thought to his own.

He spins me around. "You look really hot! I didn't know you had such a hot body! You always wear things that hide it!"

From the back, he cups my breasts. "Sorry," he says, when I give him a look. We're not up to that. He's still try-ing to get over his former lover. But I've been hoping tonight would be the night, from the moment when he told me to look hot. He doesn't know I got this body late. It comes from the gym and the pool and the track. But I never thought to show it off before, especially my knees, which have always been fat. But he says my knees look fine.

When we started dating a few weeks ago, I told Sarah I didn't like his sloping shoulders and kinky hair and large pores or acne scars or both. But I got over that. What I can't get over is the way he suddenly folds up inside like some mutant origami. The worst night was his birthday when he took me to the blues club where his former lover belts out ballads. That night someone else sang.

Lights from the party in the large house, high on the mountain, sneak through the dark woods as he stops the Ford van behind a slew of parked cars. When we get out, he says, "That's *her* Toyota!"

"Did you know she'd be here?"

"No!"

Thoughts are running through me like cockroaches. The big black shiny kind. *Is he just using me to make her jealous? To get her back?* It's a long walk from the car to the house. I try to shoo the cockroaches.

The door is open. Our host, whose height would make him a spectacle on any night other than Halloween, yells out hello. He wears a monk's robe. A small Asian employee takes our coats. The crowd at the bar doesn't notice our entrance. They'd be a nameless bunch to me even if they weren't in costume. I'm new around here and know few people besides my date.

In the large living room, I see eyes. A roomful of eyes. Eyes behind masks. Eyes behind feathers. Eyes of devils, monsters, goblins, werewolves, ghosts. Eyes of a Suzanne Somers look-alike. Stoned eyes. Roving eyes. Downcast eyes. Glassy eyes. Sneaky eyes. Animal eyes. Eyes framed by screaming red wigs, blond wigs, black wigs, green wigs, witches' hats. Then bodies. One in a skin-tight leotard. One in a floor-length gown. Several in sparkly tops. One Hansel and one Gretel. One Humpty Dumpty. Two in tuxedos. One in diapers. A pony-tailed flasher in a pinwheel hat with a big open coat. Bodies with hairy arms, hairy legs. Bodies draped in loose fabrics, off-the-shoulder sheets.

Which of those eyes, those bodies, belong to *her?* My arms press firmly against my sides. Suddenly they feel fat. The rest of me feels fat too even though Ken and Steven and Larry, my date's friends, lean in and kiss me, say I look hot. I feel eyes on me. Men's eyes. Women's eyes. I sit down on a loveseat. Lou licks his lips. I don't count Carl, the crasher. Chest hairs stick out of Carl's low-cut print dress, long blond hairs from his wig tickle my shoulder when he kisses my neck, tells me how hot I look.

I am the only French whore. My date brings me vodka. As I take a sip, I see the smile — *her* smile. Before he says a word, I know it's her. Elaine. I recognize three moles in a row down her right cheek though I've never seen her before and didn't know she had any moles. She smiles at me, then pulls him close, kisses him.

"On the lips!" he says, angrily. "For God's sakes, why'd you kiss me on the lips?"

Something wakes up in him. It's not the anger. The anger is always awake. What wakes up behind the anger is hurt. The hurt is green. I see it as green. It writhes and twists like the tail of an alligator caught in a vice.

Elaine doesn't have a body like yours, he had said in my house. She's hidden from neck to knees in something loose and white, her hair hidden under a wig. A wig like one I should've bought to hide my hair. Bad hair. Thin. Not French whore hair. Wet dog hair. Hair isn't the issue, however.

A man in street clothes brushes my date's shoulder, smirks. Did he buy that nose in a store? Is his mouth real? As real as mouths behind masks, talking, eating, drinking, laughing? I hear him murmur, "Thanks for the job, pal." My date looks angry, murmurs something back.

In my partially inebriated state, I look at the man in

street clothes and decide that people are more real when they are *truly* fake. I imagine this thought to be wisdom.

"That's Elaine's date!" he says to me. "A plumber! *I* hired *him* to fix Elaine's sink! Did you hear him *thanking* me?"

What pushes me into the next moment? Even when I don't want to go. While he elbows me from bar to buffet, he mutters, "That bastard! Thanking me! Thanking me for introducing them!" I remember when Elaine left his slippers and his neatly folded robe on his doormat. *Does that mean she wants me back?* he said. We eat slabs of smoked salmon, drink more vodka, talk to guests with voices that come from somewhere else. Switzerland? Rome? Atlantis? Mars? Hell?

I smile, laugh, shake my head, nod, look surprised, look amused. I hear words leave my mouth. Do I know what I'm saying? What they're saying? Have I a clue? Are clinking glasses clues? Who is talking to me behind a black mask? If I dig my finger deep into the fabric of his costume, will my finger hit fat? Muscle? Bone? Nothing? Are we in a movie? Who is "we"?

Elaine and her date leave early. They're going to bed! my date's eyes say. I understand those unspoken words.

Talking to monsters, devils, witches, the Suzanne Somers look-alike, the diapered man, the flasher, soon seems ordinary. "There's no music! We need music!" my date shouts suddenly to our host. Even our needs seem ordinary. As ordinary as looking hot. As ordinary as sleeping alone.

THE JACK OF HEARTS
TONY BRUNGARD

"Your nipples are like planets!"
I said this to Catherine in awe under the patchwork quilt pulled over our heads, illuminated like children by a flashlight tucked at our feet. It was 1974 and we were naked and beatifically stoned on some mellow grass. Outside on wide Clermont Avenue in Brooklyn, the two a.m. night was quiet and October chilly.

I cupped Catherine's pendulous breasts in my palms, admired the spill of brunette hair over her olive-hued shoulders and strove to remember through the smoky haze how I'd gotten here. We'd already made wet groaning love three times, her irises rolling up under her eyelids as she came.

As my thumbs stroked Catherine's swollen dark nipples, it came mistily back to me.

We'd met the week before, Catherine having come to the small college town in Pennsylvania as a nude painter's model for the students. They hired models weekly and they stayed in the room across from mine above the restaurant where I lived.

While there I'd started up a local magazine with Andy Stein and we were advertising for stories and articles in New York and Philly. Catherine and I had grown chummy and I could sense the musk welling between us and then on her last night as we kissed by Catherine's door, her hands drifted down and grabbed my ass and she pulled me into the room. Man, was she a loud moaner, and on the third or fourth time with Catherine squatting above me, I gazed over her shoulder and saw on the wall a painting of a one-eyed Jack of Hearts leering down on us. This was the symbol for the restaurant's name and I thanked God for playing cards.

The next day Catherine was going back to New York after posing for a morning class. At noon she knocked on my door and said her clit was throbbing the whole time she posed, so I groggily fucked her again and watched her floating irises drift back and knew I was caught. Coincidentally, I was slated to bus up to New York the next day to visit my friend and see a writer who had submitted a story to the magazine. So that Saturday morning at the old dowdy Port Authority, I met Paul and we subwayed up to West Seventy-second where the writer lived in a third-floor walkup. Naturally I told Paul about Catherine and that she wanted me and him to come over that night.

Spencer, the writer who went by that single name, was an urbane man in his thirties, confident and warmly responsive to the piddling edits I proffered for his story.

Later, as we left, Spencer asked what I was doing that weekend in New York and I told him we were heading to Brooklyn to meet some woman. "Somewhere on Clermont Avenue," I added.

"Clermont!" Spencer repeated warily. "That's Fort Greene." He slowly shook his head. "I wouldn't go to Fort Greene at night."

Paul and I tentatively eyeballed each other. Paul knew the city after a couple years in graduate school, so he replied complacently, "It's near Pratt. That's a big college area."

Spencer pursed his lips and nodded. "Okay. I'm just saying."

That night we wandered into Brooklyn and switched to

a G train. "I've never been on this line," Paul said uneasily, and when we exited into the pitch dark of Clinton Street and shuffled down the deserted avenues, it felt like wolves were lurking in the shadows.

Catherine looked lasciviously glamorous. Her breasts mounded under a red wool sweater like plump cushions, and though I'd told Paul I wasn't going to stay the night, we both knew I was hooked. After dinner in a small candlelit bistro, with Catherine's eyelashes fluttering like tiny exotic spiders, we bid Paul goodnight and meandered under the glow of streetlights, hand in hand, back to the fifth-floor steep walkup were Catherine lived.

Which brings me back to the cloistered quilt haven, where the musk from the dark fur between Catherine's legs was making me hard again. She kissed me with those plush cherry lips and her hand grazed down my belly to slowly, gently stroke my cock.

"Wait," I murmured into her cheek, "I kinda have to… pee."

"Hurry back," she whispered huskily, giving my cock a quick affectionate kiss. I climbed down the wooden ladder leading from her loft bed and wandered through the shadows of the unfamiliar rooms to the bathroom somewhere in the back.

It was cold in the apartment and I felt the chill on my goose-bumped thighs as I pissed in the bowl that gleamed luxuriously in the warm floral light and I noticed that the sliver faucet glistened. Then, glancing in the mirror, I saw my puckered eyelids and remembered "I am so stoned." I stupidly grinned at myself like the Cheshire cat.

I stopped in the doorway before putting out the light and saw across the outside room a painter's easel with brushes in jars and tubes of paint. Catherine was a painter she'd said. Working in "rounded, semi-nonrepresentational forms that mirror the…" something, something she'd gone on to explain. In the rectangular shaft of light I crossed the room and studied the painted canvas. Maybe it was the dope, but the red, blue and yellow forms seemed to subconsciously clarify before my eyes and I discerned the suggestion of a smirking Jack of Hearts. Yes, there was the mitered crown, and in two corners the form of a globular pulsing heart. Then I noticed the far wall of old bricks with what looked like two lengths of chain dangling from brackets with leather straps at the end. Hmm? What the hell, I thought.

As I padded back with my arms wrapped around my chest for warmth, I thought how sweet that Catherine had sought to memorialize our time together. And what a fast painter. She had only been home for less than a day. I climbed back into the loft with Catherine still humped under the quilt.

She lifted the quilt and pulled my hands between her thighs to warm them. "There's sometimes no heat at night," she explained. "Except down here," she giggled and squeezed my hands tightly.

"I saw the painting…that you worked on. Of the card with the Jack. You did that fast."

"What do you mean?"

"Well, you only left yesterday and it kinda looks like you captured that Jack of Hearts from the room in Kutztown."

Catherine squinted at me puzzled. "The one on the easel? No, I've been working on that piece for two weeks."

I tried to reason through the blurriness in my head. "But you said you'd never been to Kutztown before. How did you know to paint that card face from on the wall?"

"What face on the wall?"

"The Jack of Hearts. It's right there on the wall."

Catherine smiled dismissively. "I'm really oblivious sometimes. I was hardly there. Classes all day, and at night I just stumbled back and drew or read." She placed my hand on her liquescent cunt and then sprawled back spreading her legs. The hell with the Jack of Hearts, I thought, and I plunged into her moistness and we pumped away with Catherine's legs clasped around me for a good half hour because she had drained me before. I tried to focus on her nipples bobbing to my thrusts and I had almost willed myself to come.

Then Catherine turned over and tugged me in from behind. "Come on baby," she urged, whispering. "Come on…hit me," she pleaded sweetly. "Hit me." I looked at her round up-thrust ass and figured, well, I've never done this before but why not, and then I heard it…a throbbing distant drumming soared over the rooftops from somewhere north. An incessant African sound like Tarzan might have heard pulsing through the jungle. Then it grew louder and more insistent.

"What the hell's that?"

"Ah ah ah ah!" Catherine groaned into the pillow.

"No. Seriously." I stopped thrusting and sat up, gazing out the window. "That drumming."

Catherine turned over and squatted next to me, somewhat annoyed. "That's the drums from Fort Greene Park. They do it at night. Around the monument." Then her eyes gleamed in the moonlight through the pane. "You know there's something I like to do when that starts." She glanced over to her doorway. "There's a place in the other room. Near my painting. On the wall. I like to be…fixed there." Her warm fingers stroked over my thigh. "And then you could…well, I'll have to show you," she crooned.

Then I got it. All right, I'm a little slow. The chains and all.

I started getting freaky willies down my spine. The next ten minutes was like a comedy routine with me trying to dress and Catherine pulling at my clothes as I wrestled into them.

"No, baby," she pleaded. "I just want you to try it. It's so hard for me to really come. The pain helps so much."

Outside, walking down the dark isolated street with the drumming still reverberant in the night, I suddenly flashed on the sly malicious face of the Jack of Hearts who had followed me the past two days like a determined spirit and I wondered what other arcane mysteries the world holds for us. What in the world do men and women do to each other?

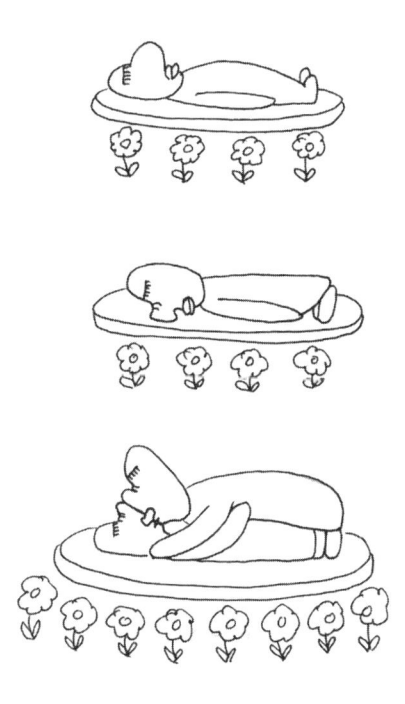

LIGHTER THAN AIR
JAMES TRIMARCO

When I first moved to New York, there was no place else that could give me what I wanted. But what I wanted must have changed, because I couldn't find it in the city anymore. I was tired of hunting for shitty freelance assignments and wrestling with landlords for heat in the winter and generally hustling all the time. I called up my mom in Florida and told her I was coming home. She was happy to hear this, so happy that she cried.

I drove the rented van down Interstate 95, past the red-brick warehouses of New Jersey and the truck stops of Delaware and the plastic-flag auto dealerships of Georgia.

In Florida things got very flat and green and hot. The sights were strangely soothing to me; the old gas stations and the people in fast-food uniforms waiting for the bus. I'd gone to New York so full of ambition: I would write books, play music, organize politics. But the color drained out of it. Nobody read books; music was a kind of popularity contest; and the problem with politics was that people were stupid. For the first time in my life, I stopped masturbating. My sexuality had gone underground.

I sat in the dull heat hanging over the traffic on the Florida interstate and wondered if it would come back, now that I was down here. I stared at the people driving around me. The guy with the ladders thrown in the flatbed of his truck, his tan face and bluesman glances. The young woman with the ponytail who opened her purse at the stoplight and poured her things out on the passenger seat. The retiree with her silver hair and expensive-looking blouse a few sizes too large.

I had never been one of them, not really, not even growing up here. But maybe, this time, it would be different.

The patterns of Florida life came back easily. I spent a lot of time with my mom, who had given up painting to focus on gardening. She grew only plants native to Florida, and legions of bees and wasps came to crawl and nuzzle on her beauty berries and scorpion tails, along with butterflies and beetles in jewel-like reds and greens.

I did all the cooking and half of the cleaning in return for room and board. I read fantasy novels by Terry Pratchett. I made no pretense of getting a job. After a month of this, however, I started to get twitchy.

One Friday night, I drove back to the Tower, the Goth club where I used to hang out when I was in high school. I drove across the bay under a sky like a picture of a storm on another planet. Soon I was in front of the massive old brick building, the sweet tang of clove cigarettes in my nose as I waited on line before a narrow doorway that rose to a peak in the center. The weathered-looking wooden doors were open wide, and a heavily pierced door guy sat with a stamp and money box, his chunks of tangled hair dyed a cartoon-strawberry red.

Inside, everything was intensely familiar. It was here, in these very rooms, where I'd caught the first glimpses of a glamorous and pleasurable escape from the ordinary world that had taken me, eventually, to New York. I climbed stairs carpeted in what seemed like red velvet. The squeak of vinyl corsets rubbing together, the rustle of a chiffon tutu. A chandelier of black plastic resin cut to shine like glass, a painting of a family with mouselike faces and lacy black neo-Victorian gowns.

I made my way into the big room with the dance floor. It was a cathedral in there, the ceilings so high they got lost in banks of synthetic fog shot through with cold beams of blue and green lightning. The sweet, moist smell of that fog wrapped me in memories of sexual exploration and psychic liberation. Strobe lights flashed to electronic booms and crashes, over which cascades of synthesizer tones played rapid scraps of melody, romantic and morbid.

I went to get a drink and smiled to see a detail I had forgotten about: a meandering river of water in miniature, its rocky banks carved out of the flat black marble of the bar. The water gurgled silently as I got into a conversation about astrology with a pixie-ish dominatrix named Tarin. Her problem, she said, was her Capricorn moon. Later, she told me she was in the mood to be spanked if I was into it. I was. We went outside and crossed a street. We scrunched over the dew-soaked grass on the way to the parking lot, where the light of the street lamps spattered over the leaves of five sprawling live oaks.

She crouched behind her car and pulled her red dress up around her ass. She wore no panties. She looked at me over her shoulder and I started into it, slapping both cheeks softly at first, building up to a few brutal spanks, and then settling back into easy ones for a while until she asked me to get rough again.

When her ass was covered with red splotches in the shape of my hands, she sighed, keyed open the door to her car, and collapsed onto the shotgun seat. She reached into one of the door pockets and pulled out a syringe and a glass ampoule of morphine. I watched the cars going by while she probed for a vein.

She asked me if I wanted any. I said no and asked if she knew anyone who sold pot. Now that I was down here for a while, I was going to need a decent connection.

"I know someone inside," she said. Her eyes dove for the floor and she laughed as though something embarrassed her.

"What, is there something wrong with this guy? I don't want to get mixed up in anything…"

"It's not like that," Tarin said. "I wouldn't say she was dangerous. She's just a weird girl. She told me she thinks she's a vampire."

"Does she suck blood out of people in exchange for pot?"

"Not like that," Tarin said, missing the joke. Now that she was all fucked up she exuded a thoughtless, accidental sort of sexuality, twisting her own nipples and hiking her dress up so she could stroke her fingers across her pussy without seeming to know she was doing it. "I mean, no fangs, no blood, no capes. Nothing like that. She feeds on people's energy or whatever. Especially guys."

The offer, if that was what it was, tugged on something irresistible buried in my memory.

"Fuck it," I said. "All right."

Tarin squeezed my arm and gave me a cheerful smile that turned downward at the corners of her mouth.

"Let's go find her, then. She's here every Friday. I know right where she'll be."

The girl was holding a piece of broken glass like a monocle in front of one eye, through which she observed the gyrations of the dancers. She stood behind a pillar at the edge of the dance floor, a small girl in a black jean jacket, tight black cargo pants, and small, featureless black boots. She had bushy arching eyebrows and curly black hair so thick it was almost ugly.

Tarin went up to her and said something, turning to point at me. Then she called me over and told me the girl's name was Miranda. I held out my hand but she didn't shake it, she just stared at me through her jagged little sliver of glass. Her eyes seemed to focus and refocus and then she shuddered all over, a bony hand splayed out at her hip.

We went outside and stood in front of the club. Miranda had an odd way of walking, her small feet padding softly on the sidewalk as though she was trying to walk through a forest without snapping a twig. We smoked cigarettes and I listened to them talk about how some guy had fallen in love with Tarin a few weeks earlier. This man hadn't been part of the culture, just some guy with a southern accent who lived in a trailer park a few exits away on the interstate. Tarin told me she thought he had latched onto the scene at the Tower because he was filled with melancholy and rage, even though you might not think so because he listened to country music and drove around in a pickup truck. Eventually Tarin noticed him following her and told the bouncers not to let him in. After they had turned him away once or twice, he tried to sneak in wearing a black leather jacket as a disguise. But they caught him anyway and then he pulled out a knife and started slashing his hands and wrists.

"It happened right here, girl," Tarin said, stomping the sidewalk. "Right where we're standing."

"I know," Miranda said, knotting her brows in concentration. "I can feel his energy."

There was a side of me that thought this would make a funny story to write up for *The New Yorker* or something. But I was sick of that side of myself, sick of looking at the world as material for some future project. I needed to shift my mentality.

"Tarin says you got some greens," I said, hoping to impress Miranda with a tough Brooklyn-style opener.

"Did she?" Shamelessly, Miranda raised her fragment of glass and peered at me through it.

"You're creeping me out," I said, pointing at the glass. "What's that all about?"

She gave a half-snort, half-laugh and slipped the lens into a small leather case she wore on a chain around her neck. She had a lot of things hanging on chains there: feathers, bottles of amber liquid, crystals.

"Let's go to my car," she said.

We crossed a road still busy with club people at 3 AM and climbed up the hill that led to the parking lot. Miranda had parked under one of the live oaks and it was dark there, like a thick forest. She opened her car door and pulled out a black, coffin-shaped leather box. She unlocked it with a key from around her neck and took out a dime bag printed with tiny skulls. She cracked the bag open and held it under my nose. It smelled great but I found myself more interested in her fingers and wrist. She told me the price was thirty-five dollars and her touch was cool as she gave me back my change.

"You can go now," she said. She was looking at Tarin, who gave me a look before she went back to the club.

A moment went by. I stared at a street light, waiting to see which of us would speak first.

"I'm glad to be back down here," I said, the words bursting out like water under pressure. "I've been living in New York for almost nine years. You can't imagine what it's like. People are clawing each other's eyes out for apartments the size of a closet. Cigarettes are up to thirteen bucks a pack. And the girls are always wanting to know if you work on Wall Street. It's really…"

She muttered something I couldn't quite hear. She seemed to always speak quietly, as though her words were for herself only.

"Their fucking eyes were all over the place," she said. "Right? Where can you go, really, to hide from them?"

I ground one thumbnail against the other. "Yes! That's exactly right," I wanted to say, and, "How did you *know* that?" But it seemed fake, like a scene from a movie.

"That must have been hard," she went on. "You've got a nest of serpents inside of you. Anybody could see that."

I didn't know what to say. It *did* feel like that, sometimes, although I had mostly forgotten this. It felt so good to have someone else say it. Desire tugged on my throat and balls; it had been a long time since I'd wanted to fuck anyone really bad. We were all alone here under the oaks, the dew settling on the scratched and dented finish on her out-of-date Camry as the first rays of the sun seeped into the eastern sky. I reached out and touched her arm. My fingers dragged along her skin.

She jerked away as though my index finger was a poker just out of the fire.

Her eyes rolled up to face me. "I have another way of doing that."

I had to pry a bit, but eventually she told me what she meant. She liked to watch people through the window, she said, and always at night. Usually she stood outside, sometimes on a stool if the window was high, and stared in at the guy, whatever he was doing. The little shard of glass was her way of taking that with her.

The whole thing obviously turned her on and I figured it was a really kinky form of foreplay, although she didn't say that. She talked about it like standing at a window was the whole shebang. I didn't think I believed that could be true.

I told her she could stare at me through my window any time she wanted. I was mostly flirting, but she came back all serious, saying it had to be that way or nothing, because she wasn't going to tell me when she was coming.

I said I liked surprises. She took a receipt from the floor of her car and found a pencil between the cushions of the seats. She asked for my address and I gave it to her. I watched her write it on the back of the receipt and hoped I wouldn't regret what I was getting into.

The first few nights after that, my eyes were on every window I saw. I was always hoping to catch sight of her. But then a few weeks passed and I guess I figured she was flaking out.

In the meantime, I needed something to do with my almost-unlimited free time, and I started making collages. I collected a bunch of my mom's fashion and celebrity magazines and started cutting up the ads. I cut a smiling housewife out of a commercial for dishwashing detergent and stationed her, mop and all, on the deck of a starship. I cut the bulging, muscular arms of a gladiator and grafted them to the rigid body of a right-wing politician. I cut the eyes from a blond TV anchorwoman and stuffed them into the sockets of a soldier from some military thriller. I liked him better that way. I stood up to examine him from a distance. That was when I saw her through the window. The light from the street lamp mixed with the moonlight to dab colors on her face, one side yellow, the other silver.

I pointed to let her know I'd seen her and her mouth twisted in anger and disappointment. For a moment she sulked, squatting among the native milkweed and water hyssop with her head in her hands.

I felt sorry to have ruined her fun but I wasn't going to pretend I didn't know she was there. I sat down on the bed and stared at her. She stood up and came towards me, walking right up to the glass. I could see her in better detail now, the small-boned hands loose at her narrow hips, her nostrils flaring in arousal and rage. Her large, finely veined eyeballs leveled in my direction, her slightly turned-up nose, her mouth like a mouth-shaped hole in all of this.

Never had I felt someone's eyes on me like that. It was like a wave of fire or sound, something I could feel, flowing over my skin. I gestured with my hand at my shirt and pants, wondering if she would like me to take them off. But she wouldn't allow me any control; she turned her head to the side and swiveled her eyes at me and I felt ants crawling up and down my ribs.

I stood there and took it as long as I could. My desire swelled and I wanted to run outside and catch her, to throw off her power in the wildest and most insane ways. I saw myself chasing her down to the beach on the back of a flaming horse, but she dived down beneath the waves and the horse bucked at the edge of the water. I saw myself swooping down on demon wings to fuck her with a spiraling muscular cock, but then she swallowed it whole with her gaping, starving mouth. Even in my fantasies she always seemed to win.

A shudder passed through Miranda's body and I was so turned on that I forgot the window was there. I took two steps forward and reached out. She was gone by the time my hand hit the glass. Disappeared, like a frightened deer at the edge of the woods.

Probably a week went by and I almost couldn't believe she hadn't come back. What else could she be doing? I considered going to the Tower and finding her there. Maybe she thought I was scared and didn't want her to come again. I could promise that I wouldn't try to touch the glass, if that was what she wanted.

But I held myself back, following some kind of unspoken rule. I kept working on the collages and eventually an old friend got me a show at a local art-house cafe. I was driving back from the opening, pulling into the little alleyway behind my mom's house, pleasantly buzzed on cheap wine, when I saw a pale, sharp-chinned face against the wooden fence draped in confederate jasmine. Her coppery black hair seemed to exude its own oil as it flowed over the shoulders of her black jean jacket.

She stood there, her eyes lowered, as I pulled up beside her. Her face was over the driver's-seat window now, like a cop writing a ticket. Her eyes raised up and met mine. Her mouth had a look that I found not quite pretty, like a little girl accusing you of a crime, the lower lip protruding, accusing.

She straightened her shoulders and became cold and confident again, with something of the lion coming over her as she watched me fidget behind the wheel. I was naked before her, totally naked, fantastically ugly and beautiful at the same time. A pleasurable sensation came over my cock, like it was being caressed in many tiny places by some invisible sea anemone possessing millions of long and subtly undulating orange tentacles.

I tightened my fist around the door handle and waited to see her body tense up in fear. But that didn't happen. She kept fixing me with her gaze, the one I'd seen at the Tower when she was first watching me through her shard of glass. It was like she was reaching out and holding the window with a giant hand, holding it in front of her eye like a shield between us.

Exhausted by this contest of wills, I let go of the handle, lifted my foot off the pedal, and the car coasted forward.

The rear lights lit her up like a mannequin in a store and she waited there until the garage door closed between us.

The murk of the club was thick around me as I paid the cover and walked past the fetish models standing in clusters around the stairs, the gossip rich as chocolate on their mouths. I ordered a vodka and cranberry and sat at the bar, watching the miniature river flow along its banks of chiseled marble, as I replayed our encounter again and again in my mind. I fantasized about having thrown open the car door and then pushing her against the fence and kissing her with the full length of my tongue, my hands strong and hard against the softness of her ass. But I hadn't done it, and then she hadn't come again for weeks, almost a month now. Finally I'd decided to come and find out what was going on.

When I'd knocked back two or three drinks and my nerve was up, I went to the edge of the dance floor and watched the goths strike dramatic poses, their long fingers unfurling like Japanese fans above their heads. Miranda was there behind the pillar, and the jealousy was like a punch to the gut when I saw her staring at one of them through her sliver of glass. I waited for her to notice me, to come over and explain herself. When she did nothing, I went over to her and spoke.

"Where have you been?" I asked.

She kept staring at the dance floor. "I didn't think you would come here. You know it's against the rules."

"The rules?" I said. "But, what did you expect me to do, just wait around forever? It's been weeks, two weeks and a few days. Did you know that?"

"I don't keep track of time," she said. "You shouldn't have come. I didn't know before. But now I do. Now it's all fucked up."

I thought of the knife-wielding redneck with new sympathy. What if Miranda got me thrown me out of here, called the bouncers on me? Could I become that kind of guy?

She pulled the shard of glass down from her eyes and tucked it into its sleeve. Then she turned to me, no glass between us. A fountain somewhere stopped flowing. They were brown eyes, that's all, dark brown eyes on a little half-Mexican girl who took care of her sisters' kids somewhere in Tampa.

"You want to buy some grass?" she asked.

"I have some left over. I'm OK."

I felt so bitter and disappointed, I would have done anything to punish myself. I started by getting another drink. No wonder Miranda didn't want to come to my window anymore. I had done it again, taking things out of the clouds and bringing them down to earth, where everything rotted and stank.

Tarin came and found me in the Tower's downstairs lounge, hunched over my sixth or seventh drink and humming along with the synthpop tune playing on the sound system. She asked me what had happened and I told her the whole story, as best as I could remember it.

"I'll just go back to New York," I said. "Fuck it. I like it down here but I'm too weak to stay. I always fuck everything up."

Tarin flashed me a smile. Casually, she rubbed her left nipple through her tight dress with black and white stripes.

"You know," she said, "you're not the first one to fail her test. She's been through just about every guy in here. No one holds up. Who can do that, anyway, just give all your power to her in exchange for, for what? Does it even feel good?"

"Sort of," I answered. "It reminded me of something better than sex, something lighter than air."

Tarin shrugged and wrinkled her nose. "I saw your collage show," she said, "at the coffee house. I've been meaning to tell you, what you're doing with gender in those pictures is so interesting! Did I tell you I was a women's studies major?"

"No," I said, "I didn't know that."

As she talked, I thought about picking up my empty glass and holding it up to my eye. Anything, as long as there was something between us. It was nice as a fantasy. But not quite as nice as her hand in mine, or, later, her mouth and neck in her car, under the oaks, while somewhere across the street, a sharp-chinned face watched through the window.

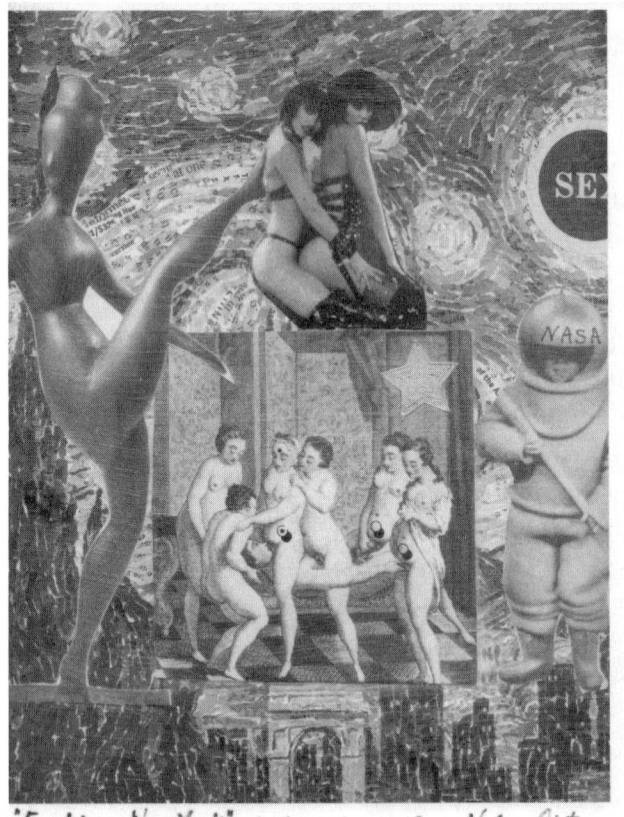

"Erotica New York" digit-collage 2006 Valery Oisteanu

MY DIARY
BRUCE WEBER

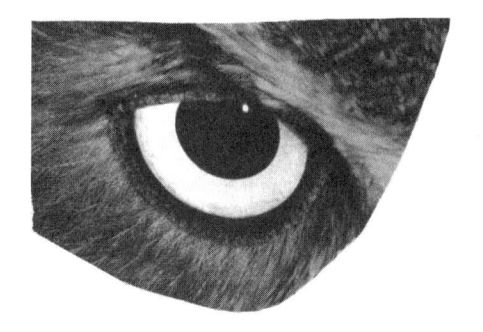

diary entry june 14th

embarrassed myself in front of janet yesterday.
forgot about her wooden leg. asked her why she
took so long to walk over to my house. janet removed
her leg and nearly cut off my head. need to be
more sensitive. wrote that down in my "help"
notebook. got heartsick remembering beulah.
despite the fact she had so many bad things to say
i adored her. probably because she gave the best
blowjobs i ever had. especially that time in the
shower before i went away on a business trip.
she'd always leave something to remember her by.

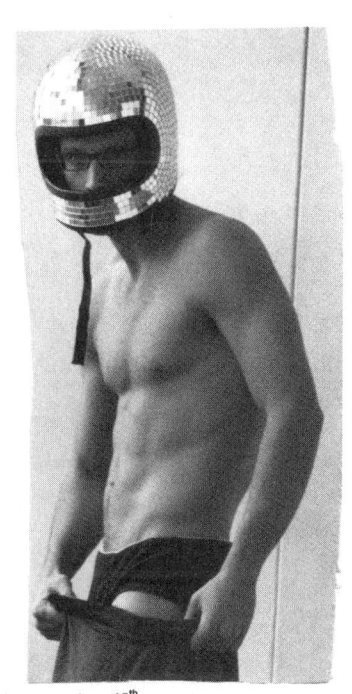

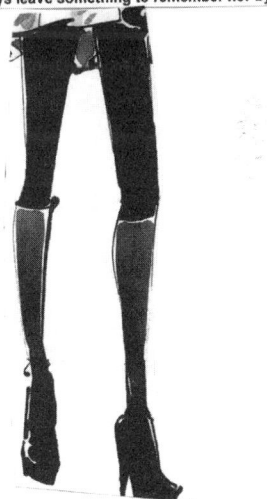

diary entry june 15th

elevated to the roof of the metropolitan museum
with my binoculars. pretended to be watching
birds. instead i studied lovers in ravines. behind
tall maples. clutching together atop blankets.
i miss contact. pornography only goes so far.
maybe lill fall in love again. maybe someone
will fall in love with me again. maybe i better
call 1-900-for-sexx again.

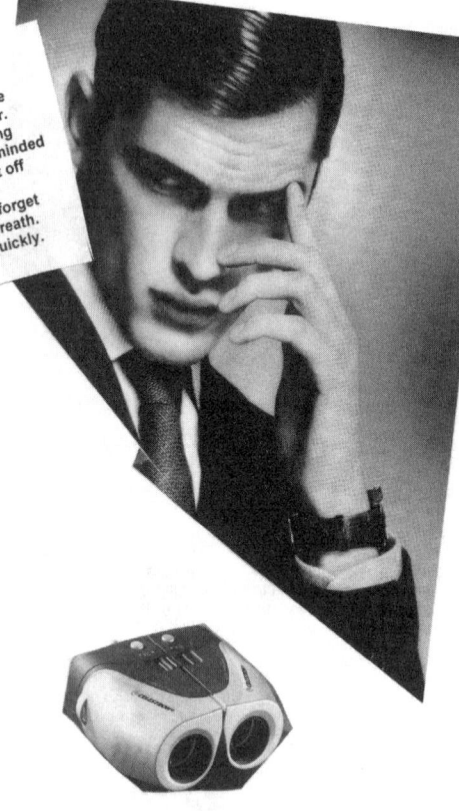

diary entry june 16th

itchy. woke up and my back was covered with hives. ate too many anchovies last night. carmine despacio invited me over to her house for dinner. we spent the evening playing scrabble and killing tics that jumped off her dog's skin. carmine reminded me about my kid sister louise. before she went off to reform school for pumelting germaine for not helping her to cheat on her spelling test. forget louise. forget these hives. forget the air we breath. just scratch me with something. anything. quickly. quickly. quickly.

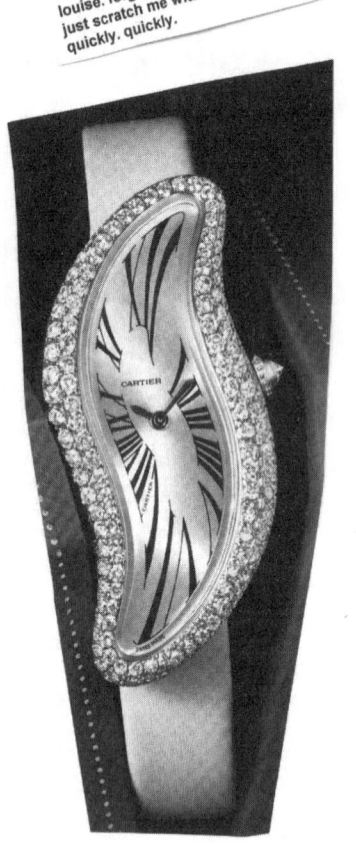

diary entry june 17th

betrayed mike this morning. the cops were asking about him and i chirped in a couple of sentences that will put him away for a while. that's good. because he won't be able to ward me off his gorgeous sister lucia. i'll send her three dozen roses. i'll write an anagram with her name. i'll leave her my life insurance policy. i'll count my chickens before they hatch. i'll defame myself in the mirror. i'll promise her eternal loyality.

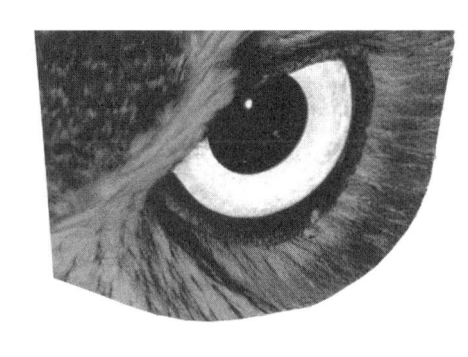

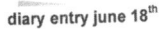

diary entry june 18th

lucia told me i'm depraved. and i started
crying. tears flooded out of my eyes like
niagara falls. and lucia rubbed by head
and wiped my face and took me in her arms
and made passionate love to me all night.
this morning she said she was going to leave
and never come back. she felt sorry for me
she said. good thing she did.

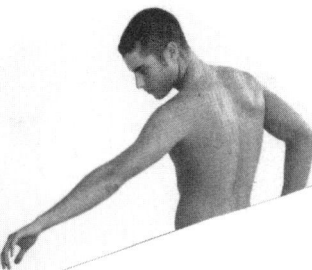

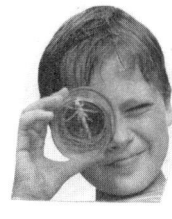

diary entry june 20th

spent the day across from lucinda's
apartment complex watching her through
binoculars. when i arrived home the police
were already there with a warrant for my
arrest. all night in jail this guy with a huge
dick kept coming on to me. in the morning
i was let go with only a stern warning. seems
lucia changed her mind about things. she
waited at the precinct for my dismissal
and we went home and made love like
wild animals. life is good. very good.
very very good.

NAMES ARE REMOVED
J. BOYETT

K., who works out, took off her clothes and gyrated on my lap in her leopard-print G-string. She had lovely breasts but her nipples were small like mine and the same color as mine. We went to her apartment "only to make out;" we went to bed "only to sleep;" then she sucked on my penis and sucked on my testicles the way I especially like. But I was almost as drunk as she was and my penis wouldn't get very hard. Even the next morning, I was so sick with a hang-over that it wouldn't get hard. In the following days she was less interested, and we never undressed each other again.

In a public bathroom in a Flagstaff hostel A. and I locked ourselves in and got in the shower together, where we made out, and she held and caressed my penis; then we had sex on the bathroom floor. She was seventeen years older than me. She said "I like it tiger-style" and I didn't know what that meant; turned out it meant doggie style. She was Irish and so maybe it's an Irish thing. Just before that, with my penis in her hand, she had said to me plaintively, "Jim, do you know where I woke up this morning? Hand-cuffed to the bed, and he was long gone. And, Jim — I never even knew his fucking name." I didn't know what to say. When I was holding her haunches and having sex with her tiger-style, I noticed that my penis was covered in blood. I would have kept going — it was just a surprise at first, that was the only reason I'd paused — but A. was embarrassed and wanted to stop.

Once, upstairs in a different country, in a long hot room, I made N. come so many times and with such interesting techniques that she thanked me — not tenderly, the way they often do, but amazedly. Anyway, that's how I remember it.

Not so long ago, I stood with J. on a leafy street in Manhattan and took her hand while she said her piece, after our second date. I'd thought our first date had gone well — when she'd said at the end that she wanted to "take it slow" I hadn't minded, because I was fantasizing about marrying her. On the second date I had been a little off, a little boring, because I was coming down with a cold; I should have rescheduled our dinner and drinks, but I'd been excited about the date. She held my hand too, our arms extended out and down; in a conciliatory voice she said, "You know, for ten years I've lived in New York and all that time I wanted a boyfriend, but now...." When we parted the wet clay of my insides had collapsed, and I only made it to the train by promising myself that I'd keep wooing her, like a guy in a book or a movie, that I'd make her love me despite herself — even though I knew that I'd do no such thing.

I remember hearing about how F. and T., when they were in high school, took off all of their clothes, and F. put his big penis inside of T.; but then they couldn't figure out what to do next, and they just lay there a while. Then they put their clothes back on.

R. brought home a beautiful Israeli girl and a beautiful Polish girl, and they were all drunk. The Israeli girl and the Polish girl started screaming at each other, and then they were crying, and then they started making out. R. ordered them to "*Get* in that bed!," and that was how he had his first three-some. I asked him what it was like. He said, "It was strange."

In the original, hand-written version of this piece, I wrote everyone's name out in full. Because it would have felt silly and pretentious to call them by their initials. Of course, I always knew that I would take their names out in the end. And I didn't want to call them something made-up.

These days, it's J. I think of the most. When I'm han-dling some girl's breasts and pubis, when she's handling my penis, I think of J., holding my hand firmly and flexing our arms out from our bodies, and of the way she said, "You know… for ten years I've lived in New York and wanted a boyfriend… but now….," and I think, This is nice, handling this girl's breasts and putting my hand inside her, but it's not that. Or some woman won't handle my penis, won't let me handle her breasts and clitoris; then I can say, That's too bad, but it's not like she's the one I'm in love with. I'm not in love with her, the way I'd like to be in love with J.

I think about J. I lie on my futon on the floor at night and sometimes I wallow in that. But I know that if I just wait, these feelings will wither away and leave me in peace. The same as with everything else. I know that I needn't fear that I'm strong enough to suffer *too* much. I feel things about J. But the odds are that, by the time you read this, I won't feel very much about her anymore at all.

FIVE MOMENTS OF MARJANE
HEATHER AUSTIN

5.

Amelia and Marjane paint wounds on their faces for Halloween — dark rings around their eyes, lips cracked and stained with fake blood. They smear eye shadow around their necks to make bruises in the shape of hand-prints.

"We look like twins," Marjane says and squirts blood onto the fake knife sticking out of her stomach. Her pregnant belly is real, but Amelia's is a volleyball stuffed under her shirt.

Their homeroom teacher sends them to the vice principal. He rubs his temple and sends them home to change. They walk holding hands, kicking up brown leaves in the gutter.

"Let's take the baby Trick or Treating," Amelia says.

They eat Mike and Ikes and the baby flips.

"Feel him, he's wild," Marjane says and places Amelia's hands next to the knife.

4.

In the back of Walgreens, Marjane pokes at the pregnancy tests with her toe, straightening them into a line. She taps her fingers against the strap of her backpack. "I've only got three bucks," she says.

"Just steal one," Amelia says and plucks one from the bottom row. She rips the tab off and fishes inside the three-pack. "Here."

Marjane slips it in her pocket and Amelia follows her out of the store. She gives her cover as Marjane squats behind a Volkswagen.

"You couldn't have waited until we got to your house?" Amelia says and jumps out of the way of the spreading puddle.

"And have my mom find out, hell no. It's turning blue. Is that good or bad?"

"Shit, I don't know, we forgot to steal the directions."

3.

At the carnival Tim spends an hour, and at least thirty dollars, in hopes of winning Marjane a stuffed animal. He shoots water into a clown's mouth making a tiger rise and rise until the bell rings. She stands at his side half in hope and half in boredom. He finally wins.

"Thank God," Amelia says.

"Who even asked you to come?" Tim says.

Marjane's prize is an ugly blue scraggily looking thing. It's her fault. She's on her fourth beer and when the guy behind the counter says, "Which one, Miss?"

She says, "How about the tiger?"

He rolls his eyes. "That's part of the game."

She picks the next thing she sees, a bear. She carries it by one arm, ashamed of it as they walk around eating funnel cake. Tim drops Amelia off and he and Marjane are alone in the car. She looks at him and the ugly thing he won for her and she decides after three months of no and maybe later, that tonight she'll let him fuck her. When it's over, she wipes up the pink mix of blood and cum from the back seat and tells Tim, "I didn't think it would be as awful as this."

2.

Amelia and Tim share cigarettes and a fondness for Marjane's long black hair. Amelia remembers how it smells of apples as Tim grinds his fingers into the seam of her jeans.

"If I ask her to have sex, you think she'll say yes?" Tim asks, giving up on making Amelia come.

"She might, but she's a virgin," Amelia says and replaces Tim's hand with her own. "Tell me how you'll do it, tell me how you'll touch her."

He whispers and Amelia comes and comes.

1.

Under a magnolia tree, the girls imagine their lives. They put fat fallen blossoms in each others' hair.

Marjane says, "I'll be notorious and bed dozens of men. I'll be a drinker and live in six European countries before I die."

Amelia says, "I'll follow you to Paris where I'll go to the Sorbonne and eat nothing but delicate pastries."

A bloom falls from Marjane's hair and Amelia bends to replace it.

"I've changed my mind," she says and pushes the white flower over the top of Marjane's ear. "Let's imagine ourselves, always, like this."

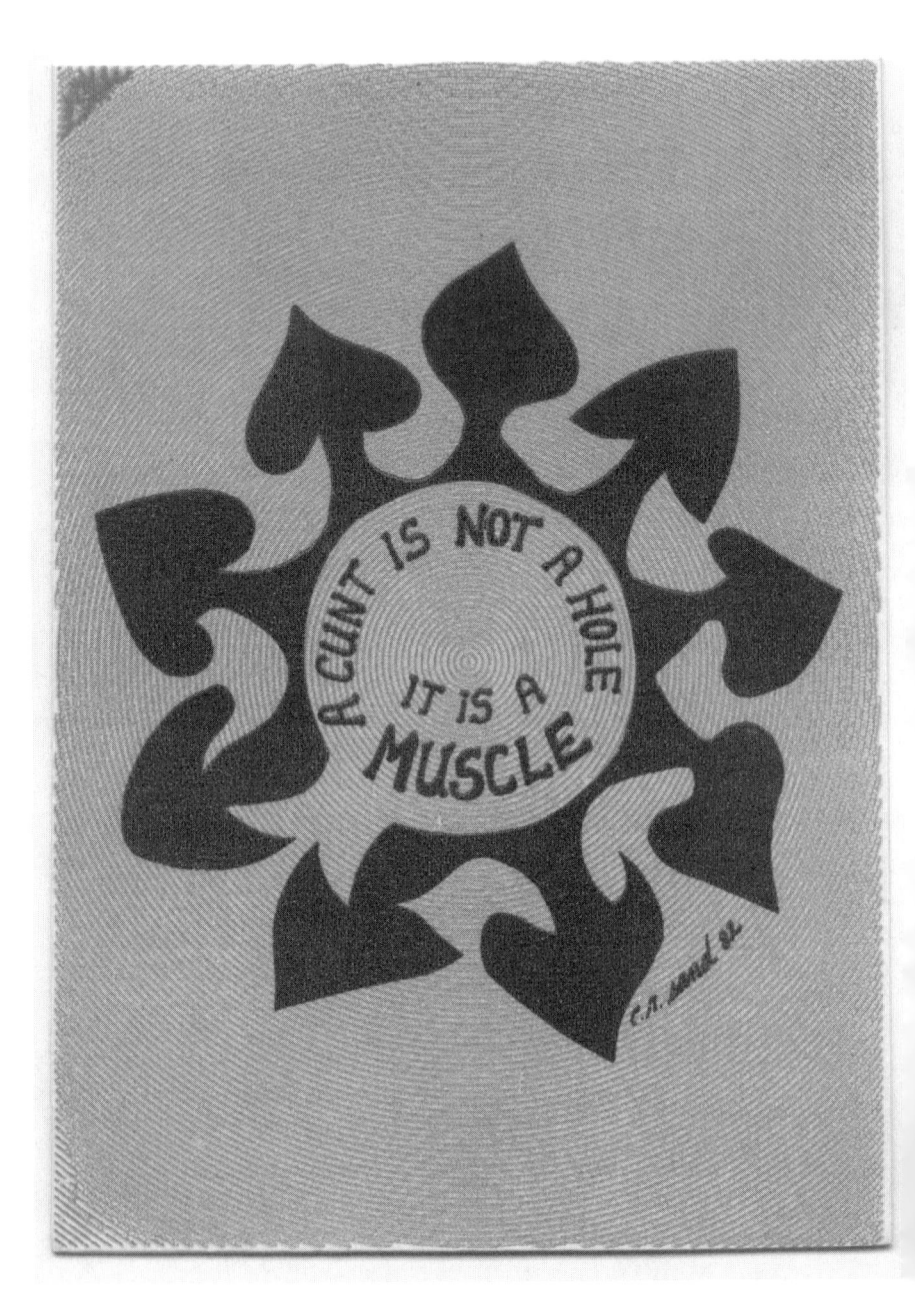

WHAT ARE YOU, SOME KIND OF ANGRY DYKE OR SOMETHING?
CHAVISA WOODS

I am only an angry dyke when I'm fucking a fag
and I'm on top
and I can't figure
how to move my hips
quite right.

When I'm fucking a woman
with my hand
I'm a just a lesbian

When I'm fucking a man
who used to be a woman
I'm queer

And when I'm fucking a woman
who used to be a man
I'm probably
really straight.

When I'm bending a trany-boy over
I'm an ecstatic dyke

When I take it
on my back
I'm a very generous dyke

When I use my mouth
on a woman
I'm
fixated on the womb

When I bend a woman over
I am a kinky lesbian

When I put my clit
against her clit
I'm a murderous lesbian

And when I let her top my ass
I'm probably really bi.

When I talk about my lovers
I'm a slut

When they beat me behind the ball pit
in high school
I was a faggot

When I kiss my mother
I am a victim

When I beat my lover's rapist
I am hysterical lesbian

When I'm saying no
I'm gay

When I'm applying for a job
I'm gay

When I first wake up
I'm grouchy and gay

When my aunt talks about me
I'm *a* gay

When I'm holding my grandmother's hand
I'm a homosexual

When they're howling at me on the sidewalks
I'm a bitch

When my grandfather's crying
I'm sick
and gay

When I fuck a married man
I'm a whore

When I fuck a married woman
I'm a hot dyke

When I swing with a couple
I'm a troublemaking
queer

When I step into my old church
I'm a satanic homosexual

When they disowned me
I was a degenerate
homosexual

When I'm getting paid to watch
I'm straight

I'm only straight for money
in hour long increments

And sometimes I'm a straight man
when I strap it on for my girlfriend...
I guess,

When I'm crossing the Williamsburg Bridge
and the sun is bursting like blood down my thighs
spread
across the horizon
I'm an art fag

And if you really push me to name it
I'm a queer dyke

But when she is calling out my name in the darkness...

When we are calling
each other
out
by name
in the darkness
we use
none
of these
words.

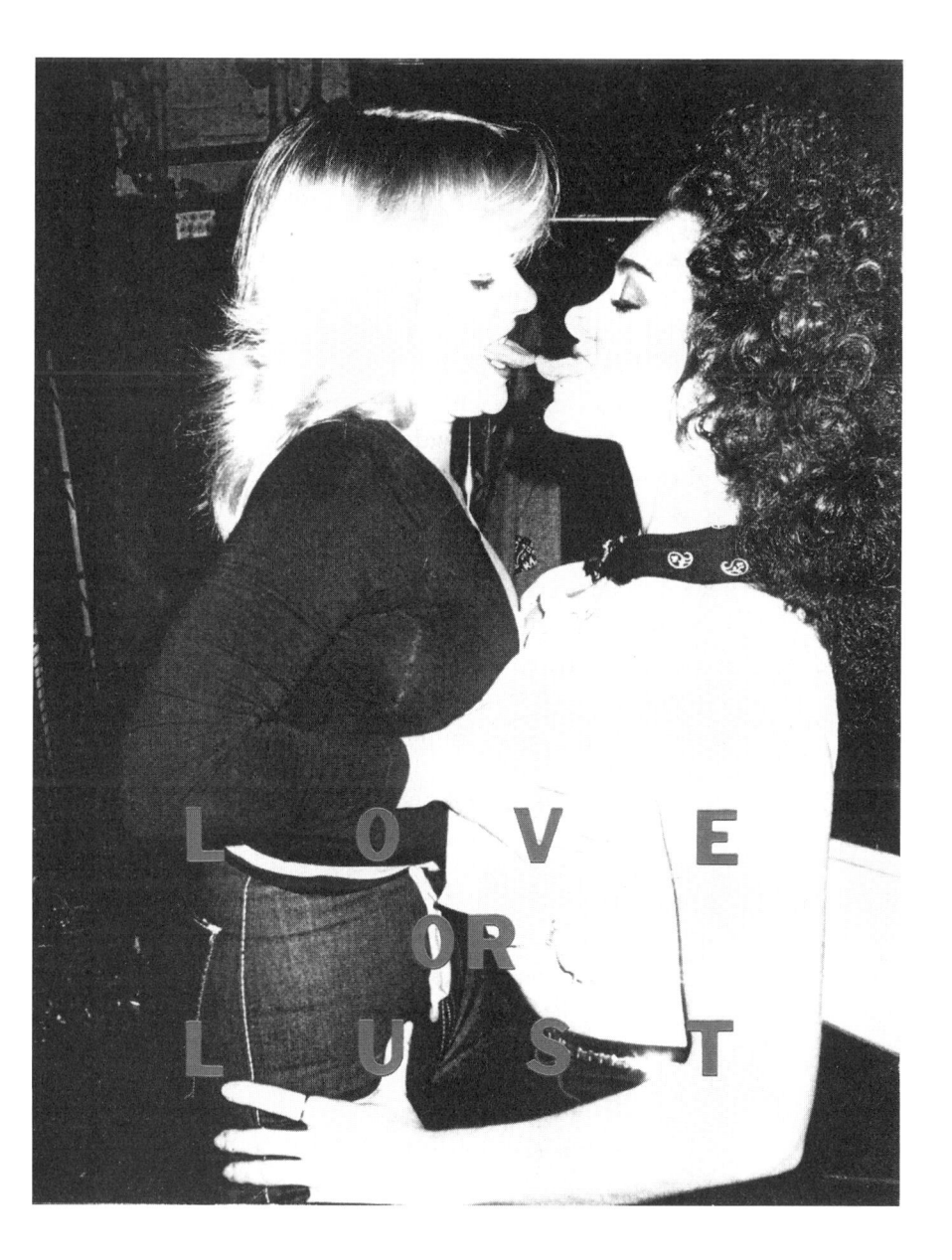

AT SALLY'S
EVE PACKER

ylvia del rio is stacked
& sits at the circular bar
in her long black spaghetti
strap dress, long bleached auburn
hair, cats-eye mascara, wide
& gorgeous mouth: a whiff of
drive-you-wild in-your-face
perfume & performance: tossing
her head, shrugging a shoulder,
arm on my arm, leg on my leg:
ava gardner, sylvana mangano, raquel
welchoverblown & hot: *i'm a pre-op
transexual* (she writes in my book)

> *a she-male is someone
> that looks like a woman
> but rally a fagit*

> (*transvestite* spelled *travestie*) — *someone
> who is a hard hard
> man who fantasize at
> being a woman*

> (*pre-op transexual*):
> *someone before she chop off
> her Dick*

in july she broke up with the boyfriend:

he doesn't
pay homage
anymore — i'm a queen —he's a liar — getting fat
missing a tooth — lazy —

what wld make you happy?
stiletto dropping a dime, hard as nail
hitting bulls-eye she says:

someone to share my life,
appreciate me — if

you can't do
that —

yr a piece of shit —
give me
my trophies

you're out —

as i go she tells me her phone number:

you can suck
my dick
anytime —

round & full & soft moon,
ny times clock reads 6:34,
very warm for january

FROM THE ASS'S TALE
JOHN FARRIS

The name of the nude joint was "Miss Lil'y White's." With a name like that, if I had been in any discernible shape, I'm sure they would have tried to keep me out, but I was still an *invisible* dog.

The decor was cedar, as if they were afraid of moths, and photographs of a petite, boyish blonde with her curly hair cut close everywhere hung in every conceivable place. What in this blonde reminded me of Peck was that she had the fresh-scrubbed look of the Ivory Snow Girl, and she really needed no clothing as freckles covered her bare skin as thickly as tattoos. I had to strain my eyes of an interested hound in the soft red glow of the place to make sure it was not she, though I was taken aback by the resemblance. It was not too far-fetched to have thought it might have been Peck as the Chicagoan had certainly passed through the Crescent City, the Big Easy, on more than one occasion in her career, and she had been certainly compelling enough to have gotten herself star billing anywhere she went. I assumed these pictures to be of Miss Lil'y herself as, along with the motif of the cedar and the photographs, there were lilies of every conceivable variety in every conceivable shade of white, including one great gilded calla that sat on a cedar lowboy in front of mirror in a lounge where table dances were offered the individual, leering customers, not exclusively male, if exclusively white, and lap dancing in which the dancer was allowed to sit facing her patron with her two hands clasped tightly behind his (her implied) neck if the tip was gratuitous enough.

It had been a long time.

A butch type in tattoos and motorcycle leather had ordered a couple of bottles of champagne and was waving over a long-limbed, pert-breasted beauty with a long chestnut mane to her table. I decided to join them before my bird began to glow.

The dancer had the lush, cushy-looking lips that parted into an easy smile that revealed her slightly crooked teeth as she spotted the hundred dollar bill the butch was waving like a semaphore. "Ah got all o' dis heah fuh you, and honey, if ah like whut you got, there is plenny mo' where dat came fum. Whereya at?"

The dancer, grinning some more, ran her tiny triangle of a tongue over what I was sure had to be the plushest lips in Royal. Royal, hell, in the Crescent City, the Big Easy. Her voice was all silk, and kitteny. "Hi there, sweetheart," she purred. "Welcome to Miss Lil'y White's. What's yo' name honey? Why, is this yo' fust time heah?"

"Sho' is," the butch said. "Ah'm fum Bogaloosa and ah'm jus' comin' out."

The butch wasn't bad looking. She had great muscle tone and fine bones though her lips were a little too thin and her nose a little too sharp. She said her name was Canine. I had to laugh. For some reason, I thought of Needle-nose, the sparrow. "Ah'ma gonna put all of dis heah money and some mo in uh great big wad in mah pants, and you kin have much o' it as yuh wont, is dat awraght wid yew, ba-by?"

The dancer delightfully grinned her assent. "Mah name is Kitty," she said.

It was a good thing I had spent all that time up on Morningside Avenue watching John and Milene work out as I am quite sure it was only that experience that enabled me to keep my bird from glowing like a searchlight as I waited for them to go through the preliminaries, and the butch had ordered another bottle and gotten drunk enough and wet enough for me to join them though, as I think about it now, it probably would have gone unnoticed in that red light. Knowing this was going to take a miracle as far as timing went, I waited until the butch named Canine had slipped her well-oiled finger into the dancer's ample rectum, and the dancer had retaliated by throwing a fierce Georgia-grind as she sucked cherries from her neck by the bowlful, before I carefully nudged the butch up on one cheek and slid my waiting thirsty bird into the dancer's willing, grateful cunt with a whoosh.

"Ooh, ooh, ooh, oooh," she exclaimed, grabbing what she thought was the butch by the back of the neck but which was, in fact, the back of my great hairy neck of an invisible bloodhound, "Canine, honey, ah, ah sho' do love yo money!"

The butch was so drunk and so excited by the passion aroused in her by the lapping action of my long, hungry tongue of a bloodhound in her ear she thought it was her own prick that had the dancer whooping like a High Plains Indian and gyrating in her lap as if she were grinding the corn and mashing the pemmican for her man's long trip to the Happy Hunting Ground, and didn't even mind when my growing boldness and complete mastery of the techniques I'd learned at the hands of the expert Woody and the divine Miss Peck and those I'd learned from watching my poor but equally well-trained donkey and his lost, lamentable lady Milene made me quite firmly boogie my way out of the dancer to ram my great ramrod of a bird up her own narrow behind. "Oh, Kitty, Kitty, Kitty," she moaned, "Yew got da grand prick of uh big dog!" And sat for me obediently, wagging her tail and barking like the canine I assumed she had named herself.

She didn't even mind when I took it upon myself to lead them into the techniques and practices that formed the five-pointed star, using my four paws and tail to bring them into the exercise, or when I howled like a mourning Irisher when I took them to the pretzel. I was right 'bout the dancer's lips, and I ground my own lipless mouth of a bloodhound against them, resting there as if I were resting my very soul on Buddha's couch, and as she shook her head from side to side, they slowly parted enough for me to slip my great engine of a bird between their incredible softness into the wetness of her throat in an exercise I had perfected on 'the street.' Using a circular breathing technique, she took in great, heaving gulps until my hairy balls were bouncing against her thrusting chin. I didn't at all mind Canine's little toadstool of a clit against my rear end, but when she tried to introduce her fist into it I had to close up shop, though the dancer did mind when I gently guided the offending appendage into hers. It was the one good deed I was going to do for the day. After all, the butch was paying for it, but she was not worried about her money now, as I was giving her as good as she got. "Oh K-K-K, Kitty, K-K-K-Kitty, Kitty," she stuttered between her moans and rebel yells, "ah, ah, ah, ain', ain', ain' had no idea it was go-go be like this, h-honey," as we brought ourselves to a great shuddering climax.

"Oh mah god," she said suddenly sitting up from where we had fallen to beneath the table and gratefully planted a kiss while examining the dancer's well-developed clit, "Honey, whut yew kin do wif dis lil' thang yew got down heah between yo' laigs oughta be a daggoned state secret. Yew, yew, yew know whut, Kitty? Ah, ah, ah thank dat fuh sa fust time in mah whole cotton-pickin laif ah done fell in love." Her gaze was tender as she looked into the dancer's eyes.

The dancer's smile was as wan as if she'd just given birth, and there were tiny beads of sweat over her exquisite lips as she leaned over to give the butch a grateful kiss. "Oh, Canine," she said softly, her hand on the butch's cheek, caressing it like a crystal ball. "Is dat fuh true?"

"Oh Kitty, Kitty, Kitty," Canine said, her chest heaving mightily, the blood rushing to her own cheeks, "ah wont yew ta know fuh sho' dat truer wouhds ain' nevah been spoken. Kitty, baby, whut kin ah do fuh yew tuh prove mah lov fuh yew?"

"Move in wif me and be mah fren'," said Kitty. "Do fuh me whut yew jus' did fuh me all da time. Tell me, would dat be too much?"

"Oh no, Kitty, oh no." She ran her fingers through the dancer's chestnut mane.

So, although they didn't know it, I had made a couple of fast friends. I knew I would have to visit with them frequently, at least until I had finished my investigations, so that they could get the big bang out of this relationship they sought, otherwise, you know what they say: 'the first time can be the best time.'

FROM GROOVE, BANG AND JIVE AROUND
STEVE CANNON

Annette was more than a little puzzled. She quickly retied the handkerchief, leaving everything as it was, and was about to drop it down in her purse when she heard a noise at the door.

She quickly wiped her behind; the shit was black. (I don't know what the broad had been eating.) Stood before the mirror pulling up her drawers when in walked Virginia. She strolled in swaying hips to the movement of the craft, her eyes slits, like she was high behind some good smoke. She eyed Annette's fine round young thighs.

Annette was wise to her eyes. She pulled up the bell-bottoms and tipped as the plane bounced, rocked and shook, moved towards the bowl and began combing her wig.

Virginia gave her a sidelong glance, dropped her drawers, lifted her skirt and sat down on the john. A quick glance told Annette that the bitch had black hair on her pussy and blonde hair on her head. "I've been holding this in since we left the airport. Feel like I'm about to burst." She splattered what sounded like a gallon of water into the commode.

Annette was always shy around people she didn't know. And… er…white folks, well, to her, let's face it, they smelled. (Of what? She never explained to me.) She gave Virginia a thin-lipped smile and concentrated on the tune going through her mind:

Runnin' thru the city goin' nowhere fast
You're on your own at last

"Man, you sure did tell that Max off, honey." Virginia finished peeing, didn't even wipe herself and pulled up her pink panties. She rubbed her tanned thighs — so unblemished, they looked like mannequin legs sitting in a Surrealist Pop-Art Trash Can. "Served him right, he ain't had no bizness telling that lie on you, honey. Served him right."

Annette glanced at her. Blonde hair on her head? Black hair around a pink-lipped pussy? Annette was having her troubles putting it all together. Virginia looked up and caught her looking at her thighs, then shot a message through her eyes. It hit Annette in the pit of her stomach, dropped to her womb and made her ass feel good. She quickly turned her head and continued to comb her blonde wig. "Damn, I'm hungry. Is there any food on this thing?" She talked to herself in the mirror.

Virginia acted as though she hadn't heard. She continued with her own line of questioning, dropping her skirt down over her twat. "You from Hoo Doo, right?"

A pain penetrated right above Annette's heart, right between her two lovely breasts. "Huh?"

Annette checked out Virginia's pinkish-brown, red face; the blue eyes and false eyelashes, and the arched eyebrows which had been plucked into crescent moons; the straight nose which might have been hooked in the first generation, and the thin, thin, red, painted orange lips. Virginia let her tongue roll slowly across her lips as she eyed Annette's hips.

"I was asking if you come from down there? You know, Gumbo?" Virginia moved closer to Annette, Annette could smell the best and worst of American beauty perfumes, colognes and bath oils emanating from her body.

Annette had to get the associations straight in her head before she answered. "Gurt Town. The projects."

The plane humped about ten thousand feet altitude, like flying over a big-titty woman. Annette held onto the wash basin. "Why?"

"Then that means you must know something about the Dark. Er… I mean mysteries —Voo Doo, the Occult. But that's what that word means, isn't it? Occult? Dark?"

"Beats me, Bones." Annette couldn't help but laugh, as the image of Marie in the coffin slipped back into her mind, candles burning upside-down, black snakes, the eternal, Sun, Moon and children of the night. Infidels. All this ran through her mind along with spirits, natural and supernatural, two heads ha'nts and curses. "Just that they kin put the bad-mouth on you, that's all."

Virginia was originally from the South. But in those days there wasn't such a thing. When she was a little baby, her father had abandoned her little ass and sailed back to England, left her to be attended by the Indians, then the Blacks took her and made her sell pussy; afterwards she went back to her own people and got a permanent position on the Governor's line. This way she didn't have to wash drawers, be humiliated and stuff, just push products instead — autos, washers, vaginal sprays, cigarettes and Dope.

But she was a firm believer in the dark forces of the Universe, the Indians and Negroes had taught her all that, but when it came to Hoo Doo and root American lore, she was just as dumb as the rest of 'em, believing that everything good came from Europe, and everything that was home-grown was rotten to the core. She'd accept seaweed from China, pearls from Africa and everything from Latin America, before she'd buy dis folklore.

So when she heard Annette put those two words together, use that syntax, *bad-mouth,* her body started aching, her loins trembled, her box got hot, and her tongue was heavy, dripping saliva.

She grabbed Annette from the rear, cupped her breasts and kissed her on the neck.

"Hey, wait a minute, bitch." Annette turned and pushed her off to the side. "I don't play that shit."

Virginia hit the floor and her skirt came up. Red splotches showed on the crotch of her panties. Black hairs sticking out the sides.

Virginia got herself together off the floor and eased up a second time, talking in a low sensuous voice, almost blurring her words. "I think that you are the most beautiful colored girl… black… I mean *dinge* that I've ever seen. And really…"

At this point she placed her arms around Annette's waist; Annette struggled to get free. But Virginia had her in a clinch, breathing hard: "All I want is to suck and tongue-kiss your bad mouth. Is that how you say it? The one between your thighs? Nothing would turn me on more than that, huh?"

Strange creatures. STRANGE. The bitch wanted to play with her poodle but had to call it something else.

Mixed emotions swelled in her chest while Virginia, as best she could, felt her breasts. She smelled like she had been dumped in a vat of perfume with stagnating shit at the bottom. Bull's shit. Suddenly the thought occurred to her, since this was a one-way trip, no coming back this way, not really, suddenly she asked herself, *why not?* And turned, shoving piles of tongue down Virginia's hot mouth.

Virginia held her tightly, rubbing her stomach against Annette's, feeling her breasts with hers, hips crushing against one another. Annette closed her eyes and was still able to see Marie in the coffin. She opened them, looked at the black roots of Virginia's blonde hair, the freckles on her neck, and felt Virginia's wet tongue on her cheeks and in her ears — sending chills down her spine, her core touching her, boxes boxing and rubbing against one another.

Still they clung to one another, Virginia running the palms of her hands over Annette's well-curved hips and fat ass, feeling up her thighs; they swayed in the middle of the floor, listening to their own breathing and the plane's drone.

Annette dropped her hands around Virginia's hips, clutched the flesh of her behind, reached down, pulled up her skirt and felt the soft flesh between her thighs. Virginia opened her eyes, closed them real fast, saw images of nightingales dancing on stairs, then felt Annette's fingers inside the lips of her cunt, working slowly, faster, then slowly, and Annette was staring her in the eyes. They were in utter communication, two bodies moving as one; Virginia continued to rub her legs, thighs and wiggle her hips. The hot gushy liquids flowed slowly down her thighs. She grabbed Annette tightly around the waist, ran her hand up and down her spine, rubbed her shoulders and pulled her even closer to her. Being the taller of the two, Virginia leaned her head down and kissed Annette on the cheeks, the eyelids, all over her face. She whimpered softly in the shorter girl's ear: "Oh, baby, baby, darling, you're so beautiful. I could just love you each and every day. Up here in the airways, down there on the ground, you're the best finger-fucker around."

Quickly Virginia was down on her knees unzipping Annette's bell-bottoms, pulling down her drawers and kissing the pubic hairs of her cunt and the lower half of her stomach, pushing her backwards towards the commode. Annette sat down, and Virginia stuck her head between Annette's thighs.

Annette lifted her thighs slowly and leaned back on the toilet, looking up at the white indirect lighting and listening to the plane, thinking about Marie in the john, Willie at the Gumbo House, watching the golden-headed bitch goddess suck between her legs.

She brushed her hair with the tips of her fingers, held her tightly around the head, and wrapped her tanned brown thighs close around Virginia's head.

It was a nutty sight to witness, Annette sitting back on the john like that and Virginia down on her knees, head down, licking the top, sides, bottom of Annette's cunt, feeling her fat round thighs, and trying to get a finger up Annette's ass. It didn't work. She got so carried away, she bent down even further and stuck her tongue up there instead.

Annette let out a sigh that the ground crew could have heard.

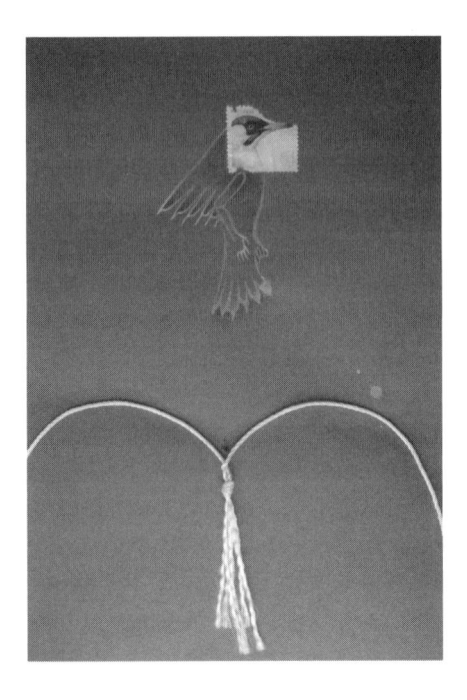

FROM THROUGH THE VALLEY OF THE NEST OF SPIDERS
SAMUEL R. DELANY

And levered out his own cock (I hope it ain't too small for these guys…), hardening when Eric saw the men inside. Some looked.

A couple of years older than Eric, one in a green workshirt with the sleeves torn off — like the boatman's plaid — grinned over the shoulder of a rangy older man — the boatman's age…? — whose pants were down around his hirsute thighs. (That's a nice cock, Eric thought.) The kid had close-set green eyes, a sparse beard you could see through to his face, broad bare feet, a tan mat of kinky hair, and a wide Negroid nose. He's black, Eric realized, though his skin was the same burned bronze as the boatman's, as Eric's. He shared a mouth with the older white guy. A smile deflected its line.

(Except for a few patches of black and white tiling, the newer, uglier, more utilitarian layer was winning.)

In his dropped overalls, the older guy wore the same kind of shirt, its sleeves pushed up hard, heavy forearms, the front open over a black T-shirt.

The bearded boatman said: "That there is Shit — " the kid smiled — "and this here's Dynamite." The older man nodded.

The barefoot kid's nondescript pants were open, too — they weren't jeans — and, as he moved, his cock slipped from the older man's butt cheeks and, still hard, fell to a downward slant. Turning, he stepped over, reached out, caught Eric's cock in his fist, and — more surprisingly — wrapped his other arm around Eric's shoulders. "My hand's kinda rough," he said, with embarrassment. "I don't wanna hurt you."

"That's okay," Eric said. "So's my cock."

"No, it ain't." Looking down, the kid chuckled. "It's a nice one." With his other arm he hugged Eric — and (Eric was about to say, *It feels good…*) thrust his tongue as far down Eric's throat as he could!

Eric hugged him back — surprised. The kid's clothes were old and he'd been wearing them a long time. Under their general funk, was a smell like sweaty leather, which Eric realized was the kid himself.

The boatman had called him… Shit?

While their tongues rolled together and around one another's, Eric saw over the kid's shoulder that the doors on the three stalls were gone.

So were the seats on the commodes.

The partitions were enameled blue, grooved and gouged, inside and out. Even from within the embrace Eric could see, beyond Shit's bearded cheek, holes drilled through the stall walls, some half-an-inch, some two-inches. Some were patched with tin squares; others had been drilled beside the patches. (Eric's tongue searched in Shit's mouth, and found no teeth at all — at least on the upper left. The surprise made Eric harder.) Among the eight men in the small room, Eric could see, a stocky Mexican sat on the last commode, barefoot like the kid with him now. (Eric pushed his tongue right. Gaps interrupted the teeth there, with — above and below — saddles of gum between.) The Mexican wore no shirt at all under a black denim jacket with frayed edges, open over belly and chest; nor any underpants: black jeans pushed to his ankles, he smiled with a wide, pockmarked face.

Eric thought: That's fuckin' sexy.

Along the trough urinal, a pipe began to hum, till, from its perforations, like tongues of glass, with small floshes, flaps, flops, and fluffles, water flushed the steel backing, to rush along the bottom.

By the urinal's end Eric glimpsed a tall black man with a shaved head. (For an instant, he thought Mike was at the urinal. His heart gave a single astonished pound, before he recognized a different ear, different head, different shoulder, thinner arm, rounder back…! On the arm below the short sleeve were black tattoos he could not make out, since the man also shared Mike's coloring. In three beats, though, his heart stilled.) Along with his stained dungarees he wore an orange and white road-worker's vest strapped over a gray T-shirt. He held his hands in front of himself, but was turned away so Eric couldn't see his cock.

Across the fifteen feet of cracked concrete by the Mexican's stall two other black guys — one notably stockier than the other — were laughing over something. Their flies bowed open — which made Eric think one, the other, or both had been fooling with the Mexican. The bigger one had a fist inside his and, as Eric blinked over the kid's shoulder, pulled out a thick cock, not as long as Jay's. Probably he'd put it away at Jay's and Eric's entrance, and only now pulled it loose again.

The kid hugged Eric tighter, drew in his tongue, then rubbed Eric's neck with his face. His beard was softer than it looked.

Beyond the kid's smell was the odor of wet stone and moist cinderblock and what seeped through cracked cellar walls from the damp — a smell, already at sixteen Eric associated with a half hour here or an hour there, sitting in some basement john stall, at a library or in a truck garage or at a bus station, because some guy finishing at the urinal had flashed him, then hurried out, and he'd waited and see if anyone else would come —

Waiting for men like these…?

The kid was strong, as strong as Eric, and — both arms around Eric's chest — his grip was tight with bone and a desperation Eric recognized….

Eric slid one hand between the boy's and his own belly, to grip his cock, which had just been up the older guy's ass. It was about three-quarters of an inch longer than Eric's — a little thicker. Holding it, Eric realized, made his own feel bigger — as, between them, the boy squeezed Eric's, with his rough hand. Eric thought: I wonder why he likes holdin' mine?

Beside them, the white guy bent to tug up his bib overalls. As he stood, on his once black T-shirt Eric saw a foreshortened dump truck, in gray, green, and more gray, before the denim rose over it. The john space was small enough for Eric to hear the suspender's wide wire snap catch a steel button.

Then the boatman raised his tattooed arm and put it around Eric's shoulder — a third arm around him. "'Scuse me, Shit. But this boy's gonna suck my dick now. You can have 'im soon as I'm finished." Taking a deep breath, Shit released Eric, stepping back, looking a little confused.

Disoriented, Eric looked left and right, still holding Shit's cock.

"Hey, Jay," Shit said. "I'm sorry. Sure." The boatman — Jay? — had *actually* called him "Shit." Till then, Eric had assumed it was a repeated miss-hearing, perhaps, of "Shim." In Florida, the security guard for Barb's trailer park had been called "Shim" and his mom had had a neighbor, Mr. Shippey, who Shim had always called "Ol' Ship"….

"Now, you — " which was Jay talking to Eric — "can hold onto *his* dick all you want, long as you're *suckin'* on mine."

Eric laughed. And the colorful, multi-headed arm lowered him to a squat.

Eric looked up at the boatman with his yellow beard and bare upper gum, grinning down. Above the boatman's jutting cock and bloated testicle, the size of a baseball really — the normal one a nodule on its side — from the john's uneven ceiling, the metal fixture around three incandescent bulbs suggested a glass covering had once softened their unfrosted glare.

Eric went forward, knees on the tile.

With his callused hands, the boatman slid his wide hooded cockhead, with its full veins, its downward curve, into Eric's mouth. It was salty — and thick enough so that, when in, it filled Eric's mouth. Eric took it deep, then backed up and, tongue thrust under the meaty hood, troweled beneath the glans — God, there was a lot in there, faintly bitter, salted, mostly dry — till his tongue pushed the frenum, which stretched against it. The big-armed boatman gave a pleased grunt.

Maybe the Mexican's tongue *hadn't* gotten to it that morning….

It felt good to get the guy's cock in his mouth.

Still gripping the other kid's dick — Shit's — in his hand (Was he three years older than Eric? Was he four?), Eric could feel Shit moving — an inch one way, half an inch the other — to position himself more conveniently. Eric came off Jay long enough to look up again and ask, "You pack that stuff in there with a *spoon?*"

"Hell…" the big boatman drawled, "I thought you said you liked it."

Shit chuckled — and stepped nearer: Eric's arm bent.

"I *do*." Releasing Shit's cock, which bobbed up an inch, to hit Eric's ear — the head was wet — Eric brought that hand over to cup Jay's immense testicle, with its smaller cousin, while four fingers of his other hand made a tent on the tile. Again Eric swallowed dick, till Jay's zipper cut at his lip.

Other guys laughed, watching, grinning. Eric grinned too — and in the dark space had a flash of Spring clarity, the afternoon sun aslant beneath the Atlanta highway — as Jay rubbed his head, the way the hillbillies sometimes had.

Eric thought: *Damn…!*

Someone said, "My kinda cocksucker, Jay," though Eric wasn't sure if the speaker was black or white.

Sucking again, Eric got to a rhythm, he could tell — from the way Jay pushed forward, his hand firm on Eric's head, the overhead grin — the boatman liked. For moments Eric wondered if he should not butt his chin into the enlarged scrotum. But after a few times — and he liked the feel of its hair against his lower face — Eric forgot it; or, rather, just enjoyed it; which the boatman seemed easy with.

Here is what, later, Eric thought:

When you're sucking a good dick, you can get so involved with what's going on in your mouth — the way something as big as, or bigger than, another tongue and of a different firmness is sharing the space, the stretch of your cheeks, the way the palate sends one with that kind of curve down your throat — it *is* different from the ones that curve up, not that I'd send someone away because of it — and the rightness it transfers to you, each thrust; of the way the thicker part toward the back — at least with a cock like this — has all the hair and also most of the salt, with someone who's been working. Scott says he doesn't like hair on a dick. But Scott's fuckin' *nuts* — ! I don't think Scott like *guys!* He'd be happier suckin' off chix-with-dix. (Imagine *two* nuts that big, in a real loose bag. I'm gonna jerk off over that…) You can live inside your own mouth, and all the world's in there with you. I guess you're aware of what's going on in the world, though it's not a third as important as what moves over your tongue, big tube with the little tube beneath, expanding along your tongue, the quarter inch you keep between your teeth and *his* meat —

Behind Eric, hinges squeaked.

Everyone in the space moved —

At least a little — and Eric knew it and moved, too.

The boatman's hands firmed on either side of Eric's head, not to halt him but to slow him, so that the motion of Eric's mouth kept on: a way to let his cocksucker know (Eric thought right there) that whoever had entered was okay.

Or, maybe, Jay doesn't *give* a fuck…?

What *would* it be like to be *that* big…?

Could you learn such strength through knowledge alone…?

At the urinal, the black guy said, "Hey, there, fella. You come for a taste o' dis?" and — Eric could just see the man around Jay's hip, when he pulled back — turning from the urinal enough so that Eric saw what the shaved-headed man in his safety vest held.

Jesus…! Eric thought — and got chills.

Who *is* that? Frack's *brother…?*

The newcomer moved into sight. Eric thought (though he couldn't be sure) it's the white guy Eric had followed into the place, who'd earlier gone into the front john. The man said: "Damn, Al, I hope you gonna shove that up my fuckin' hole. I thought you wasn't here — "

Eric reached up and got hold of Shit's dick again.

Chuckling the bald black man said, "Soon as I get my motherfuckin' raincoat on." Digging in his pants, while, hooded in its crepe cuff, a foot-plus of charred hatchet handle, webbed in black cable and all that only half hard, swung in front of him. Al pulled loose a square packet. Raising his hands (as though he might be nearsighted), Al tore through brown plastic, to pull loose an ivory condom that fell, unfolding, from his fingers. He shook it out.

"Goddamn, nigger!" one of the other black drivers said. "Dat ain't no raincoat! Al — da's a goddam *umbrella* cover!"

"Yeah — well, I need me de big ones." (Someone chuckled — probably the white guy Jay had called Dynamite.) With two thumbs in the latex collar, Al stretched it a couple of times. "Ted got such a sweet ass, I wait aroun' for this honkey motherfucker, sometimes."

The white guy in the yellow shirt already had his slacks unbuttoned. His belt dangled open, and, held in one hand, his pants drooped down one leg. He grinned around the room.

Al grinned back. "Come on, you honkey fuck hole!" Al pulled the condom on. Stretching latex wrinkled first on one side, then pulled out smooth. "Back up on dis, Ted, and le's see you do what both the ol' ladies I'm livin' with is too scared to, 'cept in the damned dark."

His own stubby cock still in his fist, the black driver said, "Well, you can't fuckin' blame 'em. I'd be scared of dat thing too."

Leaning over, gripping the urinal's rolled edge, Ted moved toward Al's end, slacks slipping further down his legs.

"You ain't too scared to *suck* it," Al chuckled. "At least de first seven or eight inches." While more guys laughed, he set cockhead in place, and, in his orange vest, embraced white Ted from behind. Black tattoos, unreadable in this ceiling light, swarmed like bugs around Al's black arms. As Eric kneeled up, again Jay's scrotum pushed into his chin. In his pants, Eric's cock head dragged across a wet spot.

Sympathetic electricity made Eric's back tingle. (No, Al's was *not* as big as Frack's; still, it was in the same foot-plus ball park.) He released the kid's cock he held — Shit's hand, covering Eric's, gave an acknowledging squeeze — and, while his other hand held the bearded boatman's hip, Eric slipped his fingers free and put them on the floor.

And something warm and rough covered them — Shit had moved his foot on top of Eric's hand. Eric rotated it beneath (the weight lightened in response), and gripped the naked foot, and squeezed. Hard bare toes grasped the edge of Eric's palm. The foot seemed too wide for any shoe.

Eric pulled his hand loose — because, crouching low, he couldn't really get the base of Jay's cock in his mouth.

"You don't use no fuckin' spit?" asked a wondering driver.

Thrusting, retreating, thrusting, Al said, "He don't need no…fuckin' spit — he keep a…fuckin' tin o' lard…up there, anyway…Or sumpin' greasy — least when… he come lookin' for *me,* he do… Spit?" His voice had dropped almost an octave. "I'd spit in his goddam ear — or tear 'im de fuck open!"

"Ted, you musta been practicin' to take dat nigger," someone said.

"Come on, Al…!" Ted whispered. His arms and shoulders rocked above the urinal's rim he gripped, the pink gone from his knuckles to the lengths between. "Shut up, and *fuck* my white ass, huh?"

"Oh, yeah! I remember what you like, motherfucker." Al was speeding up; his rhythm inflected his speech. "That's right — y'always wanna leave here… with your damn proof… o' purchase, doncha?…. Okay. Here you go — " Al dropped his face onto Ted's neck, who put his head back and grunted:

"Oh, shit…*yeah!*"

The black man, Eric realized, had *bitten* him!

Helped on by Al and Ted (Eric suspected but was not sure), the boatman's big hands tightened: he shot in Eric's mouth.

Eric pressed his face into the rough denim, taking the cock as deep as he could get it — which was pretty fuckin' deep. God, it felt good, even if he couldn't see the two at the piss trough. For moments it was as if the orchitis was a pillow beneath Eric's jaw.

With one hand and the other, the boatman rubbed the back of Eric's head; and — slowly — pulled out.

The black driver with his fat cock had come forward to wait on Eric's other side from Shit. As the boatman's cock fell free to rest beside the enlarged testicle, Eric turned, expecting to see Al and the guy he was humping at the urinal. Instead he saw the cock in the driver's brown fist — and took it in his mouth, turning on his knees to face him.

"Sweet Jesus — " the driver breathed in sharply — "this boy got a' educated mouth." Though he was uncut and thick, he was…well, free of cheese and perspiration. And he only put one hand — too lightly for Eric — on Eric's shoulder.

Still, Eric was enjoying his enthusiasm. The driver came in under a minute. Eric took him deep and held him there, while he listened to the breathing above.

Finally Eric slid off and grinned up. "You got an educated dick."

"I do?" The driver looked down, heavy brown face surprised. "Well, thank you, son. That's nice to hear. Real nice." His cock was softening. "Hey, Jay — he say I got a' educated dick. How you like that?"

As Eric kneeled back, the hood slipped forward.

"Well, I'm glad sumpin' about you's educated," Jay returned. "Somebody told me they seen you at Johnston's speakin' rally at the Interdenominational over at Hemmings. Don't tell me you gonna vote for a dumb white man like that? And vicious, besides. Nope!" Jay's forearm raised, his hand opened. "Nope. Nope! No politics in the damned john. I don't believe in it, and I ain't gonna start now."

The driver laughed, putting himself away.

A hand grasped Eric's other shoulder, slid under his arm, and pulled him up. He looked over — and smiling at him was the tall unshaven white guy — Dynamite, yeah, that's right — in his overalls and workshoes. The bib hid most of the garbage truck. "Hey, there — you don't want your knees to get sore."

"*Uh…* thanks," Eric said.

Dynamite smiled: half *his* teeth were gone — and Eric thought, this forty-odd-year-old cracker, smiling at him, with his hazel eyes and brown hair — a head taller than both Eric and Shit — could have been cousin or brother to any hillbilly he'd ever had under the highway. Still sitting on the shitter, for sex appeal only the Mexican rivaled him.

With his thumb, Dynamite pointed over at Jay, lingering now by the Mexican's stall. "Jay MacAmon over there says you might be around awhile — you interested in a job?"

(So colorful before, across the john, the boatman's biceps — thick as tire tubes — were now wrapped in shadow.)

"*Huh?*" Eric blinked. "Jay…? Eh…yeah — maybe. What kind?"

"Over in Diamond Harbor. Haulin' garbage with me and Shit." The thumb went toward the light-skinned black kid, Shit. The very wide thumb (like Shit's) did not have a lot of nail left — nor, indeed, did any of his other fingers.

(Why couldn't *I* have hair like Shit's...?) To protect himself from the feeling of confusion, Eric was about to add, *Well, I dunno*....

— when, against the wall and watching the whole room and — clearly and equally — watching Dynamite talk to Eric, Shit raised an equally big and knuckly hand to his face, dug a broad forefinger into a broader nostril, pushed, twisted, pulled the finger free, and put it in his mouth, while he watched.

Chills engulfed Eric, not just on his back, but from foot soles — as if he no longer stood on the floor but rather atop six inches of raging electricity — to scalp. Every sexual evaluation he had formed or forgotten over the six or seven minutes since he'd entered revised itself. If Eric had had any hair there to speak of, it would have danced on his scalp.

A knot of over-thick fingers, Shit's other fist hung on his dick — which, with the cuffed head protruding an inch, still looked hard. A drop glimmered on his foreskin.

(Eric thought about going over, squatting, licking it off...)

The urinal's timer turned over. Again water flushed the steel. (Fluffles, flaps, flops, floshes...)

With their unreadable black markings, Al's arms gripped Ted's yellow shirt. In his jeans, with his belt end swinging, Al's thrusting buttocks clocked the world.

Somewhere inside himself, Eric found the words, "Yeah. Sure, I..." obliterating his wariness. He hadn't intended to say them. But he had.

"You got somethin' I can write on?" Dynamite took three inches of pencil from his pocket, while Eric thrust his hand into his own pocket (I can't feel *anything*...! Glittering chills armored him...) and managed to get out the paper Bottom had given him that morning. He handed it to Dynamite.

"If you gonna be around a few months and serious about workin', show up at the Gilead dock come Wednesday mornin' — four-thirty, four-fifty. We get started by five." On the paper's back, with heavy, soiled fingers, Dynamite scribbled, then returned it to Eric.

"Thank you — hey, thanks!" Eric found his voice. "Yeah — hey! Thank you! Sure." Taking back the paper, he returned it to his pocket, then (without looking at it, he realized), because it was as if he were encased in electric armor, reached between Dynamite's legs. If Dynamite had knocked his hand away, he wouldn't have been surprised.

"Now what, son…?" The man smiled. The skin on Dynamite's neck and arms was sun-roughened and redder than Shit's. "You want some more Georgia cracker dick?" Reaching up, he pushed the pencil into a pocket on his bib, moved… toward Eric, still fingering the denim to get a grip on the man's cock. Dynamite reached for his own chest, looked down, and unsnapped one strap, then the second.

As the pants dropped again, Dynamite's hands came out and took Eric by the shoulders, bent his face down, and opened his mouth.

Then, his hands like slabs supporting Eric's back, the back of Eric's head, Dynamite's tongue went in, thickening and thinning, against Eric's own, and tasted… God, *good!* The smell was like Jay's, with a different automotive overlay.

(Regular instead of diesel…?)

Shit had moved up, too, breathing hard, waiting his turn, finger still in his mouth.

Though he was no longer picking.

Through the long kiss, Eric thought: My goddam tongue is glittering — and dropped to his knees for Dynamite's cock — thick, big, uncut — that pushed against his upper lip, then went into his mouth.

In small, upward movements, timed to Dynamite's heart, it hardened.

It had salt and — Eric got his tongue under the skin and into the circular pocket around the head — cheese. This guy was *so* good — not, Eric thought, that Scott would agree. But Scott wasn't sucking the cracker sonofabitch. His mouth filled with that cock that was — again Eric took it to the root — bigger than Jay's, if not so thick as the black driver's, while, with another heartbeat, it expanded to the size of Shit's.

Fingers like bars, rough as rust, Dynamite gripped Eric's head and cheeks. Denim bound Dynamite's thighs. Eric reached between them, under the long scrotum and moved his hand up warm buttocks, firm, flat, furry, to feel more testicles behind the garbage man, swinging into the back of his hand. Eric's fingers stubbed the firm stock moving there.

Shit had moved forward and was again fucking the guy!

Once Eric kneeled on a bib-denim strap across the tiles, as Dynamite tried to step in his big shoes and staggered…. "Damn, boy — what you doin'? Tryin' to pull me over?"

"I'm tryin' to *see*," Shit rasped, softly, roughly, on Dynamite's back. "I wanna watch your fuckin' cock goin' in and out this white scumbag's mother-fuckin' suck hole!" Yeah, he had to be black….

Eric gripped one of Dynamite's hands — as big and as rough as Shit's — as he moved to the side.

"Hey, *yeah*…" Shit drawled from above in an uprush of pleasure. "I got it, now. Good. I can see it. *Okay!*"

Eric heard shoes on the concrete behind him, then felt something press his back — a hand slid under his jeans.

"What you doin', Al — ?"

And the other driver said, "Nigger, you gonna kill that boy — he can't take that thing like Ted!"

Al said, his voice like something from under ground, "Why the fuck not…?"

Eric wondered if Ted had gone when his own attention had been elsewhere. (He hadn't heard the door springs grate.) How had he left such a small space, without Eric hearing — even if Eric *was* sucking someone off?

Apparently, though, Ted had.

"Least I'm gonna try — "which was Al's voice down behind him!

Reaching for his own waist with one hand, Eric thumbed his jeans' button out of its hole.

"See, dere — he don't min'. He wan' me to."

Someone — Al, on his knees behind him — tugged Eric's loosened pants back below his buttocks. Already Eric could smell him, added to Jay's, the black driver's, Dynamite's automotive odors. It was not the smell of the black homeless men Eric had gotten used to in Atlanta. (The plastic road vest had its own odor.) It was the smell of a man who'd been working hard outdoors, like the smell of some odd wood, sawn fresh — cedar or sequoia — that Eric was not familiar with but wanted to smell again. He pushed as if he were taking a crap — the way, just two weeks ago (*De firs' time or so, da's de* only *way you gonna get it all in, bitch. So* push, *cocksucker!*) Frack had taught him. Al entered him. "Yeah — hey, da's goin' in jus' as easy…. I *thought* it might…"

"*Goddam…!*" Shit whispered above them.

Al's arms gripped him — whatever plank it was, rip-sawed end to end — and he no longer had to work at sucking Dynamite, because Al's rhythm moved Eric's head in and out. All he had to do was hold himself up.

"Jesus, boy — what, you come in here already greased, *too?* Da's fuckin' sociable!" Since Al was supporting his own weight, it felt pretty good. "I thought it was jus' niggers who was supposed to be so greasy. Not all you nasty white fucks." Eric heard Al's grin and — still sucking — grinned with him.

No, Al's cock was *not* as big as Frack's, but, more than a foot, it would have poked from a ripped pocket by an inch or two. And did he care about the difference between fifteen and seventeen?

Three minutes later, Dynamite came.

Five seconds after that, Al grunted, "Oh. Shit… I *love* dis fuckin' nasty white shit." (Jesus, he felt really low and really good…) Then the warmth pulled from Eric's back.

Eric flinched, because, yes, KY or no, Al's pull-out stung.

"Jesus, that looked fuckin' *great…*" someone said; it took a second for Eric to realize that, over Dynamite's shoulder, it was Shit.

Dynamite had taken seconds to get hard — and took seconds to soften. Eric sucked the firm cock as deep as he could, and wallowed cum around it, even prizing his tongue beneath the foreskin to let some liquid in, till the man's hands halted his head.

The muscles at the back of Dynamite's cock tightened — familiar from Pickle — as a spurt of salt urine flushed Eric's mouth… surprising him (Pickle primed or not). Eric sucked deep again, swallowing. He kept at it, ten, fifteen, twenty seconds, hoping for more, even as he stilled his tongue. Finally, looking up, he saw the man grinning down. (Eric patted Dynamite's leg, squeezed it.) But that was all that happened. Dynamite's grip loosened around his head and he let Eric back away.

Sitting on his heels, Eric worked one foot and another under himself to lever upright, loosening Al's hands from his flank. "Oh, shit…!" He glanced back, to see Al, buttons opened around the latex sheath. "Thanks," Eric said. He was breathing

hard. As with Frack, he thought: *How did I get all that in…?*
"That was… good!" *Maybe I'm learning…. Or just stretching….*

Al drawled, "I know damned well it was." Chuckling at
Eric, he moved back toward the urinal.

Eric looked again at the garbage man —

Cock sagging, Dynamite stepped back; he too grinned
at Eric. Shaking his head, again he began to drag up his
pants, then pushed himself into his overalls.

Eric managed to stand and, looking around, saw Shit,
coming back, over uneven concrete, edging between Jay
and the driver Eric had sucked off, leading the other black
driver, a solid, dark fellow in a blue T-shirt, in his late thirties or early forties.

Shit held the man's cock — pulling him by it, it looked like.

As he followed, the second driver smiled, looking
somewhat embarrassed. (Dynamite had stepped over to
Al. They were whispering about something.) Eric was
slightly confused. But Shit reached out with his free hand
and — now — took hold of Eric's cock. The driver Shit led
stepped up to Eric and as Shit positioned himself before
both of them, smiled at Eric, and put his arm around
Eric's shoulder. His dark face was further shadowed by
bushy brows.

Eric smiled back, curious.

Holding both penises, Shit dropped to a squat and, in
his large, heavy hands, pulled Eric and the driver's penises
together, both — one dark, thick-veined, and uncut, the
other a heavy pink, over an ivory skin, circumcised, and
bullet-headed. The black one straight, Eric's slightly up-
curved, both were erect.

Eric looked down at Shit's rough, mustard nap. Already
he had a thinning spot, though he probably wasn't twenty.
Behind him, Eric could see his wide, bare feet, his cracked

blacked soles, the toes of one propped up and turned under, the pads of the other stretched behind, dirt gone shiny from walking.

Shit put the black guy's cock in his mouth. Eric felt Shit's beard against his own dick. Then he came off and took Eric's cock in his warm, warm mouth.

Shit's thick-fingered hands — bitten nails and big knuckles, both lined with black — were grubby from his work. His mouth went back and forth. Looked at from above, his nose seemed particularly broad and Negroid, and — hell — sexy.

Now Shit glanced up. He chuckled. "I wish my dick was more like one of these or the other. But it's just in the fuckin' middle."

Eric was surprised — because Shit's generously uncut cock was between half and three-quarters of an inch longer than either. It had never occurred to Eric someone could want a cock smaller than his own.

Shit went back to sucking them both.

The black driver beside him smiled at Eric. As Eric looked at his face, the full mouth opened and came forward. The broad lips kissed Eric, who opened his mouth to receive the driver's tongue, which went no further than within Eric's lips. His unshaven face turned against Eric's.

The driver closed his eyes — then opened them; and pulled his mouth away.

Eric blinked.

The driver looked stern.

(Shit's mouth came back to Eric's cock. His hand moved around to Eric's leg, where, as his mouth went in and out, the fingers flexed on the denim.)

Softly, the driver said to Eric: "Did that man you was suckin' off before piss in your mouth, boy?" He nodded over toward Dynamite.

Momentarily, Eric was flustered: "*Uh…*Yeah. A little, I guess."

The driver's body stiffened. Without dropping, his arm loosened. He moved back a chilly inch. "Dat's the third time he done that to some good lookin' fella what come in here in the last two months — it jus' messes it up for the rest of us. You'd think he was a damn tomcat, markin' his territory. And Jeb — my partner over there — *still* likes 'im. But then, Jeb is strange." He gave Eric's bare shoulder in its tank top strap a consoling pat, then dropped his hand "Well, I guess it ain't your fault. I just gotta get to you guys a'fore he do." Shaking his head, he turned away, wiping his wrist across his mouth.

And Shit rose before Eric, his chest and then the waist of his pants dragging over Eric's cock. Shit's green eyes, his wonderfully broad nose, his mouth were against Eric's face. Eric's eyes were open to see both Shit's, equally wide. Then Shit's tongue probed and rolled and wrestled around Eric's.

Seconds later, Shit pulled back to whisper: "I like how it tastes. It ain't bad — it's real nice. That nigger's crazy."

Eric was glad of the reminder different people liked different things.

The hard hand holding Eric's shoulder moved to Eric's back. At their groins, in an all-but-uncomfortable position, in which the pleasure of excitement turned into something interesting, their cocks crossed. Their scrotums hung against one another's.

With one hand, Eric held the back of Shit's neck and, with the other, the small of Shit's back. He could feel Shit's body, breathing, against his, even as he smelled him.

And breathed, thinking, for all the fucking around he'd done with guys you don't usually get *this* close to them. This was really nice.

Shit whispered: "You okay…?"

Eric whispered: "Yeah."

"Good." And Shit released his, and stepped back. "I hope he pisses in your mouth some more. Go on, try somebody else, now."

Not sure he wanted to, Eric watched Shit back up against the wall, where, again (as though he had backed outside the circle of perception of all other eight men in the room, so that the aura of isolation made him even sexier), Shit dug his middle finger in one nostril, sucked it clean, dug in the other, sucked it, digging and sucking, digging and sucking —

Surprising himself, Eric stood, stepped up to him — Shit blinked his green eyes — and opened his mouth as if he was going to tongue wrestle Shit again; but Eric took in the forefinger, with its salted crust. Shit's hands were as big as Dynamite's, with the same teeth-tortured nails. Eric saw — and a moment later felt with his tongue — the gritty forefinger. Again the kid hugged Eric — with one arm, this time, and kissed him.

The finger was now back in Shit's mouth —

Till it reversed to push into Eric's —

Then back.

Then back and forth….

Finally Shit whispered, "You taste real good." Nodding toward Dynamite, he moved his face away, grinning. "I always liked lickin' piss outa somebody else's mouth or asshole. You should go kiss on Mex. He always been drinkin' somebody's piss — Jay's or Jeb's or some other nigger's. Hey — I wanna shoot, now — I'm ready. You want it?" His jeans were up, but his cock — hard — and balls were still loose.

Eric dropped again to the tile. One of Shit's pants legs was torn, and his knee's smudged geometry showed through the rip. Since he'd have eaten out Dynamite's ass in a minute, Eric was not going to die from sucking Dynamite's crap off Shit's dick.

He took Shit in his mouth.

Shit grunted, caught Eric's head, and, propping the toes of one foot on Eric's knee, began to pump. Eric hugged his legs. The cloth was some sort of brown corduroy, Eric saw — but it had been hard to recognize, because so much of the wale was worn.

In forty seconds, Shit shot, too.

It was thick and nut like. Eric swallowed… a third of it.

Lingering, Eric sucked, hoping for piss from this one. None came.

Then Dynamite was beside him, tugging him up to cover his mouth with his own — stubble ground on Eric's face — and plunged his own tongue as far in as he could.

Eric held to his hard shoulders, a head higher than Shit's, wondering at having so quickly gotten five loads.

When they broke for breath, Dynamite stepped back, breathed in deeply, one strap fastened, one hanging. "You know — " Dynamite grinned —"I was serious about what I was sayin' before." Their uncut cocks — Dynamite's and Shit's — were the same size, with the same down curve, same thickness. Eric held one in each hand. He rubbed the hooded heads together.

Both of them smiled, missing their different teeth.

Was Shit's a hair's breadth wider? Or maybe it only looked so because Shit was shorter….

Reaching down, Dynamite gripped loosely and support- ively the complex construction the two — then three, because Eric pushed forward with his own — cocks had become.

"About that job — when Jay was introducin' us."

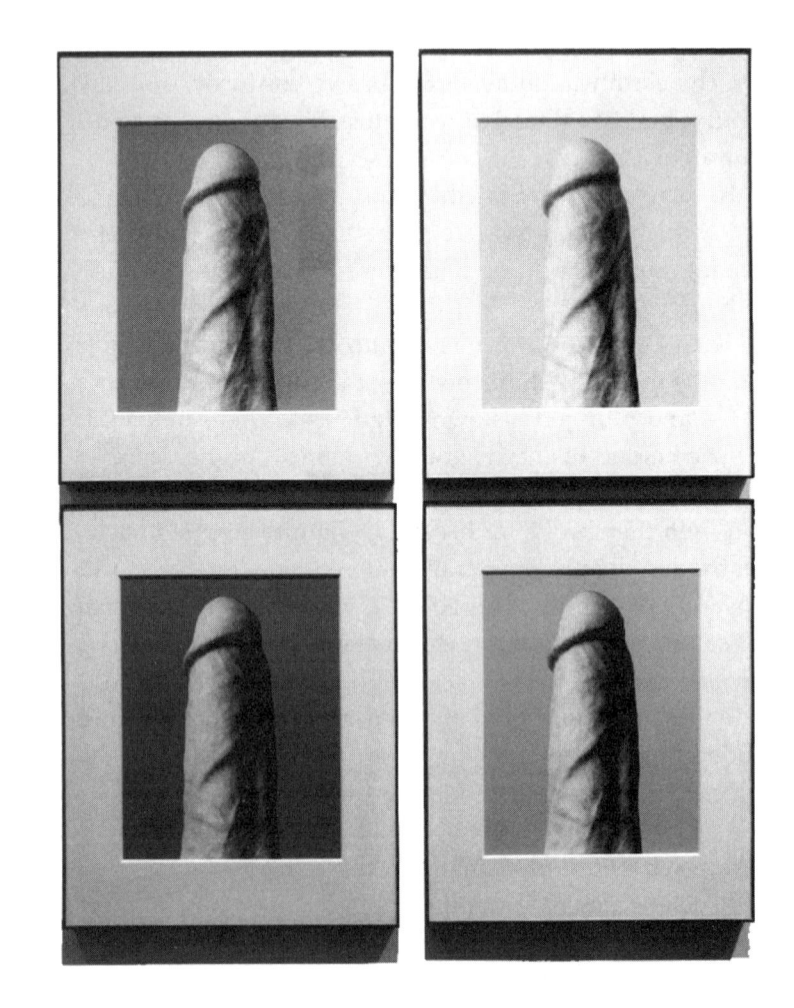

THE OTHER SIDE
LESTER STRONG

I wouldn't say it's you
in my mind's eye
as I jerk off thinking
of a young jock whose lips
brush the tip of my cock,
whose tongue and mouth
apply just the right pressure
to command the blood to
flood my loins and the
jizz to spurt in ecstatic abandon,
leaving my fingers sticky with its white foam.

But it's you, nevertheless,
you and your lithe body I caress
waking and dropping off to sleep,
you and your silky voice I hear
purring at me late night over the phone,
you and the hardened nipples of your chest I feel
caressing my own nipples into hardness, too,
you and your lusty cock I see
spearing the air in a joyous
naked dance free of all
encumbering clothes — yes,
those images shimmer within
the jock-filled vision in my mind's eye,

making my cock at last
burst forth into its cum-spattering jig
in the wild affirmation of
a longed-for union with you
somehow,
sometime,
some place.

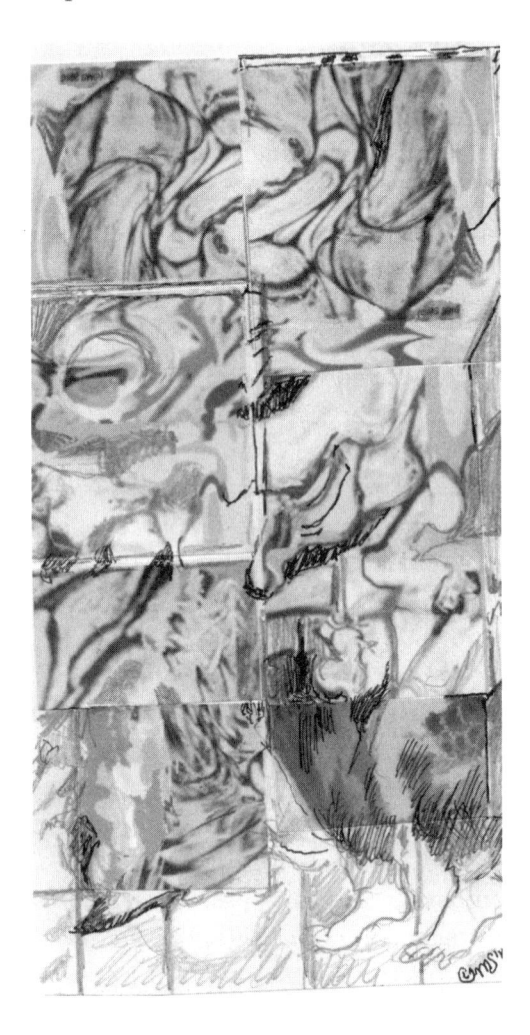

SEXODUS
TOM SAVAGE

No more McCarthy's of sex.
Our black holes can swallow Starr,
Benito Giuliani, and this
Sexless Exodus group
That wants to cut off gay men's cocks.
Sperm exodus and entry continues between the lines.
Orwell's anti-sex league has come to pass,
And pass away, it surely will,
Leaving neither descendants nor protéges
To suck its members off in the hidden dark.

I refuse to allow any Exodus
To drive the sex out of my life.
I refuse to allow the image of
Giuliani in drag into my brain, anymore.
I'd rather believe in Milton Berle as a girl
Than pretend this fascist autocrat
Will do anything for queers.
He only wants rich ones to give him money.
Those Christianized, neutralized gays still long for each other.
If they use God to suppress their desires,
Free the sky of this policeman, immediately.

Let the streets be full of sexy men and women.
Let us take off our clothes now

And force the cops to put their erections
Where their billy clubs are.

If Moses was content to dwell with a man,
It's good enough for me.
I am what I am more than that I am.
You can kiss me anywhere but on the mount of God.
But if some god wants you to mount him, who can say no?
Take your rod and cast it into Pharoah, too;
But only if he's good looking and kind.
I give you the keys to my pants.
May they provide access to the kingdom of Heaven.
Circumcised rods and uncircumcised serpents are welcome.
My uncircumcised lips demand a blowjob,
Let the daughters of Shim'i shimmy as they wish to.
Cast down or cast off rods bite.
All the cattle of castration will die
Before killing everyone else with fear.

Let us pass over and away
From this Lord who hardens people's hearts
As a test in a game.

All my life have I waited for someone like you?
Now is your time to come through.
I make this sweet offering to my lord.
Whoever touches our bodies' altar is holy.
May you come up the middle and consume me.
Let us find grace in each other's sight
Let love's fire burn our nightly bath in the mercy seat.

THE INTERLUDE
VINCENT KATZ

o shine, to be bright, brilliant, radiant. to be clear, ring loud and clear. to shine forth, be conspicuous or illustrious. to make to shine, light up: to shine.

yawning, profound. voracious, gluttonous. bold, wanton; coquettish: wayward, arch.

Jürgen sat at his desk contemplating porn. He passed a large part of his day sitting in his cubicle, avoiding work and flipping through porn. Although he always cleared his browser history, it was still possible to trace his activity, but he worked in a company with a relaxed atmosphere, there was no one breathing down his neck. Plus, he did a good job. He came in at 8:30 and left at 5:30. In between, he took care of business. There were only ten people working in the office. Sometimes, Jürgen's boss would come over to his cubicle to go over something with him. Jürgen would see him coming out of his glass-doored office, look around apparently absent-mindedly, then start to shuffle over to him. Jürgen liked his boss. He knew that *faux* absent-minded look, that shuffle, so well.

The Anus (and its concomitant ass) is living glamorous days. Sure, the ass (and its concomitant anus) has always been a source of insane pleasure, oracle of awareness

247

women and men have bent faces to for refreshment and answer to that pressing itch that never goes away. But ever since, say, the 1990s, the ass (and its concomitant anus) has really come into its own on a world scale. This is not necessarily a good thing. It means that everyone knows about it now. It is no longer within the purview of illicit knowledge, though there will always remain something wrong about it, off the beaten path.

Tantalizing because always visible, that is to say, visible from behind. Not exactly visible, but sensible, can be sensed. It projects a kind of intelligence backwards, away, but not entirely disconnected, from the face's frontward projection.

The anus is so sweet, demure.

Someone walking down the street smiles, and you see her anus. You want to be ultimately connected to that. Your whole being is being drawn into that: arms, shoulders, nose, feet, brain, into that black whole, never to re-appear perhaps. A construction by which your face is temporarily wedded to her crack, as she walks, making a squishing sound your nose and mouth contribute to.

A way of dressing that accentuates that, draws all attention to a single point.

There is something brilliant about the anus (and its concomitant ass), the way it shines forth as a point of wisdom, both given and received. It is both yawning (or the approach to it is, at least) and profound. Deep, and the knowledge given and received there is of the deepest, darkest nature. Which is what I meant, when I said earlier, it used to bestow a kind of secret information, like a mystery, entered into only by adepts and their acolytes. But perhaps, in this day we live in, if everything is known, then everything can be unknown as well, where "un-known" takes on an active meaning — un-learned, un-remembered. It will need active effort to remove these dials of pleasure from the general consciousness.

Another verb means "to teach." Sex is often realized as a kind of teaching. Sometimes, it is a terrible knowledge of something that has been done to one that now, in transference, will be done to someone else, so that they will know, ultimately, that the world is not the place they once thought it was. As with most words, this teaching can have a negative or positive spin to it. It can also be a sharing, in which bliss, experienced by the giver, is transferred, happily, to the receiver, who in turn experiences, for the first time, or in a completely new way, an ecstatic happiness.

There is certainly intelligence in the anus (and its concomitant ass). In Aristophanes' play *The Clouds,* he takes the piss out of the sophists, taking as the particular target of his ridicule, Plato's school of philosophy. In *The Clouds,* Plato's students root in the earth for truffles, "while their anuses take a minor in astronomy." (*The Clouds* also has one of my favorite lines of all time: "It is impossible for a man to stay alone in bed awake for any period of time without jerking off.") But there is a brilliant truth to Aristophanes' observation about the anuses. They do pursue their own form of wisdom. They are not entirely passive, although to the outside observer it might appear as though they only lie there and take it. On the contrary, anuses (and their concomitant asses) are constantly on the move — in a much less pretentious way than the often idiotically blabbering minds to which they are linked — and they are searching out their own happiness in their journeys throughout the world.

Kenneth Tynan wrote that at noon one day he was licking the anus of one of the most famous actresses in London. Of course, Tynan was a horrible, sadistic misogynist.

To see was to know. But to touch, to taste, to smell, are also.

Herodotos tells of the marriage of Peisistratos to the daughter of Megakles. Peisistratos did not want children with her (he already had grown sons) and therefore only had sex with her *ou kata nomon*, "not in the usual way," which some commentators have taken to mean anally. The daughter eventually told her mother, who told Megakles, who went into a rage, forcing a conflict.

But, Jürgen thought, as his boss shuffled back to his office, what is unusual about the anus? Certainly, when one takes into consideration its concomitant ass, the conjunction is something with so much personality, so much reality, in many cases displaying so much of the character of the person, that one would often rather have a conversation with it than with the face, however lovely, (and its concomitant mind) at the other end. Sometimes, the whole world seems upside down. In fact, one can easily fall in love with an ass. It happens every day.

FROM TRAIN TO POKIPSE
RAMI SHAMIR

I'm walking down the platform of the Montrose Ave. L station. My body's still leaking all over the place, in the front, in the back. I check my jeans to see if they're wet, but I can't tell. I hate the L train because you're bound to see someone you know, and usually they'll check you out to see if you're still cool or to see how much you've fallen apart since the last time they saw you. I lick around my mouth and then spit on the tracks. A mouth full of cum definitely isn't the look.

Halfway through, sitting on the edge of his bed, he told me I'm HIV positive. When I heard him moan in the late morning, I took his long dick out of my mouth and saw that it was spewing out jizz. I don't remember having any emotional reaction to what he said because I still hadn't come, and I was really high, and it was only four o'clock. Most importantly, there was still a full vial of coke we hadn't touched yet.

But when it was over, when I saw his face the way it really was, and his room the way it really was, when I felt his arms wrapping around me from behind, I got a little nervous. It's not that I give a fuck about dying, it's just that I don't want to die for him. I don't want to die for love.

I took a cab to his place because he said he'd pay for it. When I got there, I said, "hello," then went to the kitchen table where a half full vial was sitting by some lines. I did all the lines, then emptied some coke from the vial and continued. Line after line after line. He was trying to get the computer to work to play some music, and I kept going at the coke.

"Is this all we have?"

"Yeah, baby," he says coming up to me. He starts unbuttoning my jeans. He starts kissing me. "Should we get more?"

"Yeah, we should," I say, pulling away. "I'll call my dealer."

Twenty minutes later, his face is in my ass, and I'm pouring a mound of coke from the vial onto his flaccid cock. Inhale. Inhale. Go slowly on my cock, you tell me. Kiss the head, kiss the shaft. That's right, go all the way down. That's right.

"Swallow it down. Swallow it all the way down. That's a good boy."

I sit on your cock, let it fill me all the way. I wonder how dirty I am inside. I go up, your eyes go down. I go down, your eyes go up. You pull out and I lick myself off of you. From balls to head, I lick myself off your cock. Suck my dick, I tell you. I put on my Lynyrd Skynyrd hat and pull you by the hair up to the mirror. Lee Ranaldo is yelling through the speakers, *"I can't see anything at all, all I see is me. That's clear enough, and that's what's important, to see me."* I watch myself in the mirror as you suck my cock. I watch my thin body sweating, my blue eyes turning black, my face turning white. I pull your hair hard as I keep fucking you in the mouth with a limp dick that gets harder the more you work it with those pink lips of yours. *"My head's on straight, my girlfriend's beautiful, looks pretty good to me."* Looks pretty good to me.

Cocaine delivers me poorer and poor —
I am thurstin', I am thurstin' for more.

There's a part of me that hates you right now, another part that knows you hate me too, and what's left just wants to kill this thing called love. Somewhere, though, somewhere between all that, I believe that we know each other, and I believe that romance still has a chance. And right now, as I'm pulling your head back and forth with a violent movement onto my cock, this feeling, without location, without definition, as immeasurable and vast as the black space swimming between stellar bodies, is the strongest.

I spit on you. You spit right back. Really forceful like I'm useless and like you want me to know it. Then you go to kiss me. I kiss you back and then pull away to see your face. *All I see is me...* I SPIT RIGHT INTO YOUR EYE. For that I receive a hard slap on the face that makes my cock-ringed tumescent dick skip from the accompanying rush of blood.

The coke runs out. I go to sleep in your bed, and when you say, "Will it bother you if I stay up a bit?" I tell you, "No it won't bother me if you stay up a bit." Morning has come, killer of nightly things, reminder that we are nothing but the aging flesh of fragile days. He gives me a black mask to keep away the sun. As I pass out, I hear him say, "This place looks like a crime scene."

I wake up. Where are you? I'm at some boy's house. He's by my side. What's his name again...?

I told him I'd see him soon as I was walking out the door. Moments before, he rushed out of bed as I scrambled to get my things. He was right: the apartment *did* look like a crime scene. There were clothes everywhere, disrespecting the boundaries of adjacent rooms, cigarette butts in the sink, on the counter, in the multiple cups of lukewarm water, empty coke bags, empty vials, powder all over the kitchen table, his desk, his plates, and the mirror we took down sometime during the night. I decided to just focus my attention and gather the essentials, which will get me home with the hope that everything else would somehow gather itself.

I hear a car honking outside. "Man, these fucking cars! Either they take an hour to get here, or they come right away. No moderation."

Many times before, when I really needed to flee his apartment, it took three or four hassling calls to the Anonymous Car Service Company to get them to send a car fifteen minutes late. At those times, I was desperate; my eyes still round black globes, and my body still puppeted by the cocaine flowing around in my blood. At those times, I was desperate, like an animal tied with rope to a time bomb. I couldn't go outside and wait — no way — that would have been like stepping into another and dangerous dimension; but my patience for him and his apartment, the memory of him touching me and me touching him, weighed on my weak head and threatened to break it with every minute. I wouldn't be safe at these times until I got home and washed all of him off — his cum, his piss, his fingerprints. At those desperate times, the car was inevitably late.

But today, I was fine. I had already showered — alone — more to get the multiple layers of baby oil off my body than to get him off of it. He was right. The place looked like a crime scene, and we were its cadavers that momentarily got to remember the shocks of the living.

The car is green — they said they'd send a black one. A moment of panic: brief, but there. Even if I was fine and holding friendly flirtatious conversation, I didn't want to wait outside; and if this car was the wrong car I would be forced to wait outside, as mesmerized by fear as a deer trapped in the headlights. Yesterday, I marveled at how exposed the bedroom windows were. Nothing but thin transparent sheets covered them; and in the dark, all the lit up windows were like eyes, all focused on my naked body dancing around and my gesticulating hands, which moved along my ass cheeks as I performed a little dance. What if someone calls the cops and complains? What if they come and finally get me, before I even got to come? I scanned the morning horizon to validate those fears of last night, but it seemed the coast was clear. The coast is always clearer when your nerves aren't being fried by cocaine.

He was hard, and he was kissing me. I slightly and slowly returned the favor. For a moment, my lips hung on his lower lip, as if enticed by the erection, or disappointed for an instant by the inevitable ending of all things.

"You're all hard now. What a shame to leave."

"Give me a call sometime," he said, opening the door.

I always remember him — Kurt — because he looked much older in the day. He had these deep wrinkles around his eyes and his mouth, which gave his otherwise boyish appearance the brand of thirty-four years' living on Earth. That transformation from wet red hair dripping onto his gleaming torso as he sat in his chair, his dick hard — or limp, asking my lips to make it hard; that movement from a coked-out vision in the night to this one, just some HIV positive guy in boxers holding the door open for me, managed beside my better understanding of it all to fill me with a soft disappointment. Last night, you were a fantasy. Today, you are real, too real; but this time I didn't think it for more than a second. I didn't think it as I looked at his tired face, or as I walked down the stairs. I didn't think it because I already knew it.

I already knew too well that the stuff of dreams is simply the stuff of dreams, and no one ever seemed to live up to the expectation. It's as if everything was too dead with the burden of age, too desensitized by all that's happened since our beginning, to anymore live up to the dreams dreamt by those who desperately and foolishly continued to dream the great dreams of the living. The wonder of my life, of all life, seeped away enough for me to know what a huge letdown this world really is.

Without another thought to him, I got into the green car — luckily it had been mine — gave the driver directions, and watched as the familiar sight of the decayed Williamsburg skyline whizzed by me on my travel southward into Brooklyn.

That night, I dreamt of Bard. It was raining, and I remember rushing in a car, and then running across a plain of soaked grass to a barn. A heavy thunderstorm pounded the Earth with warm rain. Inside, Emily was waiting for me. When we saw each other, we were so happy that we danced around in circles for a bit. Though it was night, and heavy with rain, an outside lamp cast the window's shadow perfectly onto the floor. I was late for something, but she had waited. It felt like graduation day, and we were graduating together. I'm filled with hope and sorrow as we twirl around. The beautiful chapter of my life that was Bard ends today, but another one — beautiful because it is unknown — begins.

And then I wake up. It was 9:03 PM that same day. The night had been the day, and the day had passed by again unnoticed. Here, Emily and I never graduated together; and Bard had been beautiful, but not the beautiful that flowed through me overwhelmingly in the dream. In my dream, the sorrow over beauty lost was the sorrow over leaving behind a perfect world, where I had been happy and free in the days and nights. In real life, the sorrow I remember upon leaving Bard was like the sorrow of leaving the funeral of a greatly beloved with whom a million words had been left unspoken. I sorrowed for Bard because I could never regain it, and could never regain you; I sorrowed because I knew that the impossibility of regaining the dreams of my childhood, that the failure of those dreams, would eat at me until one day there was nothing left but the memory of dreams and how they fail when they are placed upon flesh. But here's the great question: if you don't place your dreams in flesh; if you disregard them when you see their potential in someone's eyes and someone's smile; if you look away because you know that, though the sparkle is there, the fire will not last long, because life sucks out the thunder and the flash really really quick, then what do you do with dreams? If the world can't handle dreams where are they to go? Do they travel from bed to bed, from friend to friend, from place to place, and move on quickly after they have gotten all the little they could get? Or do they just stop, dry up, because they are tired of the inevitable failure; dry up, and with them, dry you up. For what else are you but the hope and the wish of your own dreaming?

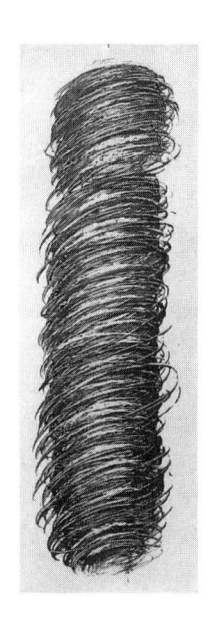

LUCKY
DEBORAH PINTONELLI

hey found his shoes three days after he disappeared. The soggy black sneakers with the white puma printed on each toe were set neatly together on a white slab of rock near the water at Belmont Harbor. They belonged to Sam Alioto from Milwaukee, a nice, good looking guy who was close to his family. His Gran was always on the other end of the phone asking, *When you gonna come home?* Gran had raised him to be the kind of boy that he was. She was not frightened of the truth. She drove a Mercedes SUV in heels, ugly furs and a rock-hard platinum beehive.

She had no problems with him, but everyone else, Sal, Mikey, Janine (his former cellmates in their mother's house where the bunk beds they slept in nearly touched the ceiling, and the dust on the massive crucifix above the dresser made them sneeze), they all did. Mommy was dead; she had no say in the matter anymore. When she was alive she only had a few words for him; *your food's gettin' cold,* or *where's your brother.* I love you was in there, too, but not very often.

Now he had Ryan McDermott and Sarah Rosemary Rabinowitz to contend with. They all worked together at Demarchelier, a little bistro off of the loop where business-men took their mistresses for *salade nicoise* and *kir royales.* Ryan had Sam wrapped, what with his Irish good looks, big dick, and killer upper torso all scribbled up with primitive

258

designs. Sarah R. was the approving little sister he had always wanted. She too had him wound, bound to her bidding like he was slave material just begging to be plucked. She had a five-year-old kid and he often found himself running her errands, taking the boy to the zoo, that kind of shit. She was very pretty, blond and petite. Nobody ever said he didn't like women. He just didn't like to fuck them.

Ryan wants you, she told him one day while they were setting up the tables for the evening.

Yeah, I know. I'm not blind, Sam said while putting miniature roses into a bud vase.

You want him?

I'm not into all that relationship stuff. I like my Freedom.

Oh, she said, as if he had passed up a free million dollars, *I totally agree.*

Sarah was into the whole third wheel aspect of their relationship; it was a way for her to forget that the father of her baby, a black dude from Texas, had dumped her soon after the child was born. Cozying up to a couple of homos was her way to make the world right for the time being. There were warm bodies involved, and neither of them wanted anything from her. Sam had told her some but not all of the details of his relationship with Ryan. She believed whatever he said. The last thing he was going to do was to tell her something and then have her repeat it to Ryan and have him get all suspicious and clamp down. Plus, when he had tried to talk to Sarah about the sexual complications, her face had gotten all scrunched and funny looking.

At the end of a night out Ryan would say, *okay, baby boy, choose,* and Sam would have to pick their playmates: short, bulked-up boys from Cicero; tall lean countrys from Peoria or Decatur; massive, silky, uncut Latinos from who the hell knows where. Pick and choose. Drive their unpaid-for cars into the hot Chicago night. Take a ride down Lake Shore Drive feeling like they could be in L.A. Or at least what they imagined L.A. to be like.

Ryan's place was near Loyola University, near the lake and clusters of beautiful old buildings that served as housing for either impoverished lunatics, or the newly wealthy. Motherfuckers were living such unparallel lives that they didn't even acknowledge each other's existence.

Boys come on in.

That was the beginning. The end of course was always unremembered, a blur of no kisses goodbye, dirty dishes, rags dipped in filth and cups and bottles and ashtrays filling up the room like lone witnesses to a centuries-old debauch. Drugs didn't just help, they made everything possible; they turned the tattered party dress into something special, the cheap haircut into a glamorous, scented halo. Sam tried to romanticize what he could, to gather up what little bit of stardust there was and savor it all on his own; the white wisp of some puppy's stick straight pubes, the brown flower of his ass turned up towards the sky as he rested on a pillow after being utilized in a funny yet possibly too militaristic scenario.

Boys, come right in. Make yourselves a drink!

Effen, Tanqueray or Bombay. Party favors. Clean towels stacked up near the sofa. Ryan knew to turn the lights down quickly as soon as they were all settled in. How many of them there were depended on the night and the cash flow. Four was a good number. Four they could deal with. After months of calculating costs they had come to the conclusion that each guest would drink a quarter to a half of bottle of booze and several beers, plus other substances. Later they only required bottled water or a soft drink. No food was in this picture. If they were hungry, Ryan would pull back the shade and point to the pizza-slash-chicken shack or the Chinese and say, *Food's good there, and there.*

The issue not discussed with Sarah, or anyone else, was that of logistics, possibly with a bit of syntactical shading, translation problems, the classic id vs. ego dynamic, and, of course, simple mathematics. Engineering? Hardly. More like the garden-variety pharmaceutical quandaries common to men all over the planet. Or maybe, finally, it was an issue more common to women than any other creatures. Ryan wanted to fuck Sam, bareback, in such a way as to produce not just the *impression,* but to solidify, some might even say calcify, his very real role as the Bottom in a bottomless non-relationship. An impregnation of sorts, the sweet union of two Midwestern boys practically made for each other.

But Sam couldn't do that.

Many non-serious excuses popped into his head, excuses that would insult and possibly even enrage his buddy Ryan. One of them was: his memory of having raped his mother's cat with a brand new pencil (eraser side in) just to see if she would like it. She did. Now, he was not anything like that cat. Sam was a traditional, all American, Blow Me Now kind of guy. Think Keanu Reeves, Johnny Depp, Ryan Phillipe. That sort of tradition. Ryan was Tom Cruise or maybe even Joaquin Phoenix.

What did it all mean? It meant that the underlying tension, the thing that went unspoken but that filled all of the silent moments of the long days they spent working or playing together, was this dilemma and how to solve it. Sam's idea was to simply avoid the whole matter. Ryan's was to harp at it, in word or deed or, far worse, subject his new best friend to a silent treatment that could last days. Silence and no touching, no silverybrowed smiles, no holding hands in the tanning booth or at the movies. Not one loving text message or arousing email, no displays of nudity, nothing. Then Sam had to come begging, dick in hand, saying that he would try, really try, to change.

This particular conversation played itself out for days, a whole week.

By change you mean that you'll do it?

They were fixing Ryan's bike flat, which had occurred near the curve at Oak Street, just in view of the W hotel.

We could get a room at the ghetto W right now, freshen up, spend the night in each other's arms.

Panic settled into Sam's sore muscles. What he would give for a hot bath with one of the massive bath teabags the hotel provided. That and a good bottle of wine, a couple of excellent movies, one of them raunchy. Ryan stared hard. Sam's eyes moved away from the light blue in them and out over the darker blue of the lake. He felt like crying. Why did things have to get ruined this way? They were having a stupendous day; it had started at dawn with a big breakfast and then hours of riding and swimming. It made him feel like he was a kid back home again, happy to be out of his mother's dank house and into the sunny Wisconsin streets with his bicycle as his trusty steed.

Unless you're going to disappoint me. Like you always do.

Just then they both spotted the hostess from Demarchelier rollerblading south. She stopped and they forced some fake smiles and chitty chat until she got going again. They watched her skinny butt fade into the downtown distance.

I don't think that is quite fair to say that I always disappoint you. Why are we together all of the time if I am such a miserable failure?

You know what I mean! You are a coward because you won't help us move forward with this thing.

They had to talk in code; the lakefront was extremely busy, people of all sorts swarmed around them. They moved the bike into the underpass. There they had to whisper so that their voices wouldn't echo.

You can't really love me if you want to force me to do something I don't want to do.

Bullshit! You are the only person on the planet I care about and *who has ever refused such an offer.*

Oh that sounds just great. Who are you, Hitler?

Hitler. Yeah, I'm Hitler.

The conversation had gotten stupid, mostly because both of them were afraid the other would leave. How depressing would it be to go back home alone, after such a day? Sam would have to give in, that was all there was to say, so he said it. Ryan's pupils expanded. A light sweat broke out on his forehead even though it was cool in the underpass.

Oh, baby, you are not going to regret this! And I have something special I saved for this occasion.

They checked into the hotel using the name of their friend Alec to get his employee discount. The suite they got had a tinted view of the lake, a living room, and a huge tub that Sam immediately started filling with water. The tea bag floated on the surface, trailing scent and little pieces of spicy petals and herbs. Ryan soon went home to get fresh clothes and other necessary items. Before he left he kneeled down by the tub and kissed Sam on the lips, something that he rarely did. *I love you,* he whispered. Sam pretended to be meditating, and said nothing.

He dozed and soaked, emerging wrinkled and perfumed after about an hour to receive room service. There was a bottle of Veuve, a white rose in a silver vase, and a note saying For you, *lover*. I'll bring another with me.

Lover. Jessica Alioto's son, Angelina Alioto's grandson, was about to become some rich Irish brat's whore. Ryan only worked at the restaurant to impress his father with his willingness to do *anything* to earn an income. As Sam stood at the window sipping champagne, he imagined himself as a character in a John Fowles (or was it Henry James?) novel, tortured, with too much self-respect. He decided to take a sunset ride to Belmont rocks, see who was there, and then return to the hotel before Ryan did. It was possible. He finished the bottle, put his riding clothes back on, and headed north.

Once outside he was glad to be out of the air-conditioned room and into the velvety dusk. Now along the lake path there were fewer people, hardly any families, mostly youngsters laughing and horsing around. He smelled pot smoke coming from Oak Street beach and heard the tinny vibrations of somebody's car radio at full blast. He shouldn't be riding in the dark having had so much to drink, but it was okay, he would take it slow.

Twenty minutes later as he pulled into Belmont Harbor he saw that the rocks were already in full party tilt with the baby boys dancing, some still in their bikinis. He noticed the party favors being passed around freely, and a tub full of ice and plastic water bottles that he knew were filled with other things.

That was the thing about the lifestyle; each decade brought its own form of forgetting. Each one was frighteningly similar to the last. The warnings passed down were heeded and then finally ignored. The new day brought with it minds so youthful they were barely formed, and not much in the mood to listen to common sense. Sam was only thirty, but at that moment he felt very old.

He wondered what would happen if he just disappeared, if he simply absented himself from Ryan's life, quit the job, changed his vitals. What sort of guilt could the man lay down then? It would be so simple, and in the end, he did not love Ryan McDermott, he simply worshipped him, as a man who lusts after a fine car or some other luxury wants only to possess the thing of beauty, not marry it.

He laughed too loud and too long when he saw the pretty face of someone he had not seen since spring turned into summer. The face waved, then motioned for him to the group he was with.

Yo Samuel, you been away too long!

It was Lola Farina, the incredible drag thing from the drag Mexican place that had closed over two years ago. What was She doing back in town?

Oh no, Sam thought, *I'm into it now.*

Into what? A short evening, nothing special. He would make excuses to Ryan when he returned. Only a bit of time, just a taste, that was all he was after.

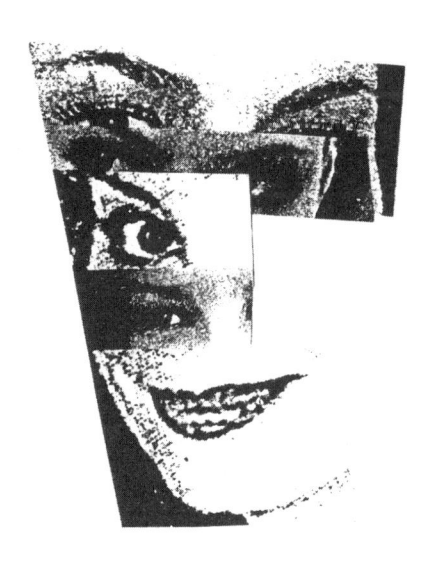

MEN & CARS
DIANE SPODAREK

I like the way men look when they look under their cars. I like to get a tall beer and stand on a corner and watch men sit in their cars, start them up, find out they don't start, get out, look at the car, then go to the hood, open it up, look in, go back to the inside of the car, start it up again. Get out again, look under the car, look at the ground, look at the spill on the ground, look all around, sometimes at their companion, if they are with someone; if not, look for another man in the vicinity to share this moment, then there are two or three sometimes four men looking under the hood or looking under the car at the ground, sometimes they stare at the spill on the ground together and then they look at each other and they get that look. I like that look. It's somehow familiar, I can't put my finger on it, I can't really say what it is, but it just gives me a funny feeling watching them, the men and their cars, although I don't really think it has anything to do with the fact that I'm from Detroit.

THE SIGN
SUSAN SCUTTI

They shook hands and after she remembered the sensation, a current of energy flowing from him into her. His hand felt dry, the skin rough, calloused, his grip the right amount of strong. A small flame flickered in his eyes and she felt a sudden stir, a quickening in the warm movement of her blood, a brief tingling between her legs. She sensed that he recognized her as she did him. Yet here they were, meeting for the first time at a dull party, being introduced as if complete strangers.

They'd seen each other many times before this first handshake. They belonged to the same gym which was housed in a squat building leaning against a taller one in the southwestern quadrant of the theater district. Once they'd run side by side for 30 minutes on separate treadmills, each listening to the same music traveling to their ears on white, rubber-coated wires connected to a small device the approximate length of a heart. When he turned, briefly, to see who was jogging beside him, he had exhaled a full panting bouquet and she had caught the pleasant scent of his breath. Turning she'd taken him in with a running glance. His hair was cut militarily short and his face, with a good nose and complex brown eyes, looked austere yet somehow emotional. Moments later, changing the speed of his treadmill, his well-shaped hands reached forward to press the buttons on the machine and again out of the corner of her eye she watched him, noticing the reddish brown hair along his arms. Side by side they ran on their separate treadmills, keeping speed. He continued to run after she herself stopped — he kept his steady pace while she bent to stretch the muscles in her legs. Walking away, she glanced at the back of him, sweeping her gaze from his feet to his head, lingering momentarily on each of the separate shapes made by his parts — the calves, thighs, buttocks, lower back, his shoulders — and then she noticed a small scar.

On the back of his neck at the base of his hairline a scar showed just below his short haircut and as she stared at this scar she no longer heard the music traveling to her ears along two intertwined wires. Fascinated she paused, eyes wide, her chest expanding and contracting with deep, post-run breaths. The abnormally white, raised skin of the scar, shaped like a thickening moon, stood out against his tanned neck and staring at this small scar, this crescent-shaped mar in his perfect surface, she heard only the sound of her own breath moving in and out of her. What happened to him once, what pain had caused a scar? Staring, unaware of anything but his running figure with a small white scar, she felt the soft thuds of her heart in her chest, she felt the sweat slowly running down between her breasts, she felt a dampness between her legs. She wanted to touch it, this small white caterpillar crawling up his neck into his hairline, she wanted to feel it beneath her fingertips.

Abruptly, the spell ended. Startled she heard the steady tempo of music in her ears, the vaguely metallic scent of the gym filled her nostrils once again and his scar, his running figure no longer held her suspended like a splash of sunlight on a wall. Yet the next time she saw him at the gym, she remembered this scar, and looked for it. Seeing it, she felt relieved, and each time thereafter it was the same; she searched for the scar as if through this sign, this mark signifying pain, that she knew him. The link had been formed, a neural path laid, and each time she thought of him she thought of his scar and she felt herself breathing, she felt her heart beating, she felt the dampness and sweat. And seeing a scar on someone else she thought instead of him and felt her breath, her heart, her wetness, and once, seeing a yellow worm crawling along the soft mud in the backyard of her sister's house she thought of his scar and felt wetness then, too.

And when on that night of their formal handshake at a dull party, when he turned and she saw how his collar sticking up over his sweater covered his neck, when she searched but did not see the scar she felt unmoored. Where was the scar, the sign that told her he understood pain… is this really *him?* The absence was palpable; she felt both nervous and cold speaking to him in a soft voice above the collective sound of other peoples' uninspired conversations. She looked into his complex eyes and wondered about the scar, yet continued to talk with him of other things. Eventually they left together; parting with flirtatious laughter on a littered street, both remarking how good it was to meet at last, both assured they would see each other soon at the gym. Walking away, she felt roused by the thought that shortly she would see him again although she did not know when.

Humid, dreary days passed, days that soon accumulated into weeks. Somehow the trajectories of their separate lives did not intersect, their patchwork schedules did not mesh, they did not see one another at the gym. Disappointment flattened her spirit like an iron. Eventually, a cool evening with vague rain interrupted the humid streak and as she crossed the street, stepped up onto the sidewalk outside the gym, he opened the heavy glass door. Glancing up her eyes met his and they paused, each smiling shyly, then both spoke at once, exclaiming their surprise at not seeing one another sooner. As he talked, she pictured his scar, imagined the scent of his breath and the hair along his arms, and the careful, feeling way his hands touched the necessary buttons on the treadmill, and she recalled how she had felt his energy flow into her that time at the dull party when he shook her hand.

Walking with him away from the gym, a cool rain fell against their faces and together they ran to a small cafe around the corner. Later, listening to the sound of rain drumming on the windows in his bedroom, she found the feeling of his rough hands along the smooth parts of her body calming. There was nothing rushed in his way of touching her, of stroking her, she liked the wordless sounds combined with excitement. She extended her fingers to his face, then reaching around, she touched his hair and the back of his neck and at that moment she heard the soft sound of his breath in her left ear. The sound of his breath was also a sensation, she felt the warmth of his exhalation on her face, her ear, her neck and she gasped as he entered her, his hand briefly touching her lips. Searching with moist fingers she found the small, moon-shaped scar at the back of his neck and touching it she felt her own gentle release.

YOU WILL NEVER BECOME A CHORE
GEORGE SPENCER

Laundry is the morning. Prosaic mid-day: there you are sleeping on the lush pillows of noon near the cotton candy machine. What is night? Fireflies, heroic mice pulling the moon the wrong way. And O your sugar thighs, mouth of bitter sweet sorbet. And candy nipples. Life's no more a diet. I search for you. You left. We were once surrounded by berry-laden bushes and premonitions of smoothies. A stream passing by. It caresses the mossy rocks, licks half submerged logs and whispers in its sibilant way: *bring you ice cream.* Me, I want to be near your painted toes. We'll be happy dreaming about absurdities. Love is a scented handkerchief. You make me see double. Love is rampant. Love has three cats. Sadly love goes south.

FUN AND GAMES
DAVID L. ULIN

n L.A., there's a guy who calls up women on the phone and asks what kind of underwear they have on. He claims to be a student at a prestigious university, but when the women press him about which one, he can never remember the name. If they're willing, he gets them to describe the feeling of the fabric on their flesh, the way their panties sometimes ride up when they're out walking or when they get into their cars. When he's finished asking questions, he thanks each woman for her time.

This same guy also hangs around in laudromats, checking out the pretty girls, hoping they'll drop something frilly and intimate, so he can take it home. He's got a personal collection of nearly a hundred items, from bras and panties to garter belts, corsets, and the occasional chemise, and he can describe in detail the original owner of every one. Sometimes he fondles these prizes when he makes his calls, and, every now and again, he even puts them on.

Once, after a particularly stimulating phone session, he pulled a pair of black lace bikini panties over his head and walked into a neighborhood liquor store. The clerk, thinking it was a hold-up, emptied the cash register and handed everything over, but the guy just counted the money and gave it all right back.

"What the hell," he says, "it's not like I'm a criminal. I'm just an average guy, trying to have some fun."

MAN JET OR EROS IN TRANSIT:
FRAGMENTS FROM A TOUR DIARY
JONATHAN LETHEM

I packed as many curved shapes as I could for my voyage — cds, a bag full of Krispy Kreme donuts, my Mets baseball cap, some Slippery Elm eucalyptus lozenges, foam earplugs, and also put my clothes into a suitcase with wheels. Where I was going was frighteningly linear, and I had reason to believe circles, ovals, pillars and tori and the like would be terribly necessary in the days ahead. The popular notion is that touring is a fantastic opportunity for sensuality, a cornucopia of fleshly distractions. In fact it is a chilly, rectangular space. Airplanes are the future. To love you will have to love a jet. I hoped my rounded objects would help make me ready to do so.

My driver made the first mistake on the way to the airport, trying to outsmart a jam on the Brooklyn-Queens Expressway by taking side streets. We exited at McGuinness Boulevard to find the chaos of other thwarted rebels trying to reboot into the mainstream of traffic. First lesson: in the future you stay on the highway. The old way out is now the new way in.

I boarded the jet. Dogman called on the cellular while I was still on the tarmac, pretending he could see me against the night sky. Dogman likes to conflate various levels of experience for amusing effects. He regarded my travel as a good sign, a sign that I was due to have some fun. "Your dick is bigger than ever," he said. "Don't forget that." I indulged his flattery, but what I know that he doesn't is that the big dick in two dimensions is microscopically thin when viewed from the front. He's seen a billboard for the future, one which blocks his view of the future itself. The sentiment is appreciated, but it's another example of Twentieth-Century thinking. In the future my dick, like anyone's, will have to work the margins, and in that pursuit size is no help at all.

Airplane food was, as I feared, all squared. I cut off the corners and slipped them into the airsick bag.

At the first stop an old friend from my former life took me aside. I could tell he was curious about my assignment, but there was very little I could safely say. He clapped me on the back and spoke in a whisper. "All I have to say, man, is hope this all translates into pussy." I didn't have the heart to tell him he'd misunderstood the problem. Not only doesn't it translate into pussy, it doesn't translate at all. This movement through the sky, movement through time, it isn't a language of any kind. To find love here involves letting go of language.

Stewardesses were sexy, Flight Attendants are not. But to go where I am going I'll need to learn to find them sexy. I've developed a theory. The sexuality of Flight Attendants broadcasts on a channel back in time — men in the 1950's are, I think, still being aroused by the energies coming off the bodies of the Flight Attendants today, which accumulates in the bodies of Stewardesses in the past. The Stewardesses in the 1950's are therefore growing more sexy with each passing year.

On the plane again the next day, I readied myself by listening to Islamic music on the Discman, changing my clothes under the thin blue astronaut's blanket, performing a series of limbering exercises in my seat without disturbing the travellers to my right and left. I was briefly amused to imagine that this might be the same set of preparations engaged in by a terrorist, once long ago.

I called Dogman on the Airfone. He is beginning to understand that my landings and takeoffs are beside the point, and mean no more than does my time on the ground. What happens in the air is the point.

Today I made the leap, and transformed myself into Fifties Man. It is he who will be able to find love on the jet. I did it by the simplest possible operation, entering a portal left behind — accidentally? Who knows? It began when I noticed in the lavatory a thin slot in the wall marked for "used razor blades." Really, what an astoundingly obvious clue. In the airport later that day I was able, miraculously, to purchase a stainless-steel shaver with flat, double-edged disposable blades. Then on the flight today I excused myself, and shaved in the bathroom. It was Fifties Man who emerged.

It was then that I began to notice the airplane's curves.

When you love a jet you love it all the way. The passengers are beside the point. And the crew, helpless to stop you. The black box won't tell your tale. You love it from your seat, without the aid of the oxygen mask, often without moving your seat out of the upright position dictated by the FAA for landing and takeoff. Oh, you might slip off your seatbelt to make room for your erection. You might go that far. But loving a jet leaves no mark on the turbines, no fingerprints on the wing or tail struts. We go into this future in a passive ecstacy, knowing our place. Knowing our size against the sky. I think in the next world all three hundred and sixty passengers could love a jet at one time and not cause a shred of turbulence. But I'll wager I was the only one today.

In the hotel that night I found my reward, the home version of the vast love I'd found in the air. It was the airplane's mortal namesake, set flush into the smooth plastic wall of a Jacuzzi. I fitted my penis into the stream, cupping my left hand around it from underneath to guide the rush of bubbles. The jetstream coursed, boiling me in bubbles. The water rushed me forward, hurrying me out of the past and into the future. I came obediently into the foam.

I couldn't believe how much you liked me. I was so wet on that ride to see you.

GOOD FOR ONE

IT WAS A BUS THAT GOT ME FROM DC TO PHILLY, AND THEN I HAD TO TAKE A SEPTA TRAIN AT EAST MARKET TO GET TO HIS PLACE IN GERMANTOWN. HE SAID IT WOULD BE EASIER FOR HIM THAT WAY.

I hadn't eaten in hours, and all you served me when I got to your house was bourbon on the rocks. I started to wonder. You were drinking bourbon every time I saw you. Did you need to be drunk to kiss me? I wanted to be sober because I wanted to remember every minute of you adoring me.

Karen Lillis

EXCLUSIVE: A STATEN ISLAND WOMAN
MIKE TOPP

Christina Aguilera arrived wearing a strapless cocktail dress looking true, truer. I peered over a bodyguard's shoulder and into her cleavage at the risk of entangling my eyebrows and jacket, cut, apparently, from the same bolt of fuzzy goods. Christina is drop-dead gorgeous, with a wonderful personality, lives in the moment, and she imparts that same happiness one might have experienced in ancient times at the sight of some choice goats' paunches roasting over an open fire.

Without a man, she may be lonely. Has her art been enough to sustain her, or does she look to Twitter for gratification? The music of Christina is like the sound of an autumn gale sweeping down the Val d'Aosta. Her artistry is, in my opinion, and despite a certain tendency to mannerism, the closest thing to perfection.

I last saw her in Paris when we were seated round the peanuts and had ordered our drinks — "Deux Scotch" Christina had said to the comprehending and indifferent waiter. Christina gave me a brief resume of her "recent whirlwind and lightning concert tour." From Cooperstown to Harper's Ferry, with a brief side trip to Davenport to perform with Marilyn Manson, who is evidently beginning to find favor in Iowa — she held nothing back. She still maintains her usual discretion in that she has revealed to no one that I sometimes wear Wonder Woman underwear. From my observation of her behavior in public one could only benefit by her proximity.

Youthful vigor, a bronze tan, increased stature, a powerful jaw, a head of at times clean hair, and a boyish exuberance. As my niece, she has been a total delight, and I have never held it against her that she identifies herself sexually as a gay man. Only recently I made her a chain of paper clips to wear with her sweaters, instead of the usual pearls, and she shyly shook it lightly so that it danced back and forth.

Christina and her entourage are glorying and unrepentant. Her hangers-on include Pearl Hurlburt (nail concern), Cynthia Bonita (massage), Delza Arana (voice), and Alice Bridgewater (personal trainer). They siphon off the money of the performer. When I sat before Christina Aguilera and her four friends, one seat over from Britney Spears, and two from Paris Hilton, my lover, I felt I was in the New York of old, with the magic of El Morocco, the conversation of the Algonquin Round Table, with no sheepish emanations expressed from Taylor Swift, sitting in front of me, on Beyonce's shoulders, or Lady Gaga, one seat to the right, who arrived late with Hannah Montana.

The usually scruffy living room had been transformed into a sumptuously inviting salon, its centerpiece a kind of rose window of God knows what. We all sat there, the Queen and I, the stars, the different ISPs, the gossip columnists, the adoring eyes, the jealous looks, amid some leftover turkey and rosettes of pale green mayonnaise. Everything was there where it should be. I re-entered the TV and peace reigned in the desert of art.

JIMMY DEAN: MY KIND OF GUY
JANICE EIDUS

immy and I met at that really famous artists' colony, the one that's been around for a hundred years. I was there to paint landscapes; Jimmy, to write a play. He announced this at dinner, his first night there. He'd grown tired of film acting, he said. He described scenes he'd been forced to play all wrong in *East Of Eden* and *Rebel Without A Cause,* scenes he'd wanted to play tough, but which the director had made him play sensitive, and other scenes he'd wanted to play sensitive, but the director had made him go all steely and macho. "I want to be my own boss," he said, downing his third glass of red wine, "to write, direct, and star in my own play. And don't worry, it'll be a real work of art," he added, as though any of us at the dinner table that night would have doubted his artistry.

I was the only woman at the table. That was because, out of the twenty-or-so of us in residence at the artists' colony at the time, there were five gay men, all of whom had major crushes on Jimmy, and all of whom had made beelines for Jimmy's table. "Jimmy is our idol," they'd informed me, the night before his arrival, "with those soulful eyes, that perky nose, that rebel mouth. We believe that in his *heart,* he's one of us — whether he really is or not." The five of them, plus Jimmy, equalled six, exactly the number of chairs at the dinner table. But there was no way — on Jimmy's first night at the colony — that I was going to sit at one of the other tables, trapped next to Olga, for instance, the photographer known for her pictures of human fingers and toes. After all five of the men and Jimmy were comfortably seated, I squeezed in a seventh chair. I wanted Jimmy. I intended to have him. Not for eternity. Just for my stay at the artists' colony.

All week long, before Jimmy's arrival at the colony, the five men — each of whom I had become good friends with — had argued over which of them Jimmy would sleep with first. "Me, first, definitely," insisted Gregory, in a state of near-rapture. "I'll win him over with my music." Gregory, a composer, was smug because his works had been performed by The New York Philharmonic. "No, me first," argued Paul, belligerently. Paul was a poet who wore round, clear-framed eyeglasses that slipped down his nose. "Remember, guys," he added, "I'm the film buff in this crowd. Jimmy and I will *bond*." They were all wrong, but I never said so aloud. It would be *me* first.

Jimmy Dean was ambivalent, ambiguous, tortured, talented, tormented, gorgeous, and non-committal, and I always click with those guys right away. We see in each other the same swirling, relentless inner turmoil that devours our souls, the same wild desires that drive us so hard, but that are too huge, too scary, even to name. "We have no skin," a former lover once said to me, "there's nothing between us and everything else." I don't know where that former lover is now, of course. I never expected to be with him forever. I never want forever — with anyone. I'm not that kind of girl. And none of them are that kind of guy. We know that perfection can't last. But we wouldn't exchange our one perfect moment together for a lifetime of anything less.

And I was right: When Jimmy's eyes met mine across the dinner table his first night at the artists' colony, we clicked, clicked, clicked, like a TV remote control gone wild. He just kept talking, though, like nothing out of the ordinary had happened, regaling us with some dishy anecdote about Natalie Wood, Sal Mineo, a bathtub, and a French poodle. He didn't miss a beat. I could tell that not one of the five men sitting at the table with us had any idea what had just happened. After we'd all finished our beef goulash — the colony chef's special, prepared in honor of Jimmy's arrival — I got up from the table and walked outside into the warm summer air, strolling purposefully through the dark woods back to my studio. All I had to do was wait. I sat in my chair in the center of the studio, staring at my own moody paintings hanging on the walls. Moments later, I heard Jimmy's knock on the door. The artists' colony rules strictly forbade residents from conducting love affairs on the premises, and even rebel-without-a-cause Jimmy followed the rules. So he and I hopped onto his motorcycle and drove into town. We booked ourselves a cozy room in a charming Victorian-style hotel, where, within moments, we ended up naked, entwined, on top of a postcard-pretty, four-poster bed.

And in that bed, all night long, Jimmy said all the right things, the things a girl like me just loves to hear. "I don't know who I am," he whispered, staring into my eyes and stroking my lips. His sultry whisper made me even more desirous. Our lovemaking grew wilder. He clawed my back, drawing blood. He cried out, "I'm in agony. I want this, but I want that, too. Hold me," he commanded, "tighter, tighter, even tighter, really tight, *hurt* me," he said, flinging himself across the four-poster bed. "No, no, let *me* hurt *you*," he changed his mind, and then, "No! No, let's not hurt each other, let's just lie here and cuddle like two innocent schoolchildren, okay?" He grew insecure. He sat up. "You like this, don't you?" he asked. "Oh yes," I answered. I grew nervous: "Jimmy, am I a good lover?" "You bet," he sighed. We knew how to drive each other crazy with lust, how to play on each others' fears, how to reassure each other tenderly, over and over, all night long.

After that, we spent every night together for the rest of my stay at the artists' colony. We always went back to the room with the four-poster bed, other than one Saturday night, when, just for kicks, we went to a sleazy motel on the highway. By the time my residency had ended, I'd completed over a dozen landscapes, one of which — the most violent and ambiguous — I gave to Jimmy as a parting gift. Jimmy was scheduled to stay on at the colony for two more weeks. He kissed me at the bus station. "My play is almost finished," he said. I nodded, kissing his fingers in farewell one by one, wishing that Olga, the photographer, was there to capture with her camera my lips on his beautiful fingers.

Sometimes, after lovemaking, Jimmy had told me that his play was about a Brooklyn cabdriver named Antonio who yearns to be a boxer. Other times he'd said it was about a young girl named Antoinette who yearns for the love of a tough guy named Tony who won't give her the time of day. Honestly, it didn't matter to me what Jimmy's play was about, or whether he was even writing a play. It also didn't matter to me that — after I'd left the artists' colony and had returned to my gloomy Manhattan studio, where I began a series of black-on-black urban streetscapes — Jimmy began to spend his nights on the four-poster bed with Gregory and Paul, and even with Olga, on one or two occasions. Jimmy and I hadn't had that kind of relationship: it hadn't been about possession, 'till death do us part, meeting the in-laws, houses with picket fences, children, and grandchildren. The only thing that mattered to me then — the only thing that matters to me still — is that Jimmy Dean was my kind of guy.

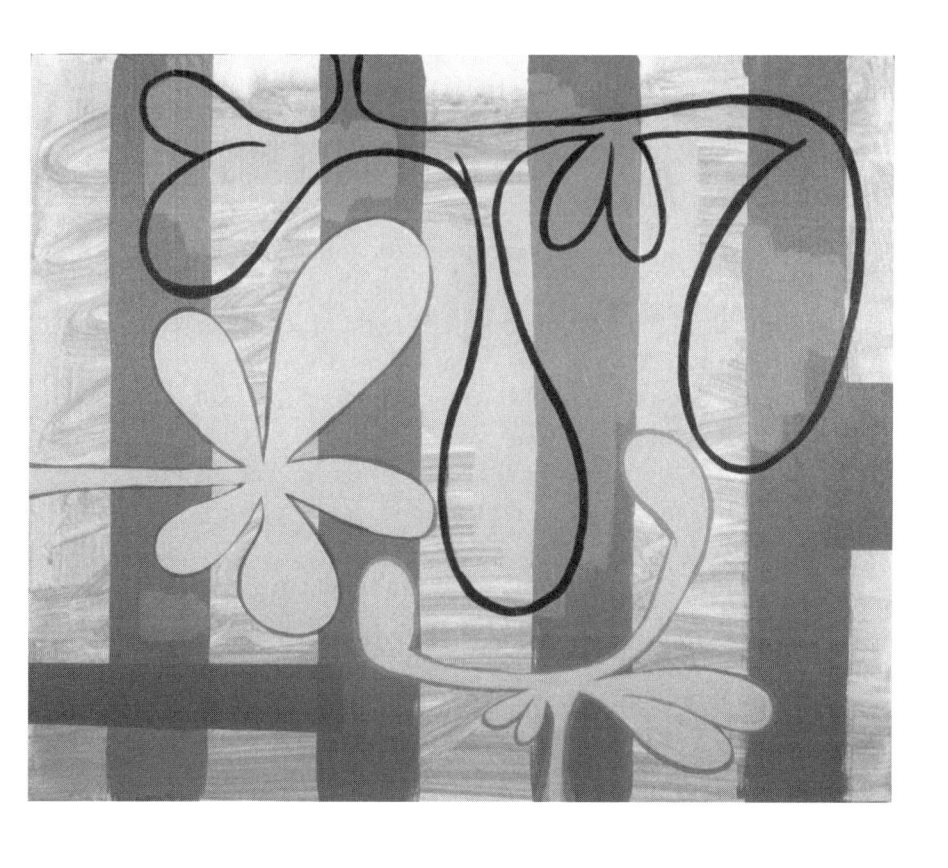

HARD-UP, HARD-ON, LIMP DICK
DAVID HUBERMAN

There I was, once again, hard up as usual. However, this time I was on a movie set in a low-budget film playing the role of the notorious Green River Serial Killer who supposedly killed over forty-five women. This B-flick was based on a true story where the killer finally gets caught, though some people believe that the murderer is still out there, doing what serial killers do best.

San Diego reminded me of a giant exclusive suburb. It is a place with lots of space for its well-to-do citizens to live their suburban fantasy. Clean, airy and rich. I stuck out like a sore thumb with my Semitic features and poor choice of all-black clothing.

People kept asking me what it was like to play a serial killer. How did I approach the role? My reply was always the same. Having had my own mommy dearest, I let the abused child in me take over. After years of therapy, I woke up to the fact that I was damaged goods.

No wonder I could be so abusive to people around me. I picked up the same defective behavior pattern from the parent who abused me. There were times when I could be very nasty to people, especially women. As an actor, my karma had put me in the role of the ultimate abuser. I was perfect for the part.

One day on the movie set, the director introduced me to the actress who would play my latest victim. She was a twenty-two year old, slim built, long-legged brunette with a short pixie-like haircut and spaced out eyes. She was victim number eight. Her name was Victoria. We talked a while and she asked me if I wanted to smoke a joint with her. I told her that I stopped getting high a long time ago. She just gave me a vacant smile. She told me she smoked at least seven joints a day. It was my turn to smile and not say anything, figuring that if it worked for her that was fine by me. Maybe smoking a few joints might help her relax into the role of my next victim. She seemed to be attracted to me. She kept looking deep into my eyes. Then again when you're hard-up like I was, you start to imagine that women who are just being friendly want more than just saying hello.

The director changed the schedule so that my scenes with Victoria would be filmed the next day. I wasn't feeling too well and I told her I was going back to my motel room. As she was gloriously puffing away, she asked me the name of the motel I was staying in.

"It's the Quality Motel on Highway 52," I said. I felt I could have said the Bates Motel and it wouldn't have registered with her. As far as I was concerned, she was on cloud reefer. I left her, thinking to myself that she was nice enough, but was lacking confidence. That was the reason why she smoked so much dope. Then again you should never go by first impressions. I had learned the hard way not to judge a book by its cover.

Later that evening I was in for a surprise. It was the fifth day of filming and I felt horrible. I was constipated for three days and I thought my bowels were made of concrete. The director also had a problem similar to mine. He believed that since San Diego shared the same water supply with Mexico, health officials treated the water to prevent diarrhea. Unfortunately for me and my director, the treated water seemed to have had a heightened effect on us.

It was late evening and I was in my motel room constipated, naked with a hard-on. I started to jerk off while watching Will Penny, the old TV western show. It was my favorite late night program. Now don't get me wrong. Will Penny had no erotic effect on me. The fact is, since the show had no sexual appeal, it was just easy to jerk off and watch TV at the same time. Besides, I was in pain and jerking off was a good painkiller.

I was just about to cum, when all of a sudden, someone started knocking at my door. My first reaction was that the maid had come to my room, but what would she be doing here at this hour? The next question I asked myself was: do beat-up motels have room service? While I was thinking about this, the knocking didn't go away. After about a minute or two of being dazed and confused, I finally answered the door.

"Who is it?" I asked.

"It's Victoria, I came to say hi."

For a second I forgot who she was. Then I remembered. Lo and behold, Victim Number Eight. What the hell is she doing here? I said to myself.

"I'll be right there, let me get decent," I said. I put on my underwear and a T-shirt to hide my big belly. I opened the door and let Victoria inside.

"Hi. What happened?" I asked.

She looked the same as when I first met her, except she was carrying a bottle of white wine.

"I brought this wine for us. Do you have any ice?"

"I don't drink," I replied.

She put the bottle on the table, then turned to me and

said, "I thought maybe you wanted some company." She winked at me.

I didn't know what to do. I sat down on my bed and looked her over from top to bottom, but before I could say anything, she said to me, "I see you have a hard-on."

I looked down at my crotch and I could see my hard-on sticking out of my underwear. I didn't know what to say. I was in shock. It had been a long time since any woman noticed me in a sexual way.

Guys like me, who go for long periods without sex, can get really twisted. I still didn't say anything. Emotionally, I wasn't prepared for this situation. I sat there frozen, motionless, yet I watched her every move. She jumped onto my lap and we began passionately making out. I almost came from dry-humping her in that position for what seemed like an eternity. I was so happy just making out with a woman that I didn't try to initiate any other sexual moves.

Finally she asked, "Do you have any condoms?"

"Yes," I said. "I have some in my wallet. Let me get them."

I got my wallet and took out my ancient package of multi-colored condoms. They were getting so old that the colors were fading.

By the time I returned to the bed, Victoria was naked. Life was looking up for a change. But I still wasn't feeling well. I was so constipated that I barely could walk. The situation was starting to take its toll on me. I panicked and I rushed putting on the condom. I was deadly afraid that I was going to lose my precious hard-on. It was Murphy's Law versus the Power of the Libido. By the time I got on top of her and entered, I was limp!

My huge hard-on had shrunk back to its original pee-wee size. The condom just sort of floated off. Needless to say, this went on all night. In the morning we were both exhausted from having bad sex. Frustration was our common denominator.

Victoria finally got off the bed, went to the bathroom and after having her morning joint said, "You were the third guy who couldn't keep a hard-on for me. What's wrong with you guys? No wonder there are so many men becoming serial killers. You never hear about women serial killers."

I just nodded my head. I understood. She was angry and I didn't blame her. All I could do was just nod my head. After all, there isn't much a man can do when he's constipated and has a limp dick.

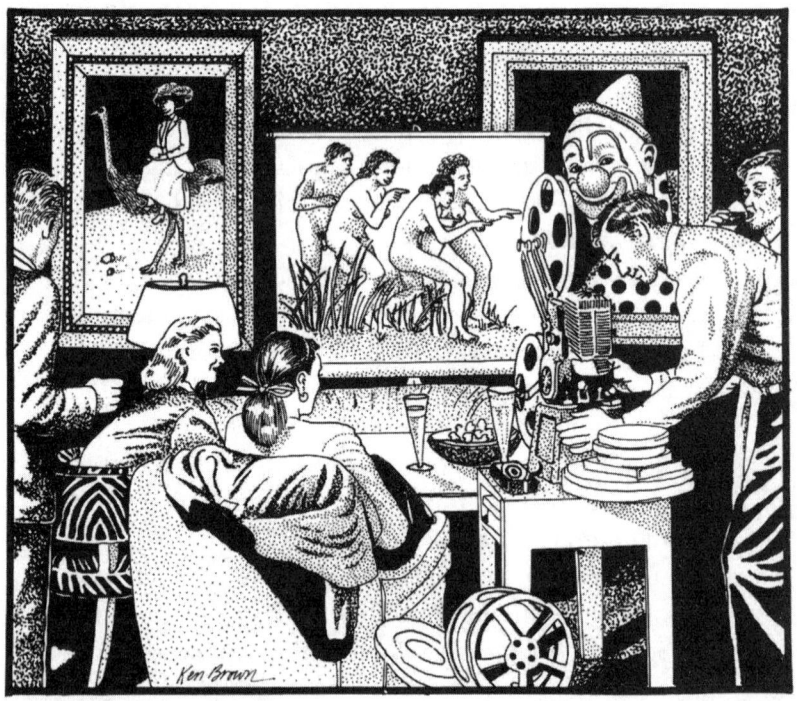

HOME MOVIES

FUSION ARTWORK CENTERFOLD
SHALOM NEUMAN

Life's experiences are inextricably linked to our senses. We see, hear, touch, smell and taste almost without cognition as we navigate through our daily lives. Our senses heighten our awareness thereby enhancing whatever it is that we are experiencing at any given moment in time.

There is no experience that so encompasses the senses as sex. The more of our senses that we incorporate into our sex lives, the deeper the erotic arousal. The same could be said for art. The more engaged our senses are with an artwork the more we can both comprehend and appreciate the work.

This methodology of merging the senses is dominant in the work of the fusion artists whose art is represented in the centerfold of this book. The common denominator in all these pieces is the artist's recognition that in order for the art to translate into this 21st century it must make use of every artistic genre available — painting, sculpture, video, sound, action and movement, the written word — and combine (fuse) these individual methodologies into another genre that by its very nature is limitless.

These are artists from all corners of the globe who refuse to be limited by artistic convention and have made a lifelong commitment to breaking down the conventional barriers, breaking away from the "purist" traditional methods of artistic expression, enhancing their work with technology, and thus being in the "now" instead of in the "then." By incorporating technological innovations such as kinetics, video, light, projection, computers, motion detectors and other assorted electronics these artists not only reflect our multisensory world in their work but have expanded their toolbox as well. The media they use to create has now exponentially larger allowing them virtually limitless creative possibilites.

They understand that without fusing the disciplines and availing themselves of technology thereby allowing the viewer to experience the work with all of the senses (rather than relying solely on the visual), they would be merely repeating the past and not forging ahead into the infinite future.

ARTISTS AND TITLES

1. Shalom Neuman, Czech Republic / USA, "Double Exposure — Marilyn and Barbie," 2009.
2–3. Doron Polak, Israel, "Bodies," 2010, Installation Performance.
4. Medeiros-Venturi. (Photo: Bernard François).
5, 8. Edwood (Edwige Mandrou), France, "Les Culottes de Ma Mére," 2010, Installation Performance. (Photos: Bernard François).
6, 9. Maria Clark, France, "Ovotestis," 2010, Installation Perfor-mance. (Photo: Bernard François).
7. Joakim Stampe, Sweden, "Bottles I Drank 2009," 2010, Performance. (Photo: Chuyia Chia).
10. Kika Von Kluck, Brazil, "Sacred Yoni," 2010, Performance.
11-12. Keiko Kamma, Japan, "Impure Innocence," 2010, Fusion installation.

13. Rosa Naparstek, USA, "Baby Love My Baby Love," 2010, Fusion artwork.
14. Shalom Neuman, Czech Republic/USA, "Unholy," 1999, Fusion artwork.
15. Ingo Lie, Germany, "Echo," 2010, Fusion artwork. (Photo: Roland Schmidt).
16. Taisuke Morishita, Japan, "Automatic," 2010, Fusion artwork.
17. Milan Knizak, Czech Republic, From the cycle "Clothes painted straight on the body," 1965–1991, Performance.
18. Joceyln Fiset, Canada, "I Love You," 2010.
19. Carrie Beehan, USA, "Singer in New York," 2008, Performance with Fusion artwork.
20. Shalom Neuman, Czech Republic/USA, "She's the Man of the House," 1985, Fusion artwork.
21. Nicola Frangione, Italy, "Sound Sex Vertical," 2010, Fusion artwork.
22. Joanne Pagano, USA, "HE TrUsTS YoU WiTH HIS thinner skin," Collage, mixed media, 2010.
23. Liu Guangyun, China, "Civilization Games," 2005, Fusion artwork.
24. Liu Guangyun, China, "Lotus Ham," 2003, Fusion artwork.
25. Jongwang Lee, South Korea, "Ecstasy," 2009, Fusion artwork.
26 Hernani Cor, France, "No More of That," 2010, Performance.
27. Gabriel A. Levicky, Czech Republic/USA, "From the Nice History of Mirrors — Hunger," 2010.
28. Joakim Stampe, Sweden, "Untitled," 2010, Performance. (Photo: Chuyia Chia).

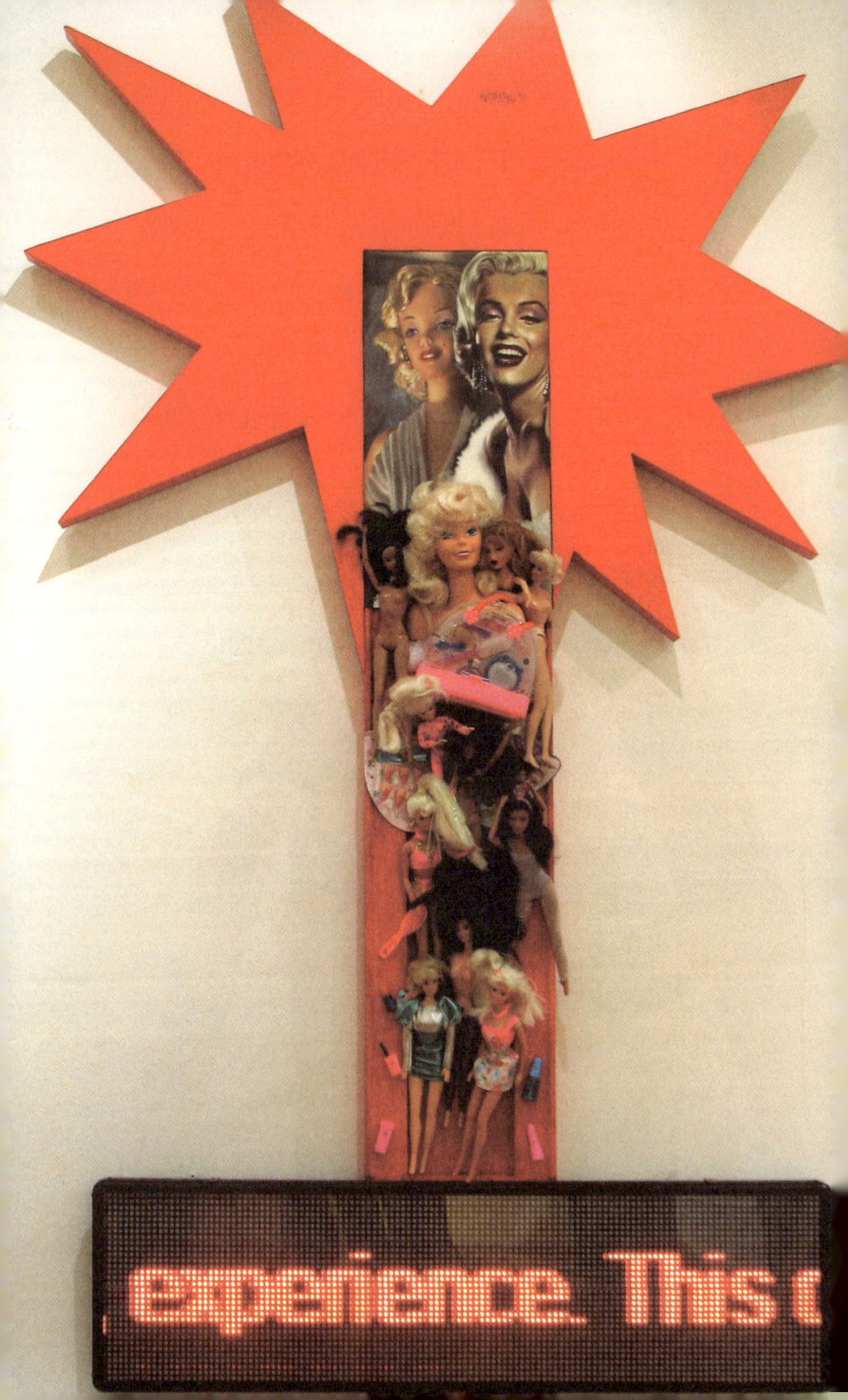

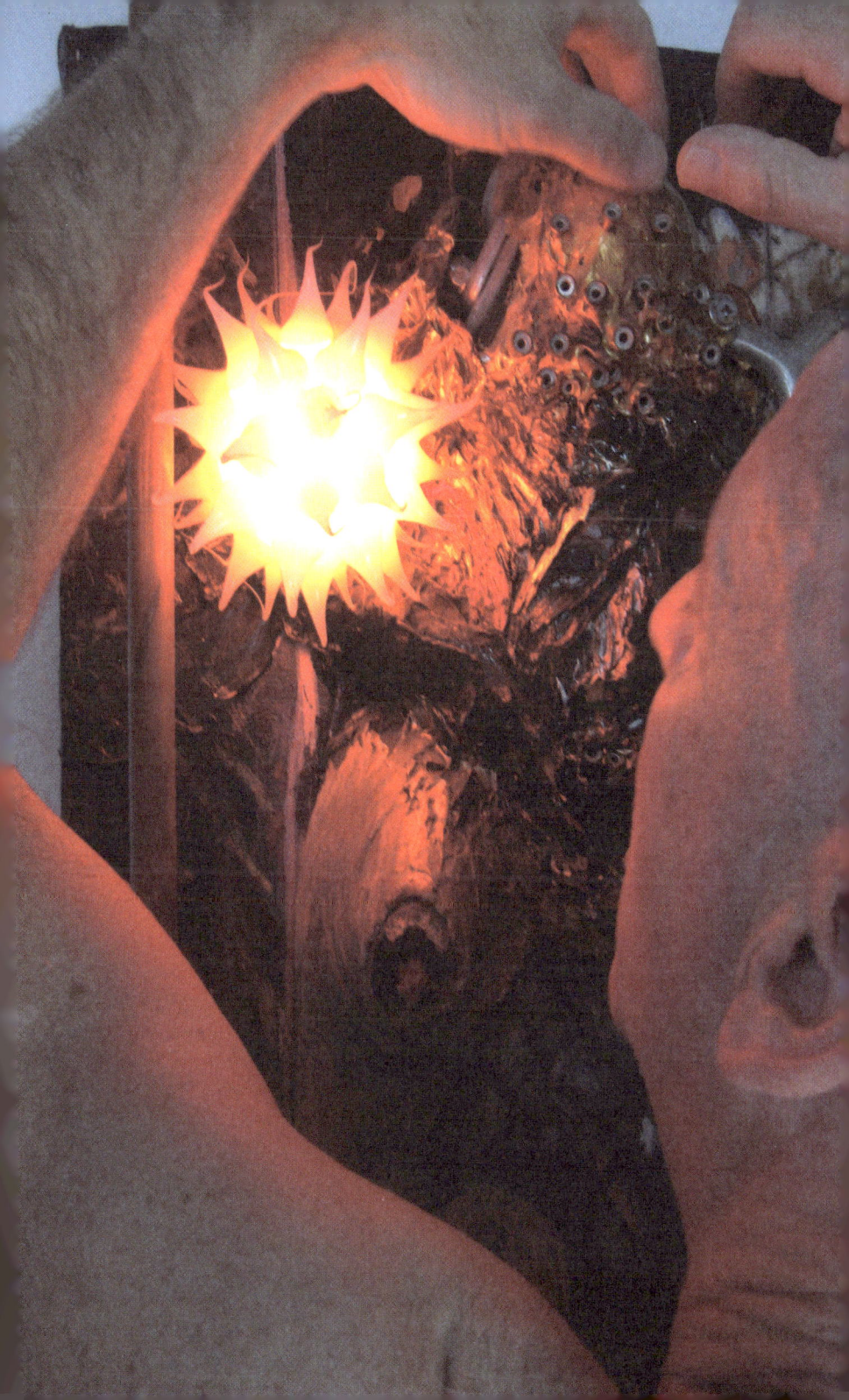

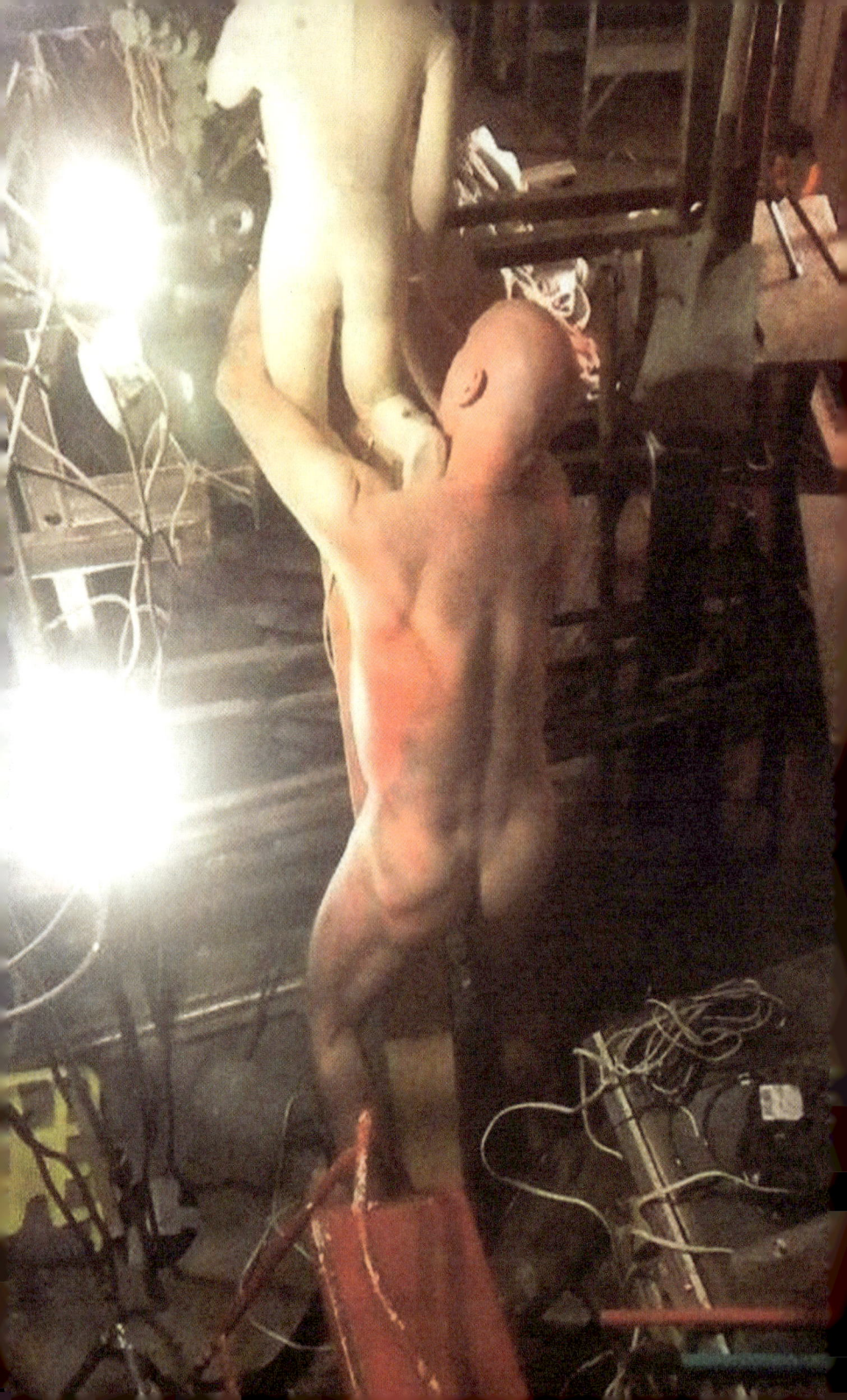

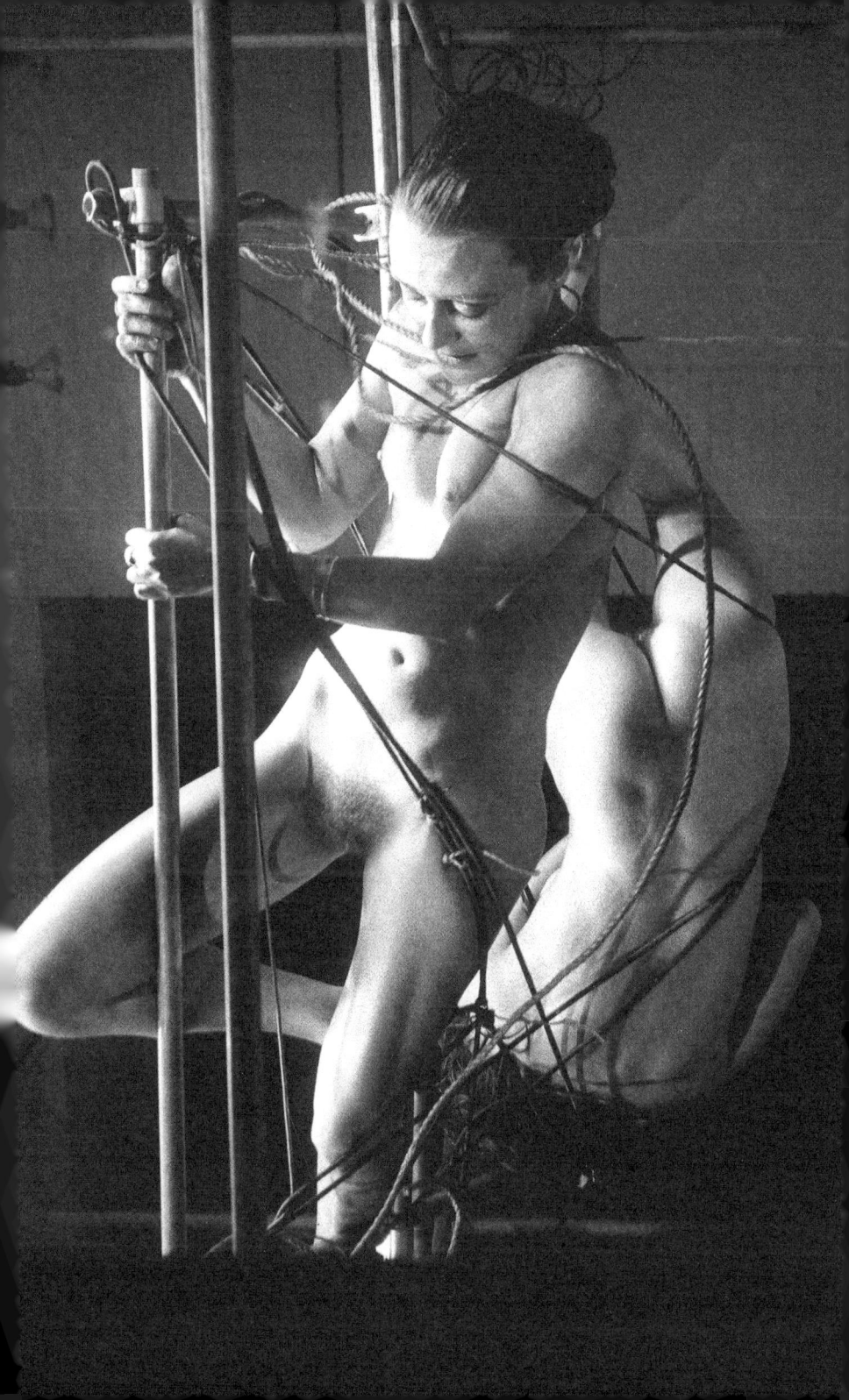

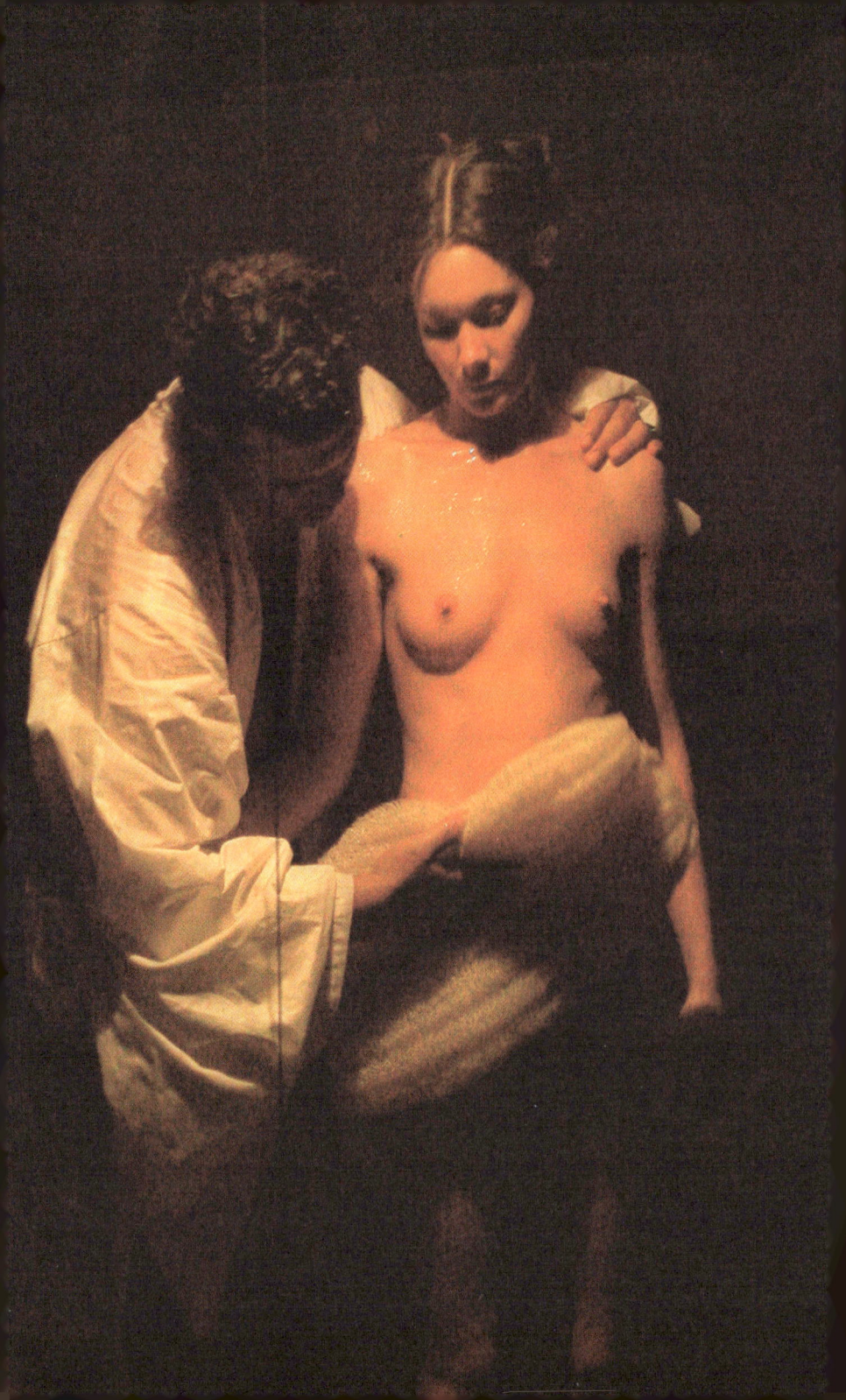

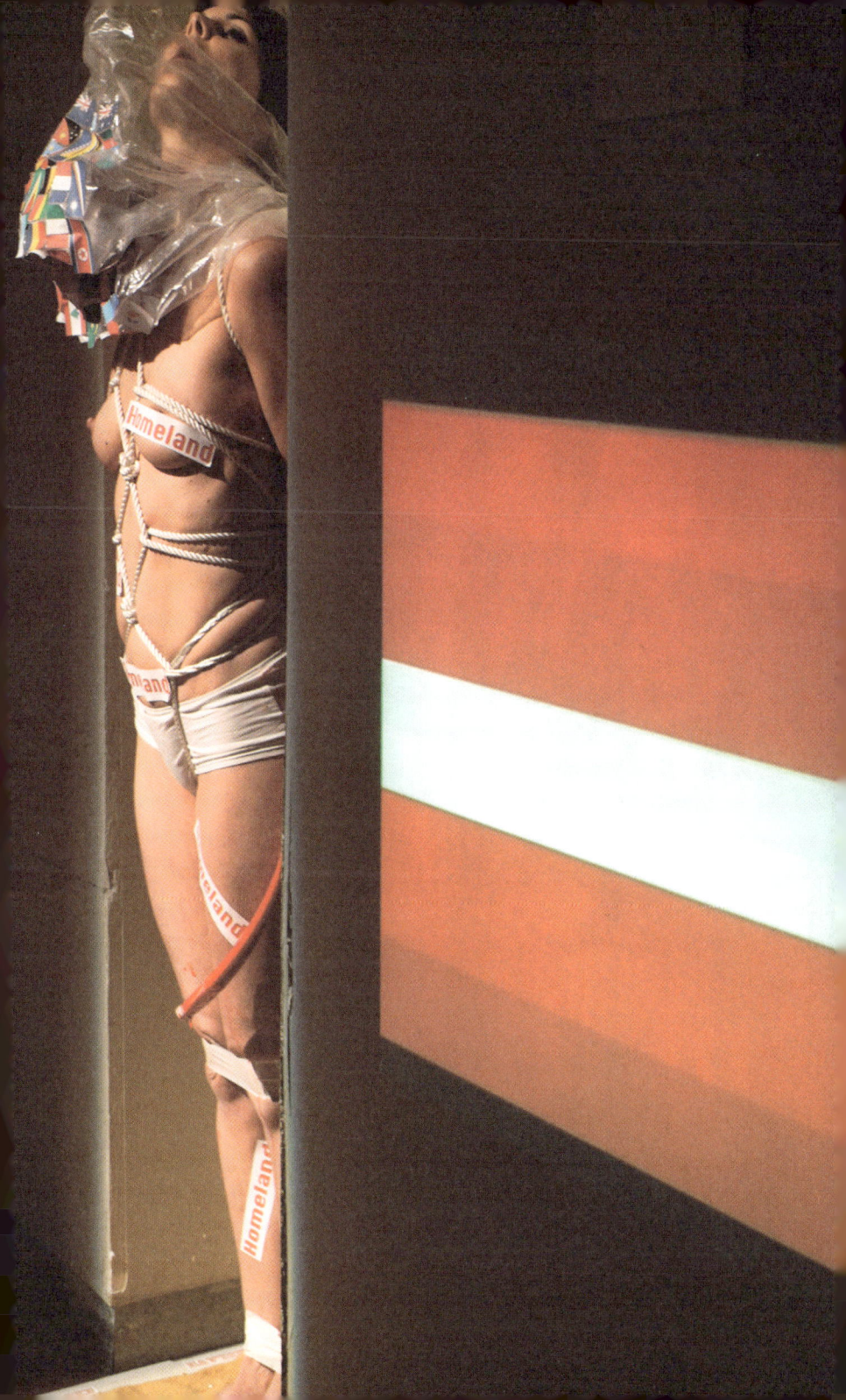

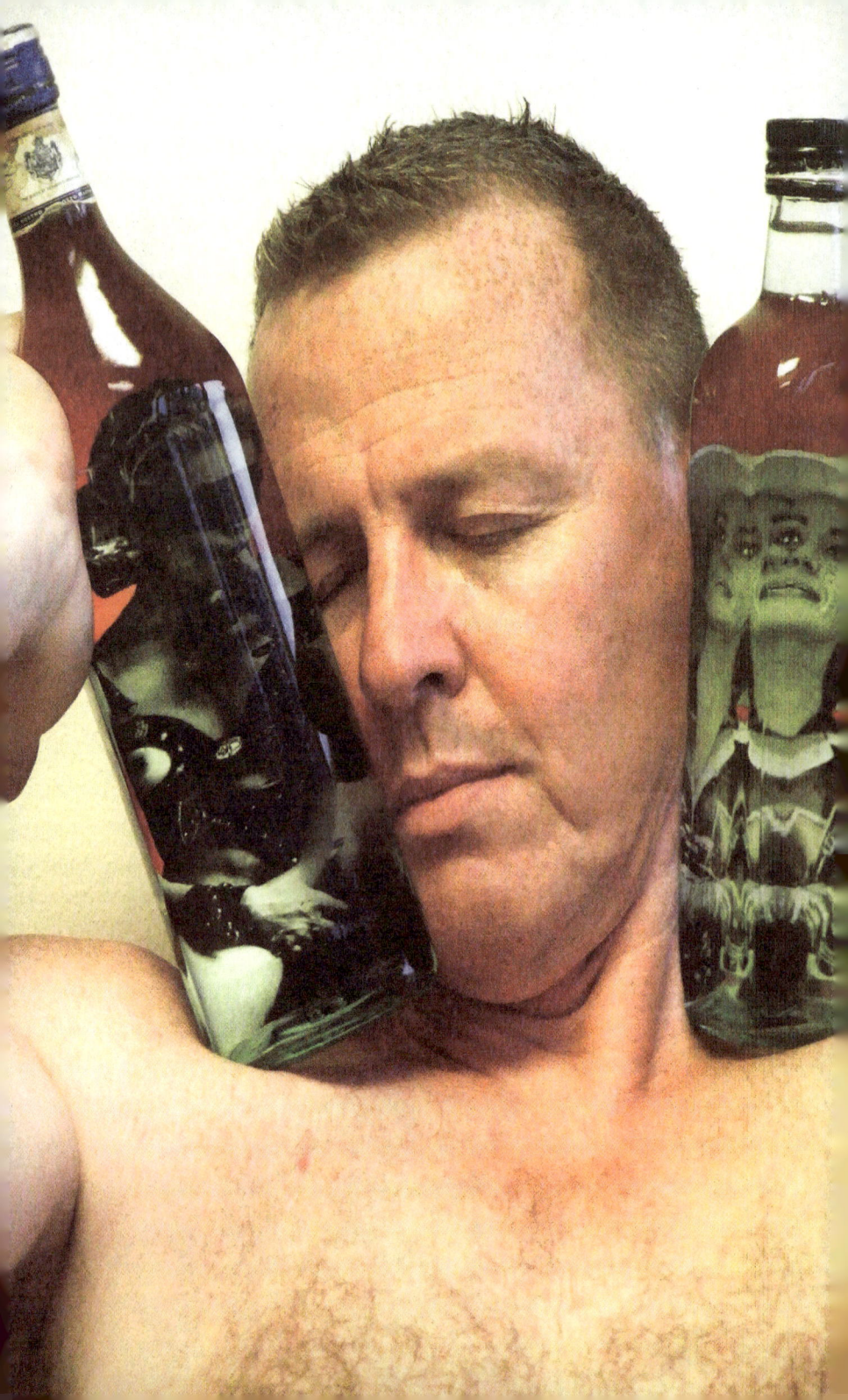

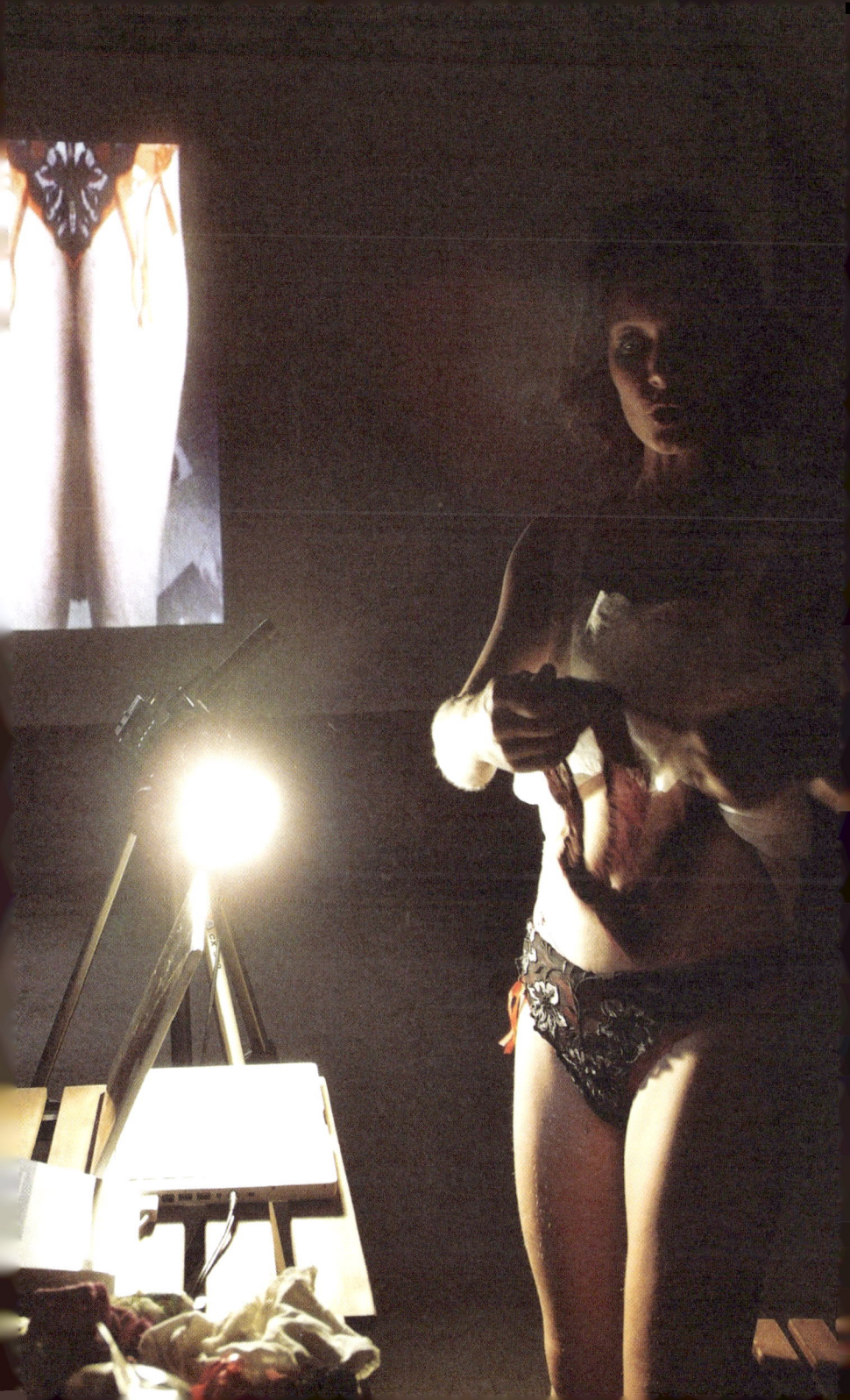

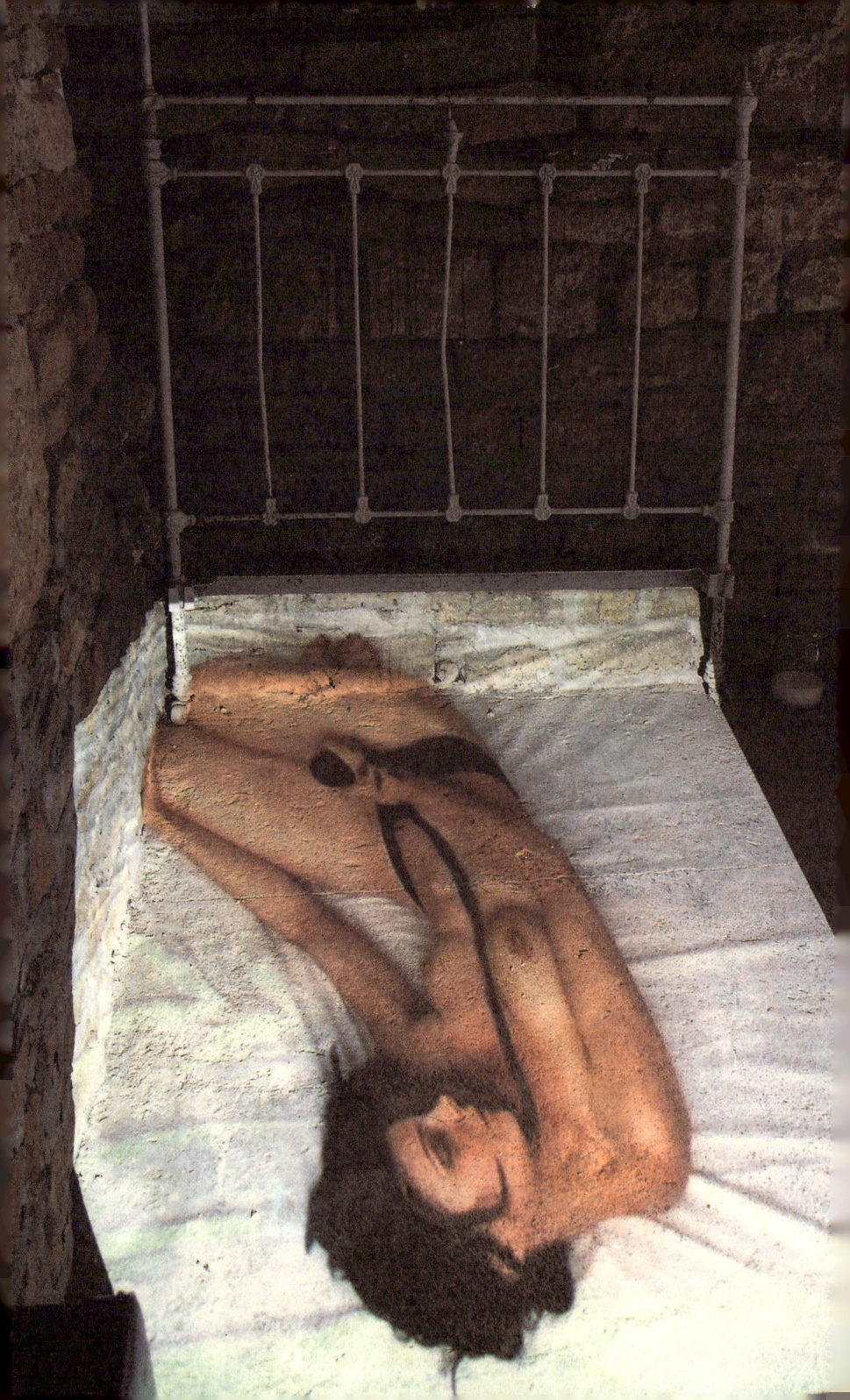

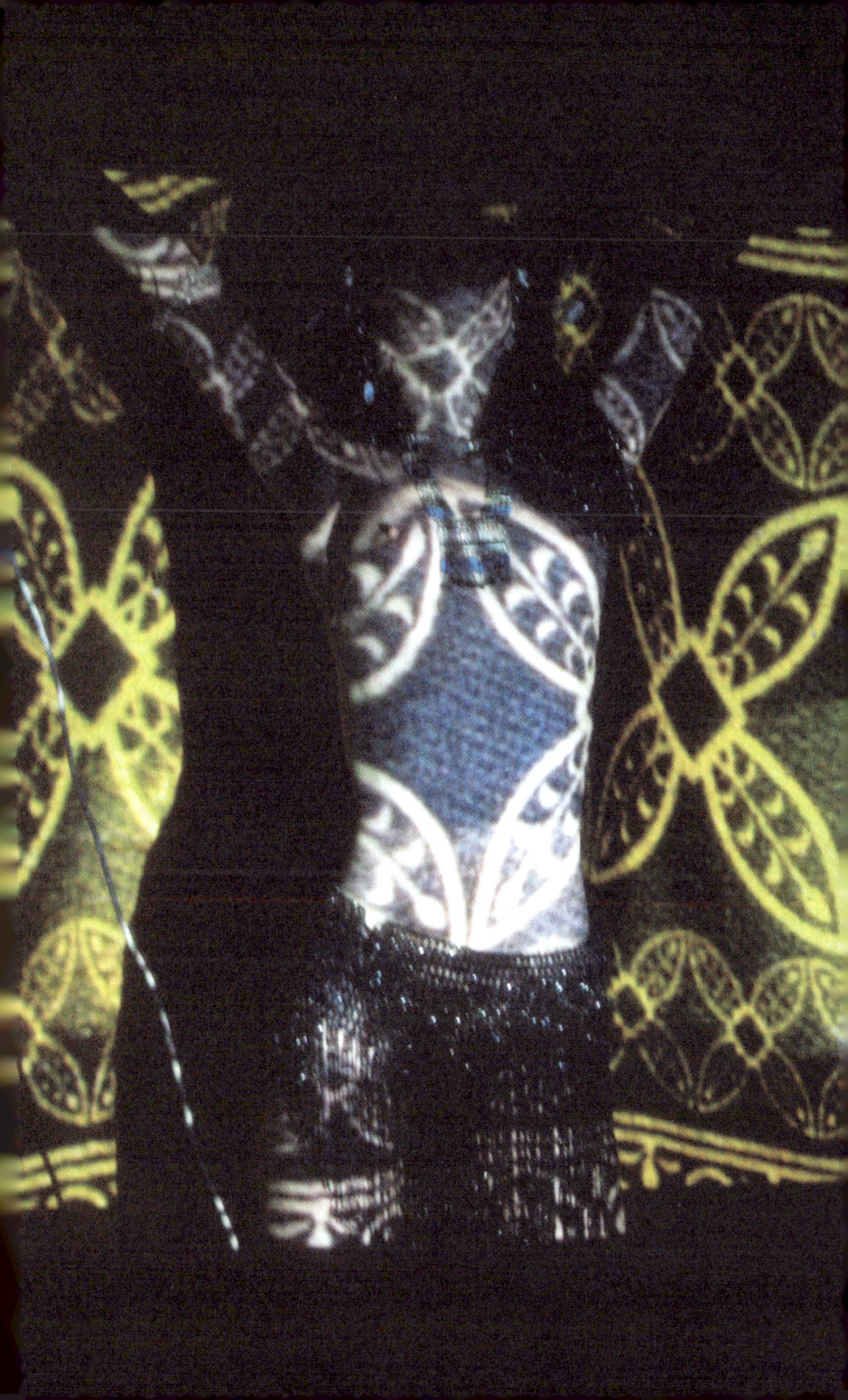

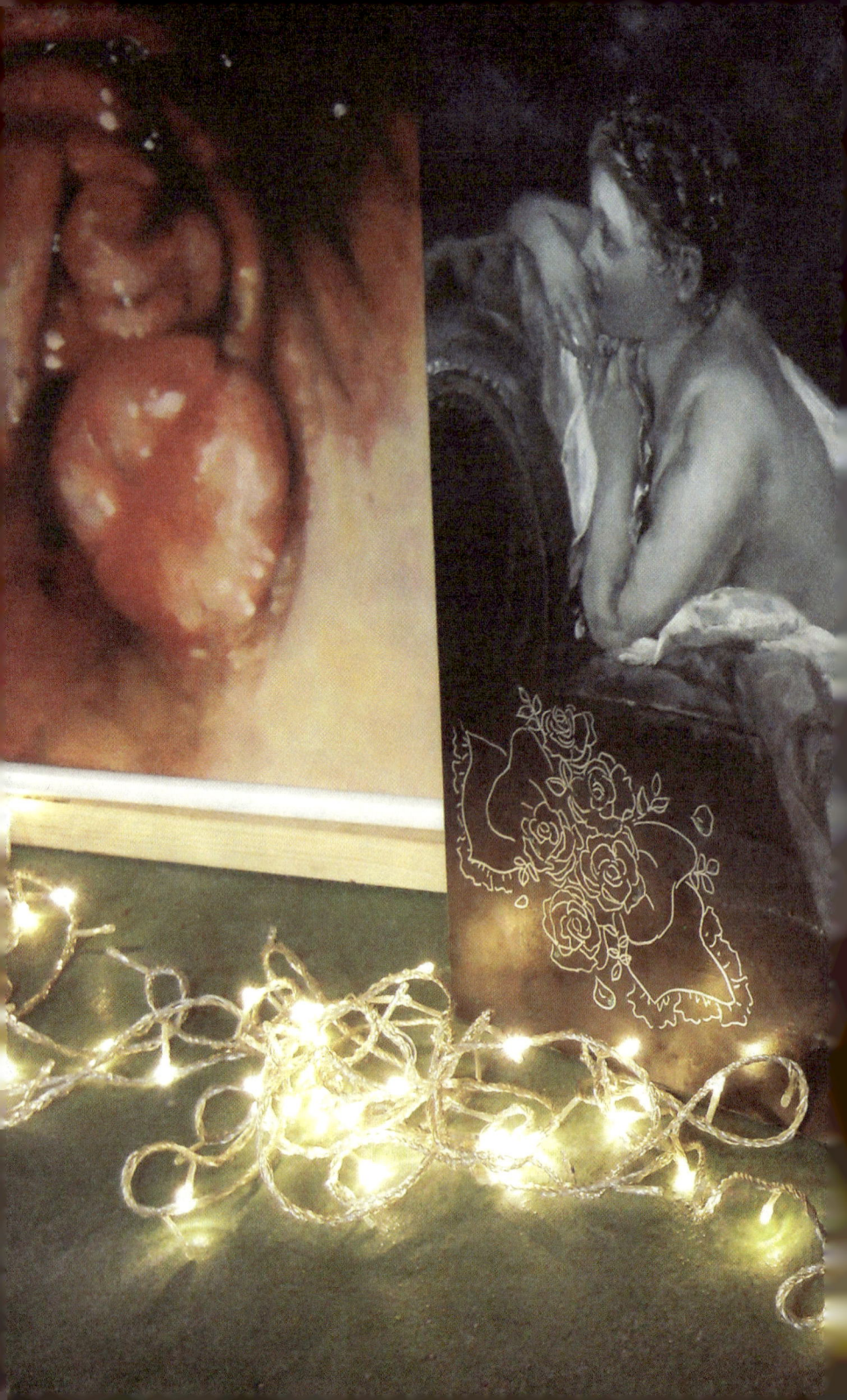

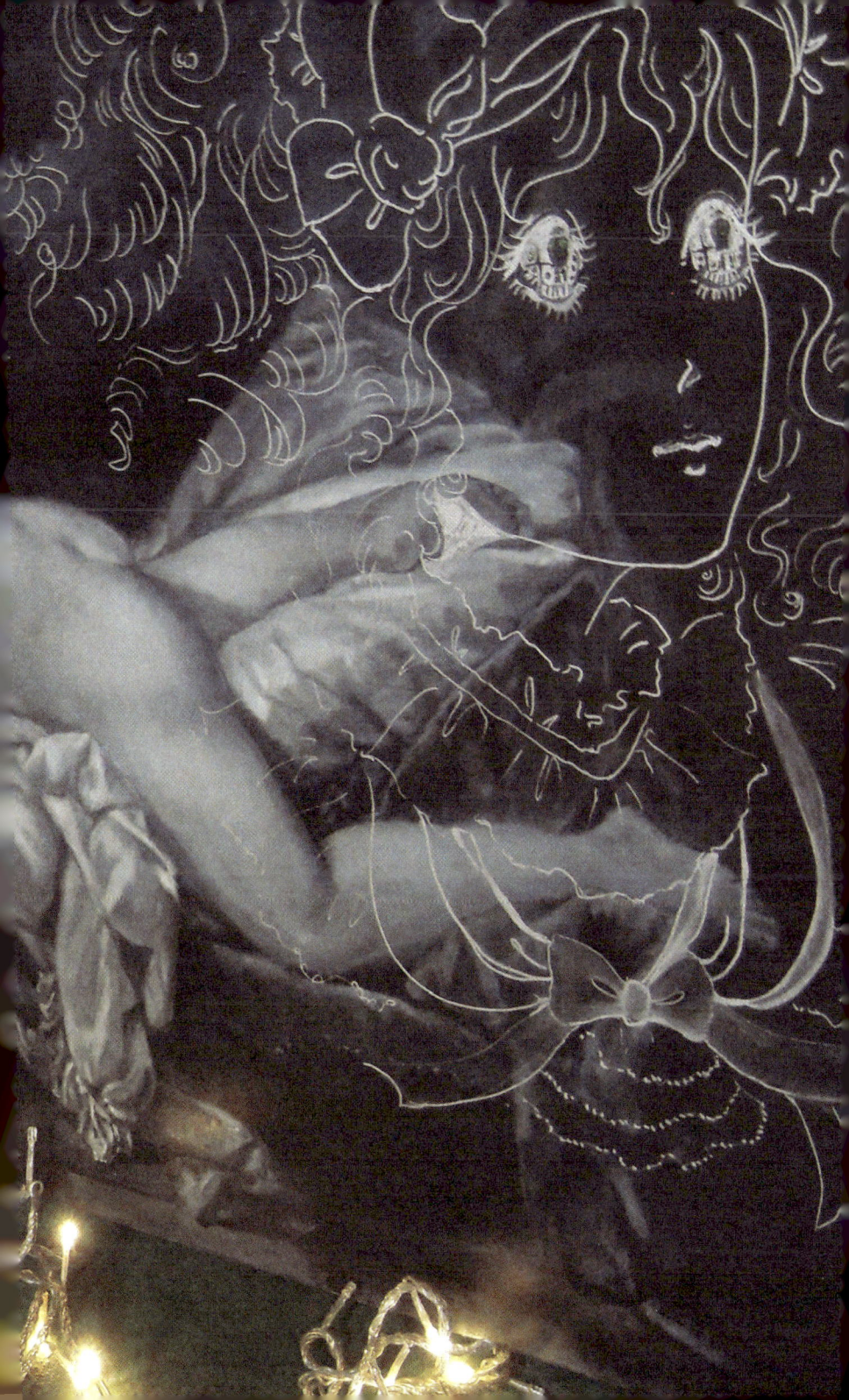

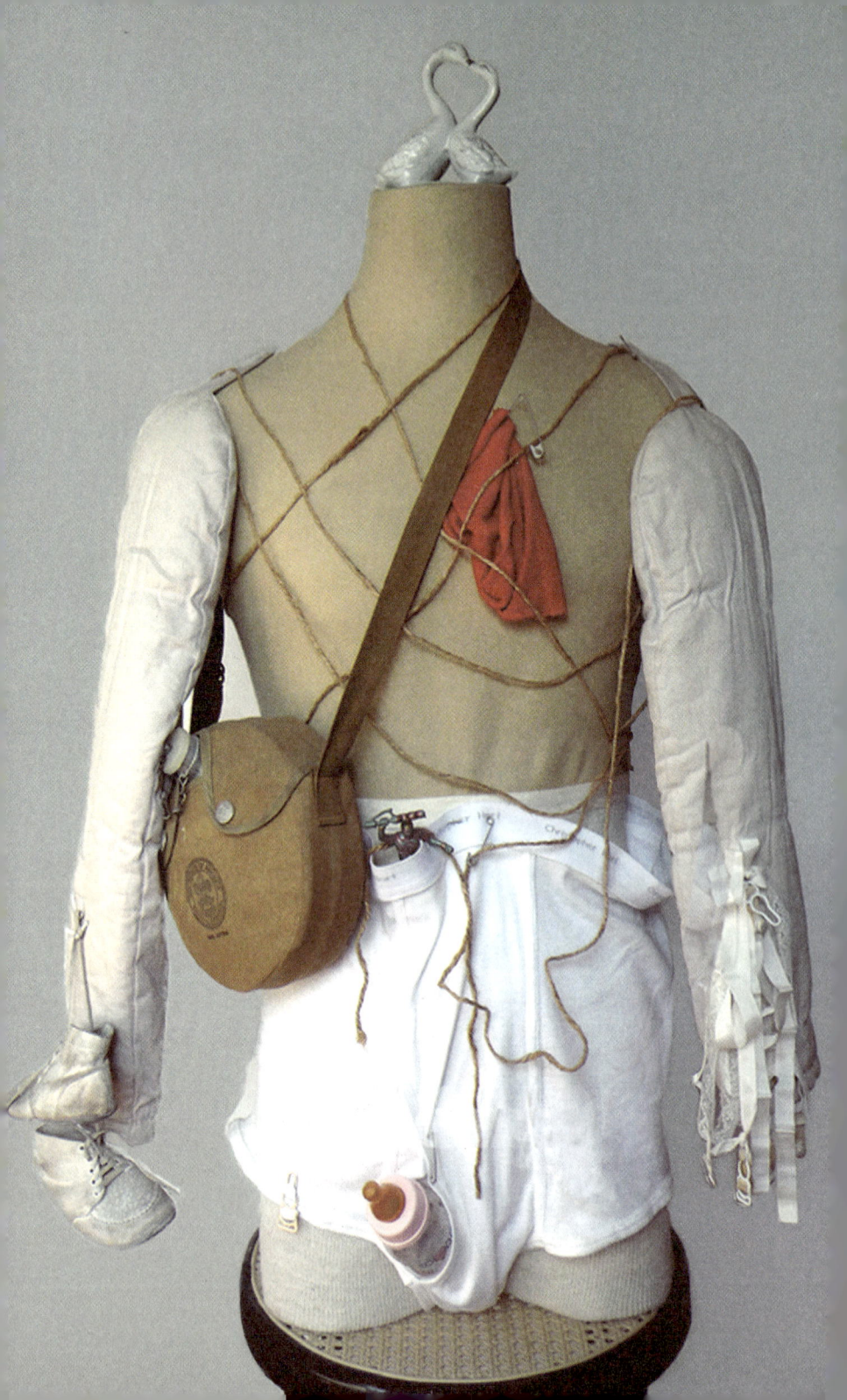

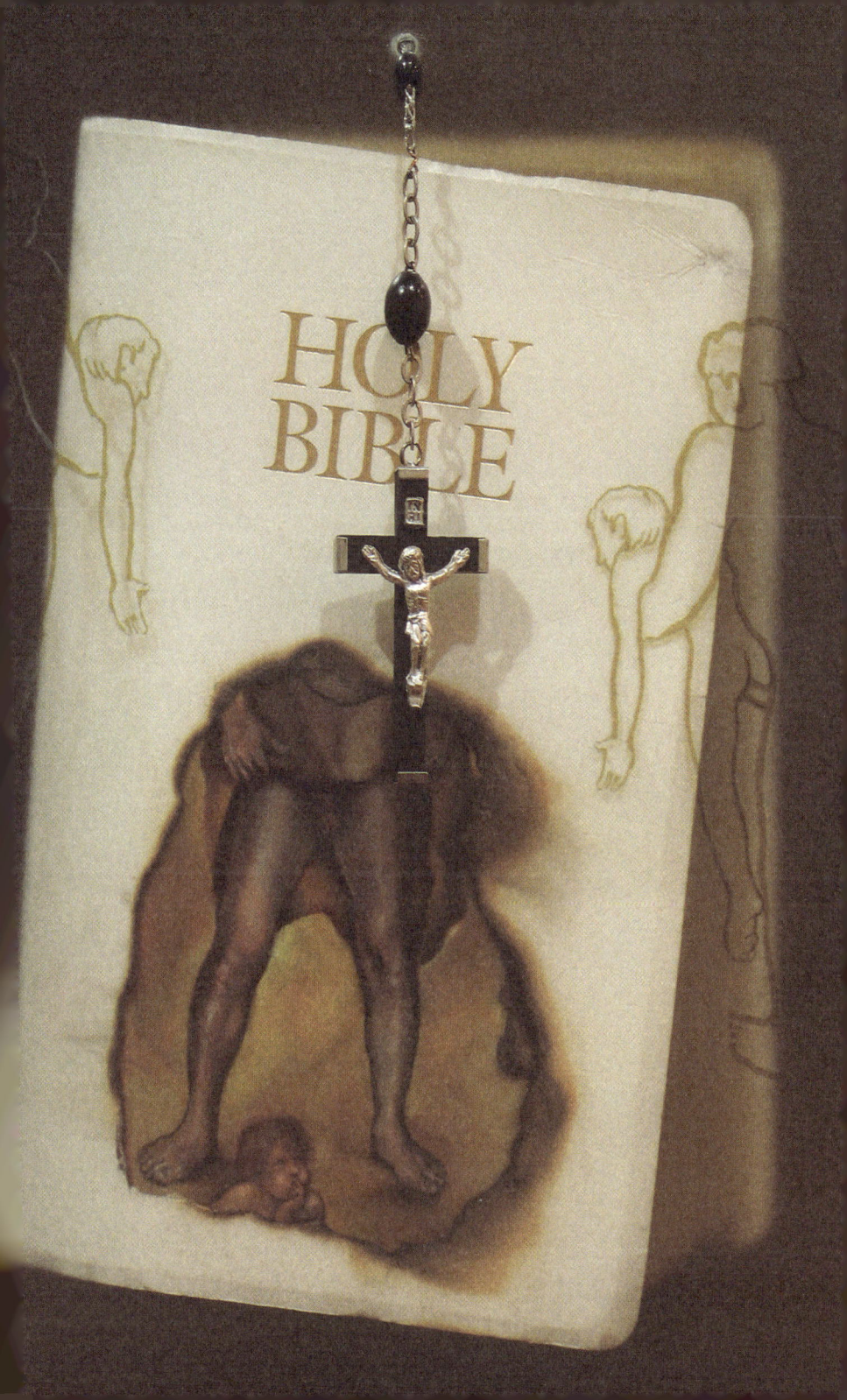

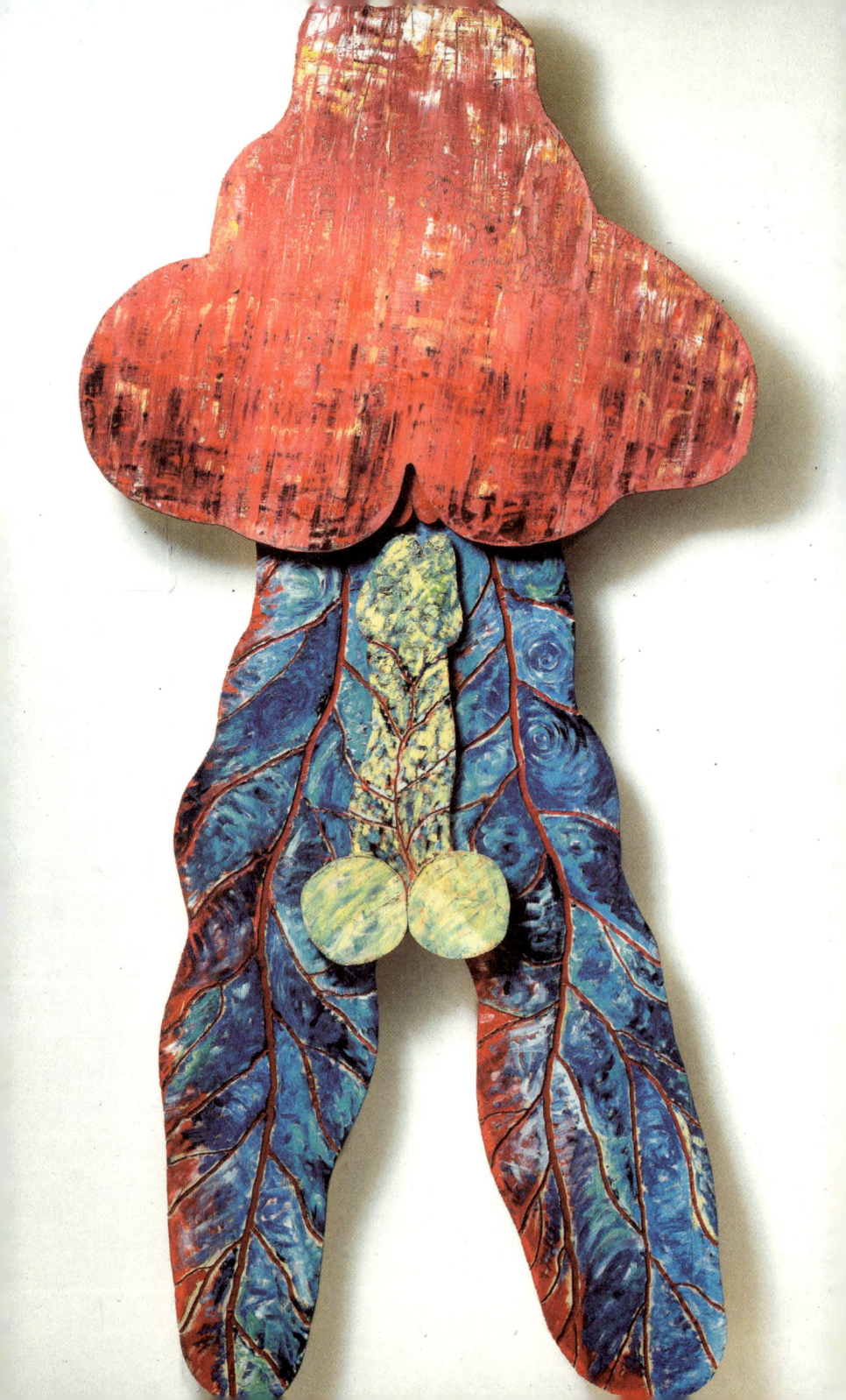

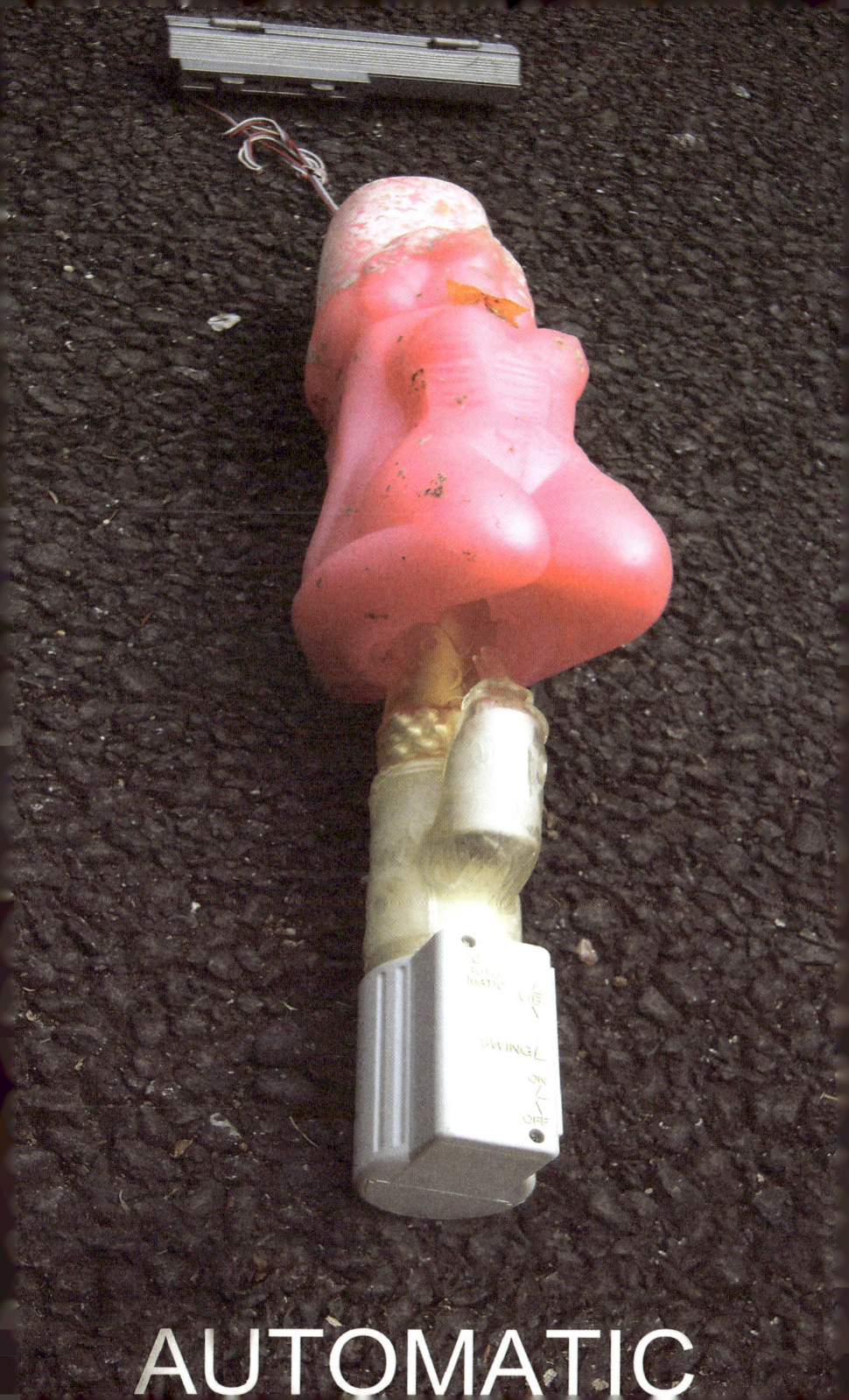

AUTOMATIC

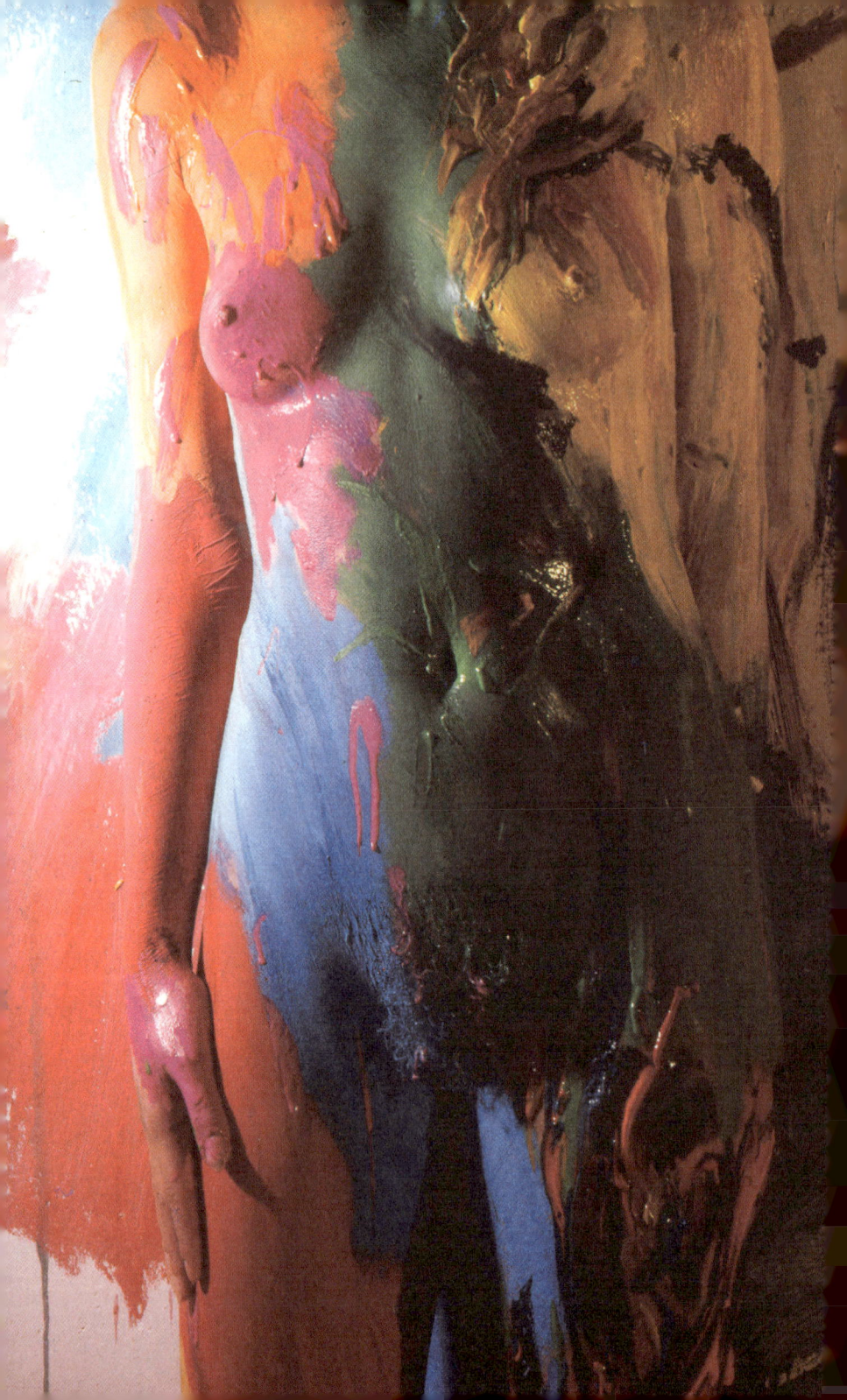

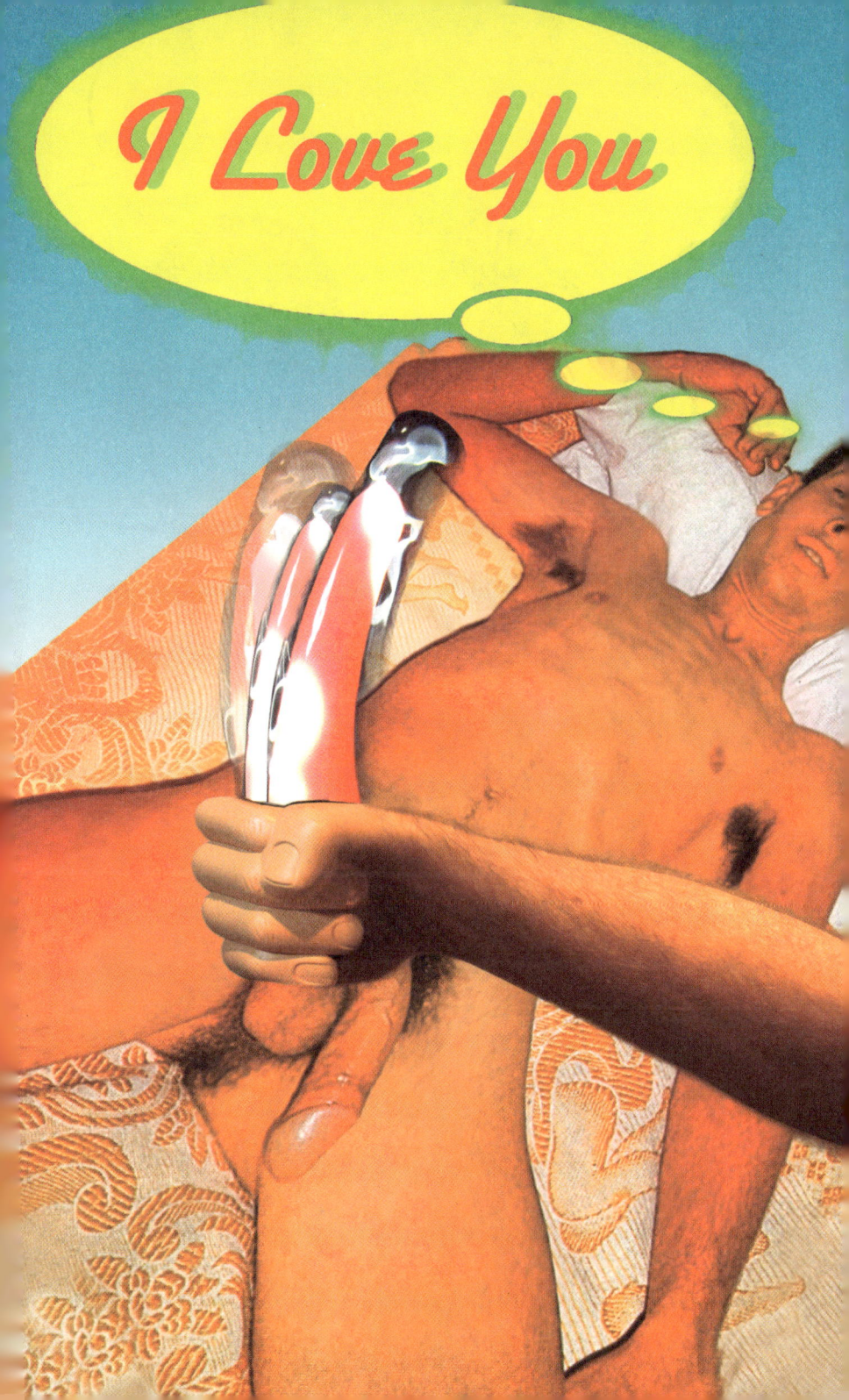

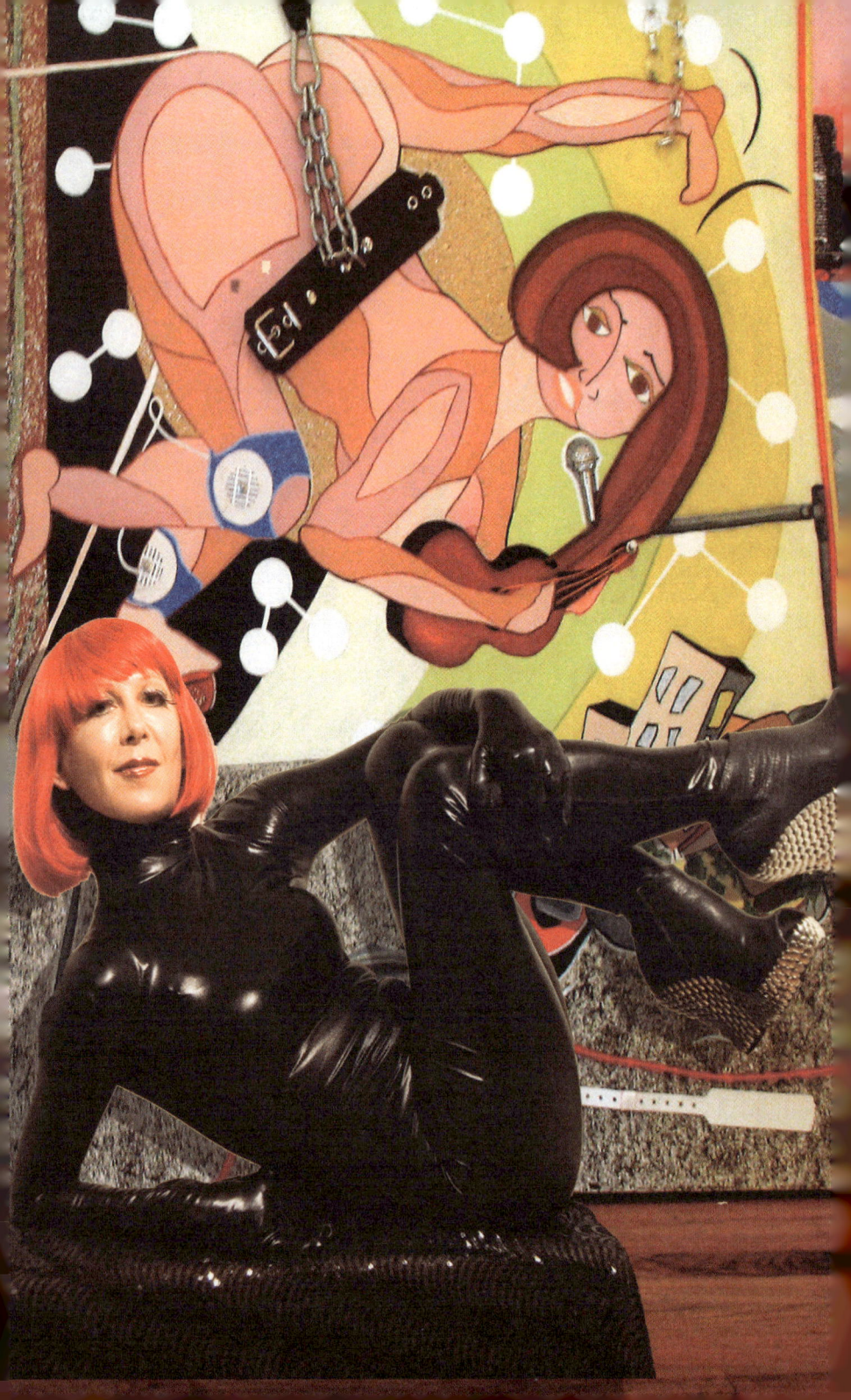

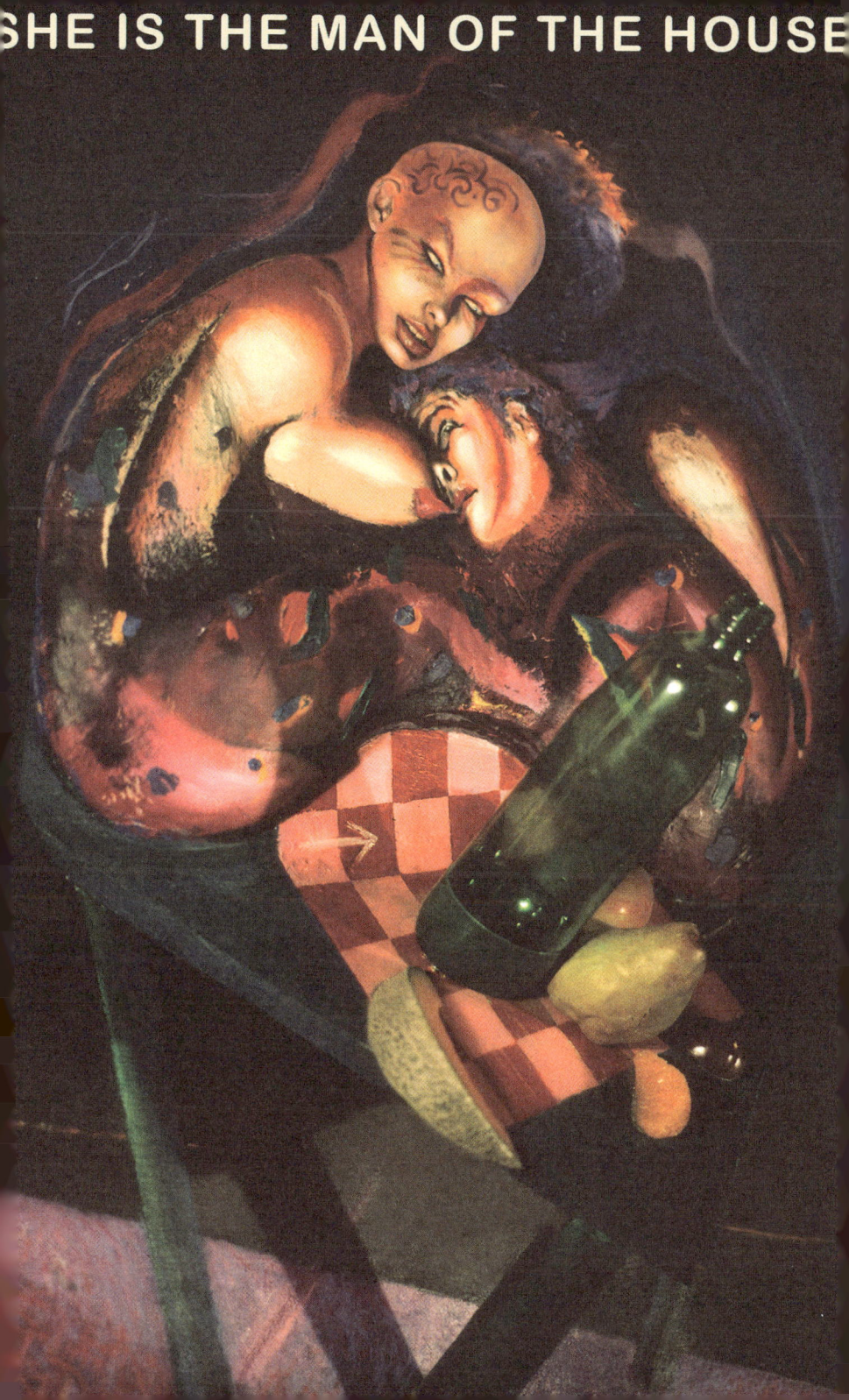

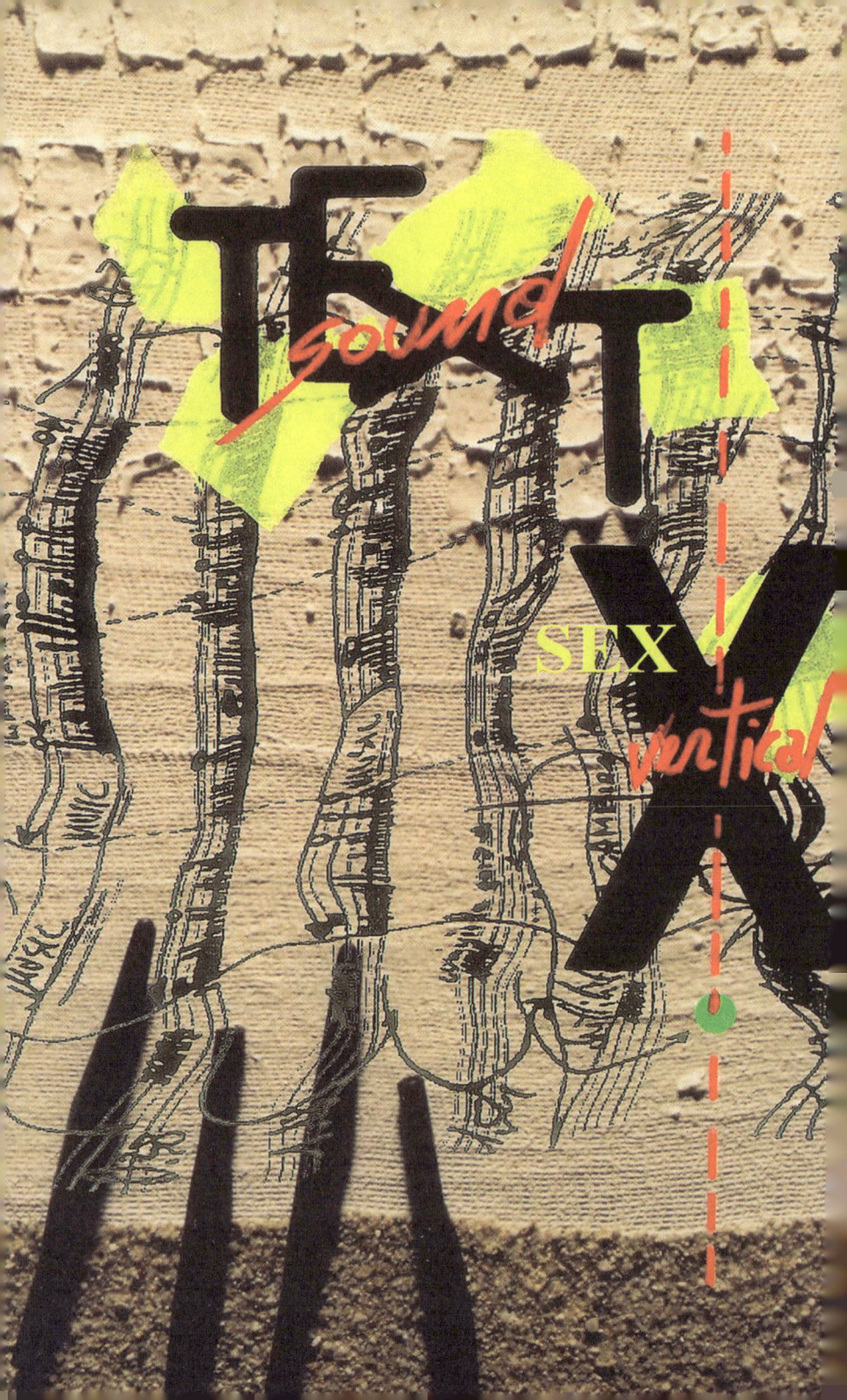

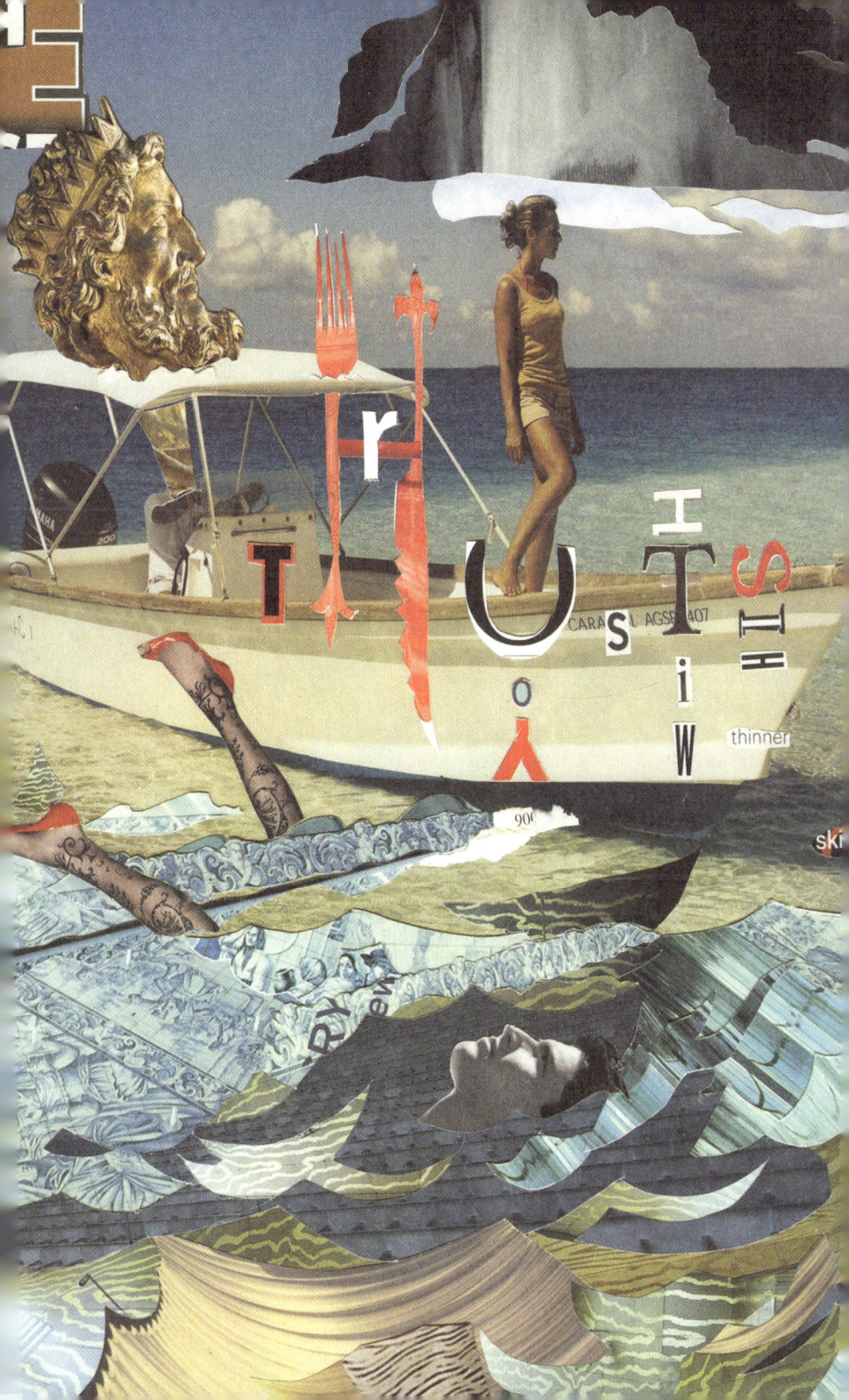

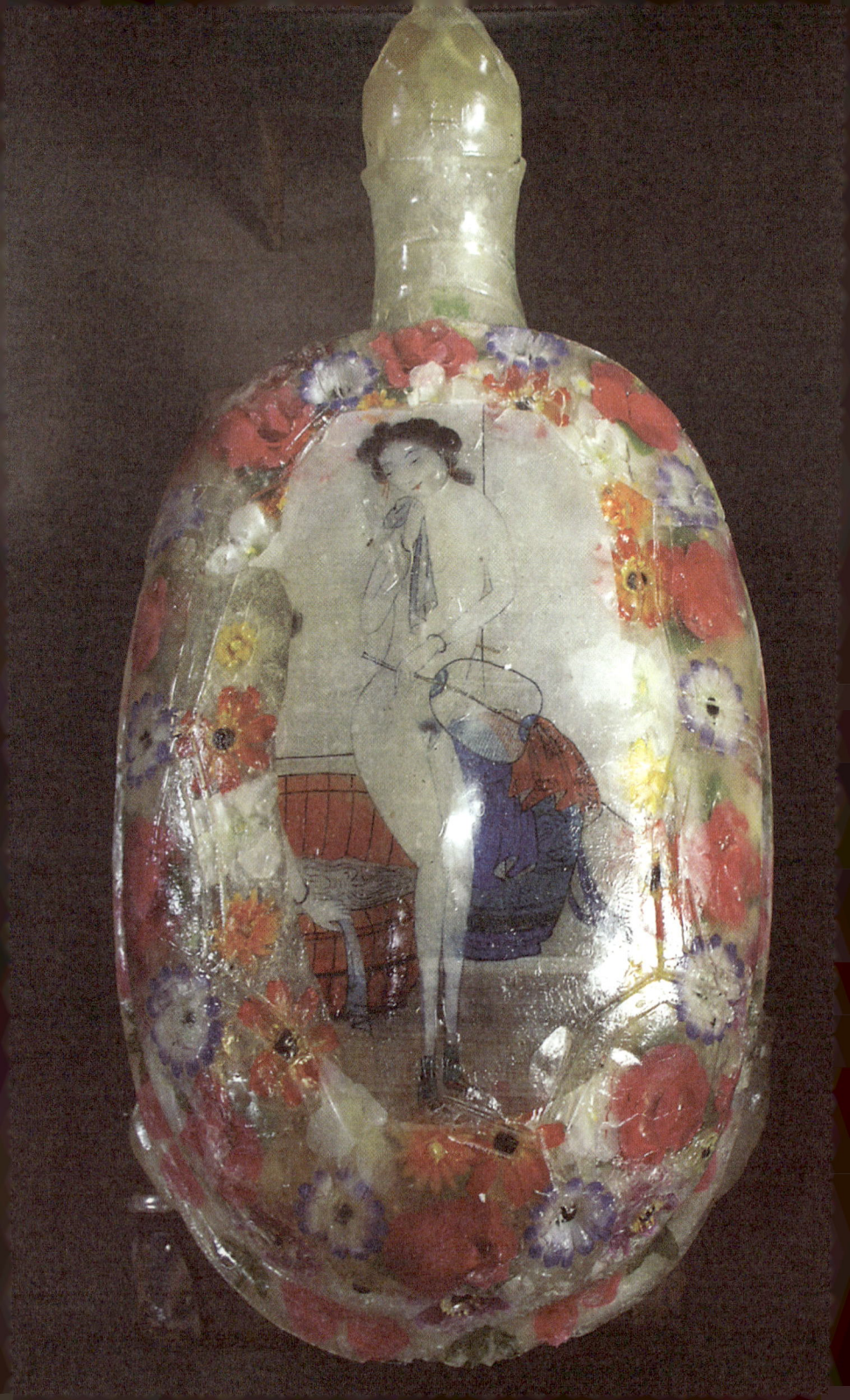

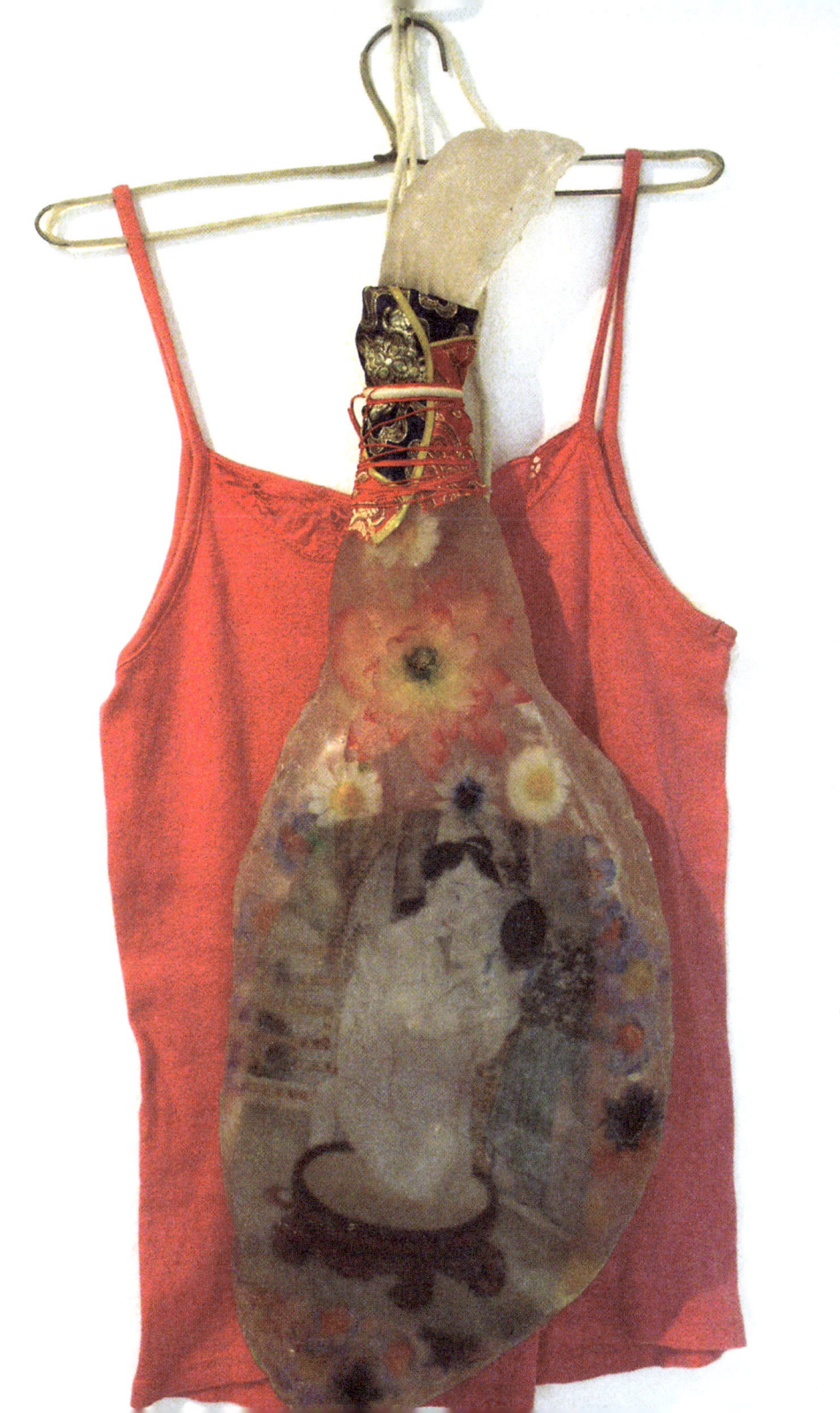

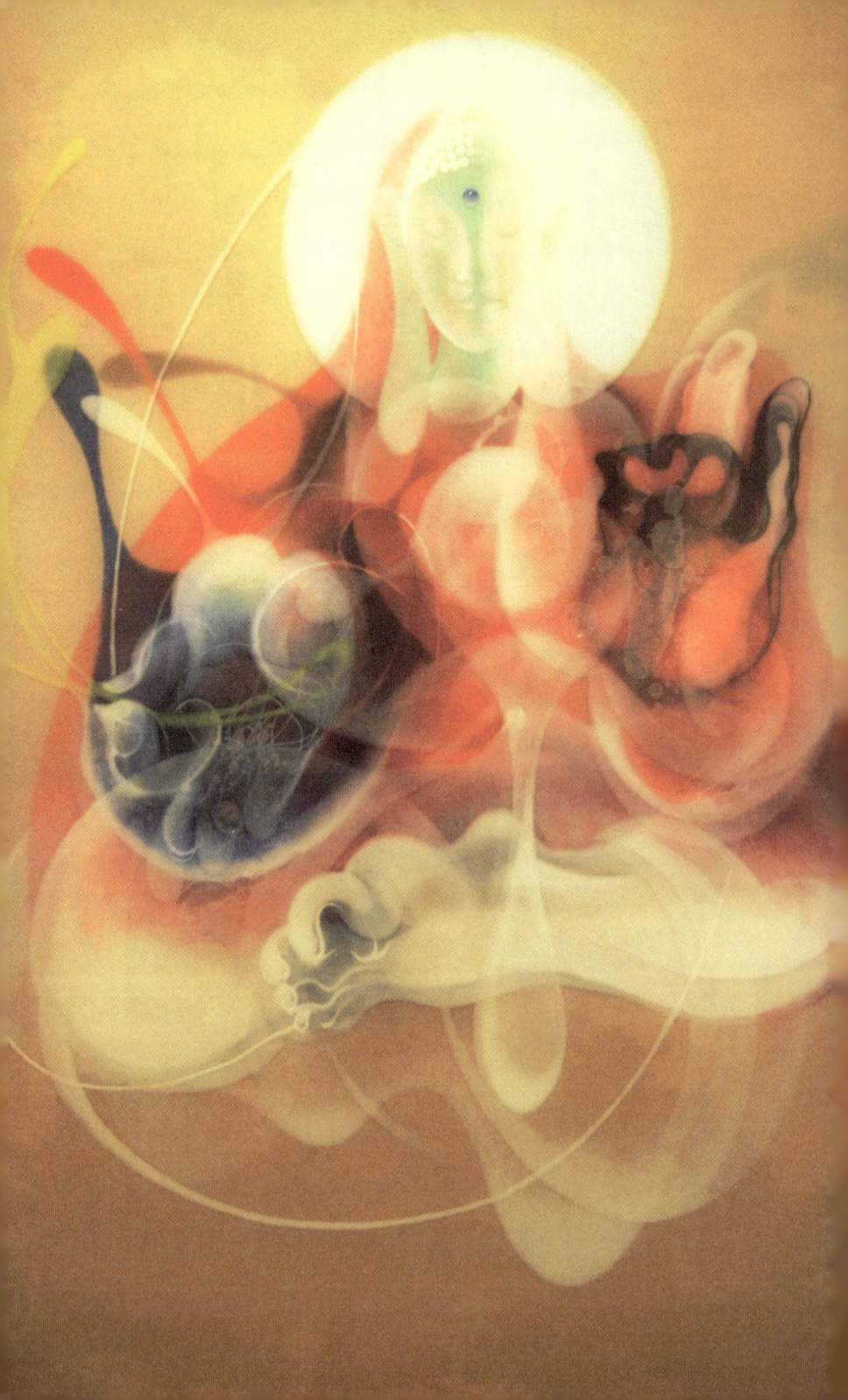

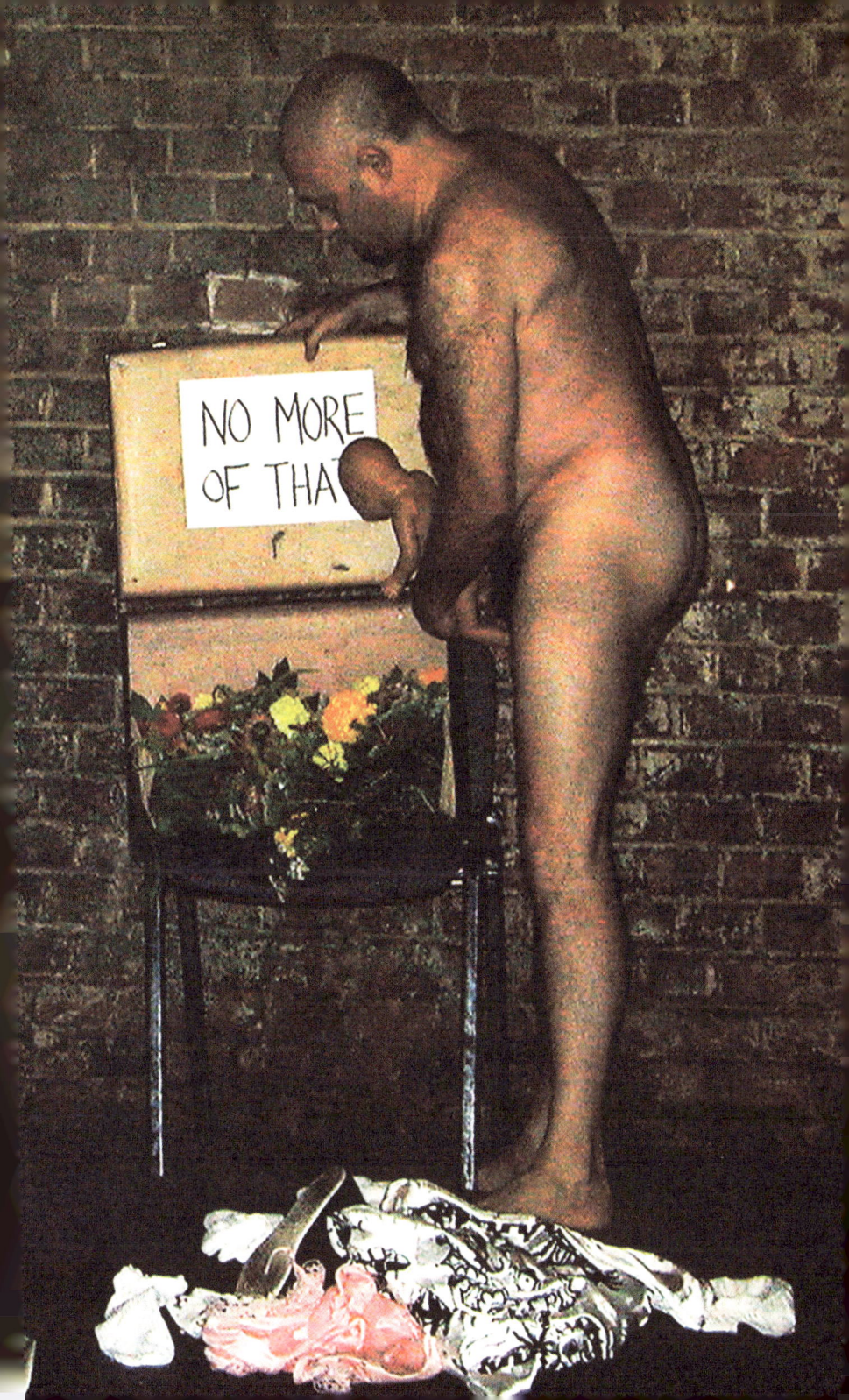

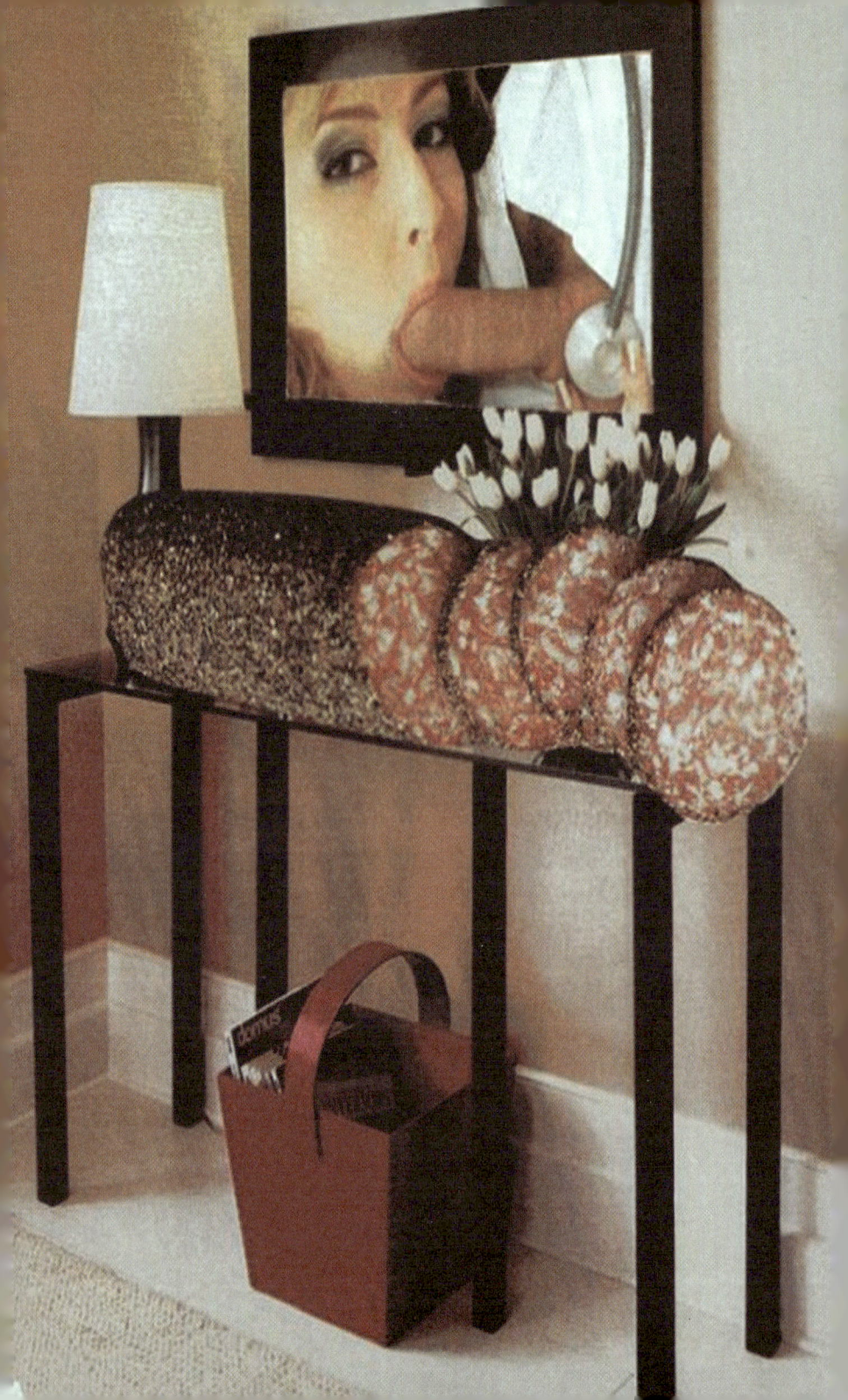

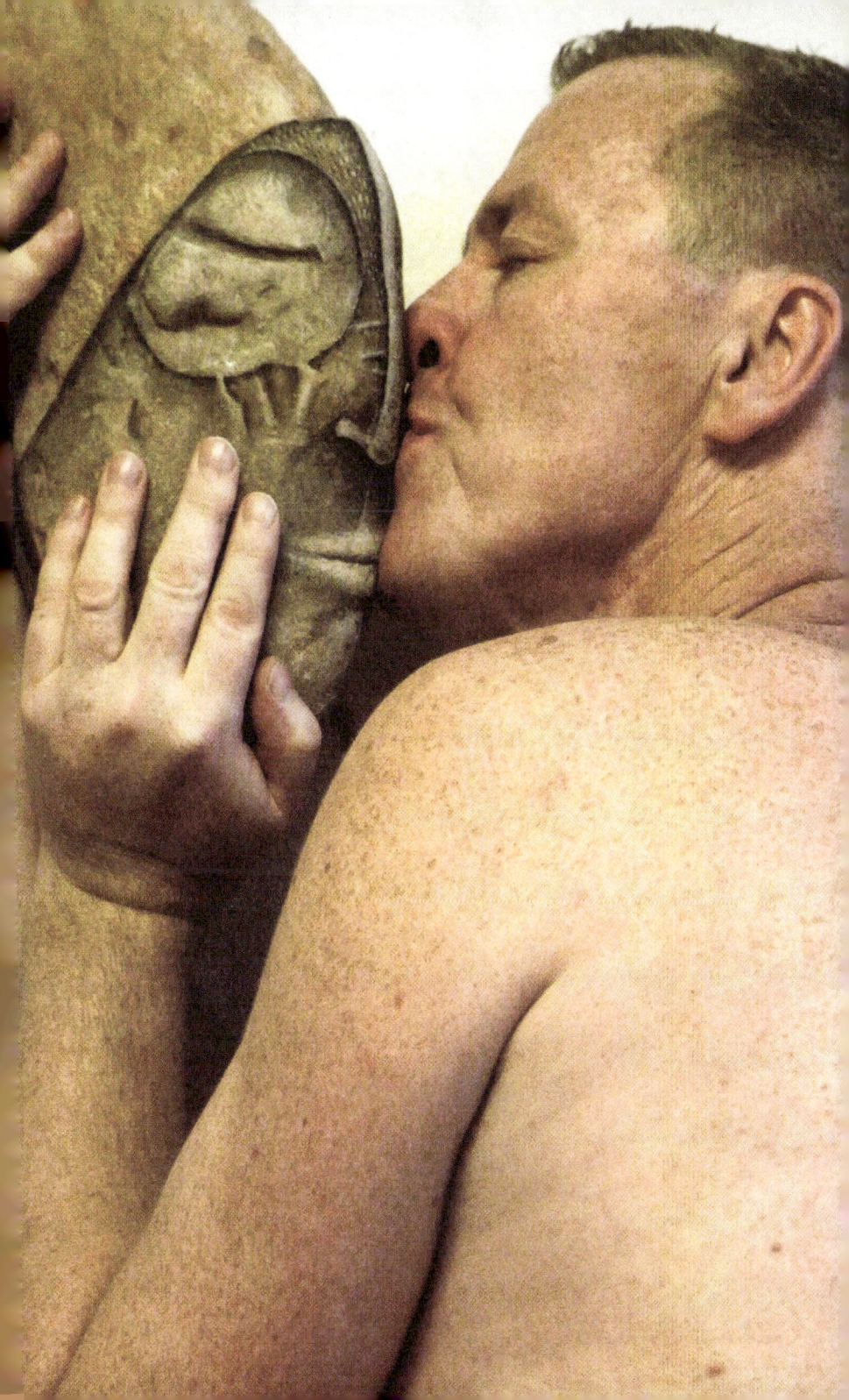

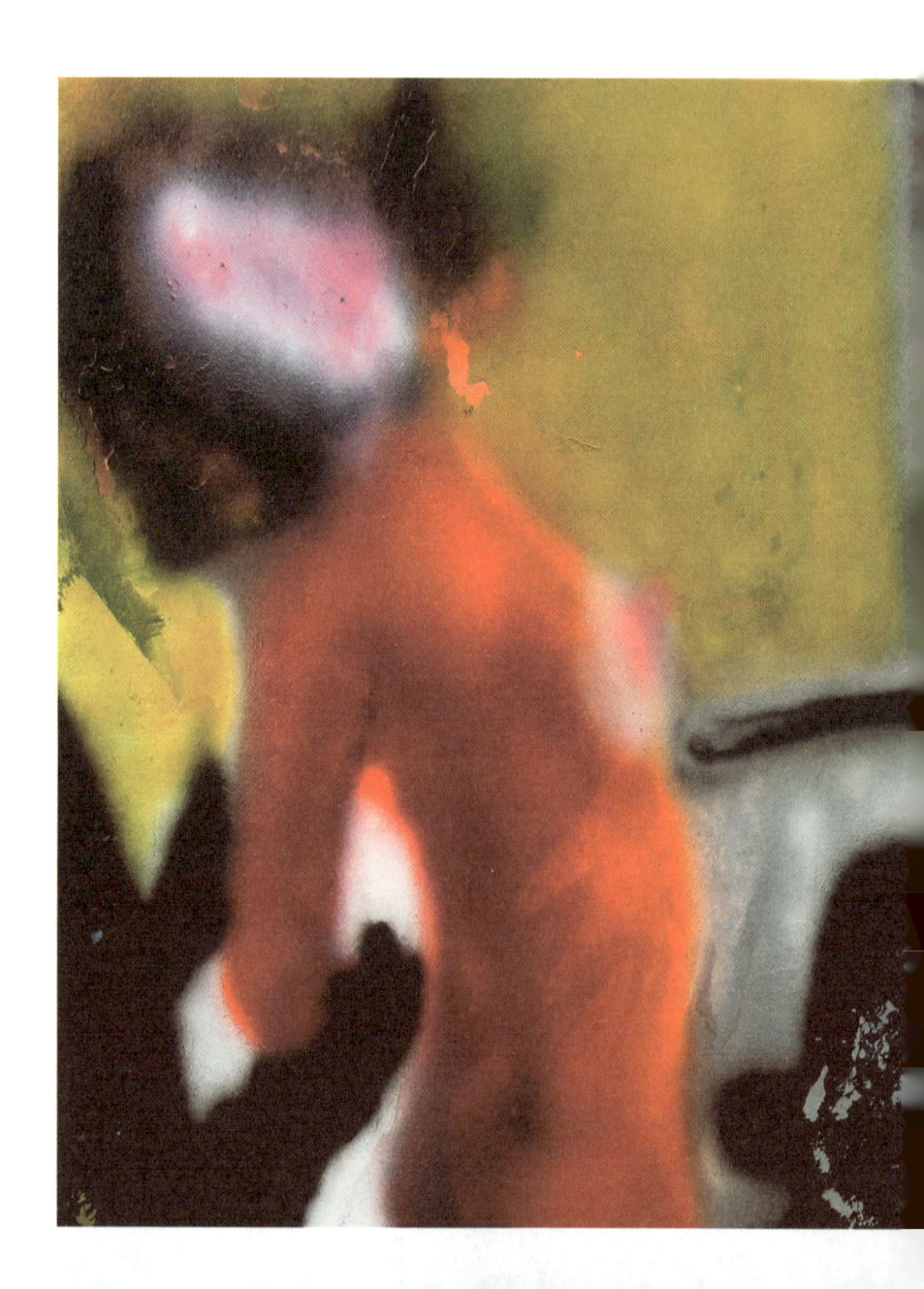

FROM SUICIDE CASANOVA
ARTHUR NERSESIAN

The outlying wings of the dilapidated motel are bordered by a splintery balcony. I park toward the far right end of the wooden structure and flip off my car lights. This flophouse is an insurance company's nightmare. A small spark and the entire place is in embers.

Still combating the five Bloody Marys she had downed at Charlie's Steak & Grille, Jeane starts, "I don't have time…."

"No one does," I battle.

"It costs too much."

"I make enough," I mollify.

"Les," she leans forward, "I'm married!"

"Just stay in the car." I go into the central shack. Ma and Pa Kettle are camped in front of a TV set that has no off button. She looks like an ashtray; he resembles a liquor bottle.

With minimal words — one day, no luggage — lest they offend their antennaed god, we do the keys-for-cash exchange. I sign the registry: Jethro Bodine. Maybe they'll read it during an infomercial. One struggles to remember what mankind did before TV. Back to the Jag.

"Come on," I say, opening the car door. I hold Jeane in my arm and escort her to the room. She doesn't have a clue. Her head flops against my shoulder. I unlock the door and flip on a light. There is a telephone on the end table and an old TV against a wall. With the necessary furniture, clean walls, and no unbearably bad odors, the room is servicea-

321

ble. Jeane turns on a lamp, I turn off the overhead. I sit on the old queen-sized bed with her, gauging its springiness. After kicking off our shoes, we're back to square one.

Slowly, while we kiss, I curl up in the director's chair of my fantasy: In the prior scene, Perry Cruz had extorted this virtuous wife and good mother with nude photos of her daughter. Perry needs to believe that she is doing this not because she wants to, but because she has to. It is not so much that I want to believe I am forcing her, but to attain turgidity, I need to believe that my will is inexorable — I have to be a fiend with single-mindedness of purpose, and she has to be one of the unsuspecting innocent. Otherwise, my erection engines will stall and I'll start to lose altitude.

Action: As I grind my crotch into hers, I remember her character: She is married, a mother of two, a career woman. Her motivation: She is offering me her body in place of her daughter's innocence. I kiss and rub her, and slowly stroke her thighs down to her midsection and stomach. Inevitably my fingers prowl along the outer area of her moistened panties.

Soon I push aside the thin fabric and I am fingering her tenderly, stroking along her pubic mound. She is moaning and opening her legs wider. Looking at her closed eyes and panting little mouth, I can see she's having her own fantasy. Probably *Bridges of Madison County* crap. With most women, sensations are emotions; a touch means they like you, a fuck — total vulnerability — is love.

Without taking off my pants, I unzip and rub my hooded bob against her blossomed rose, spreading open her moisture, flicking myself along her bulged clitoris. It's as though a dam has broken. She's wet all over. With my pants still on, I enter her gradually. She lets out a back-of-the-throatism that resembles a soul fluttering.

"Should we really do… this?" I ask remorsefully. She doesn't respond; I ask again.

"Yes! I need it, but… but I feel so guilty."

I pull out punitively.

"No! Fuck me! Please!" It's better than any of her old films. Working it back in, I lap up her bouquet of facial expressions, perfect silent tulip lips surrounded by dainty baby's breath of exquisite winces, articulate floral gasps. On to the next fabulous sphincter of hell: "Have you cheated on Eddie before?"

"I'd rather not talk," she mouths more than mutters.

"I need to know," I demand, as I stridently drive my thickness into her. She reaches around, grabbing the cheeks of my pants-sheathed ass, and moans, "Yes!"

"Yes what?" the interrogation commences.

"Yes, I cheated!" Her closed eyelids are like the mouths of tight little fish, and again I have to catch my breath.

"More than once?" I begin again.

Yes, her mouth forms, but only a bubble appears.

"How many times?" I toy.

"A couple, for goodness sakes," she replies. Now she is trying to turn her head, trying to hide her abominable shame in the contours of an old pillow.

"Were they good?"

"Yes, yes," Jeane pants. I give absolution by worming my forked tongue into her creamy, silky mouth, but she won't have it. As I'm slamming myself against her cervix like a wrecking ball, she squeezes her legs, pushing me back, retaining a modicum of control. I flip her over on her stomach, yank her knees out from under her, and plug the tip of my cork back into her. Her right hand slips slowly downward. Her surreptitious index finger strums her string as I continue to bang away. When she is close to eruption, I pull her plucking fingers from her nub and say, "Now, did I say you could do that?"

"Please!" She desperately tries to touch her fuse box.

"Who fucked you?" I push.

"Nobody!" she shoots back.

"Where'd you meet him? At work?" It's confession time.

She shoves me backward and spins around, angrily looking at me. "What the fuck's the matter with you?"

For an instant I am powerless. "I'm sorry, I guess I lost myself a little."

"I guess you did," she replies. Then she lays down again.

After a pause, I reenter and resume gradually, building up to our former pace.

"Fuck me!" She orgasms as she screams insanely through walls not much thicker than cardboard. "Fuck me! Goddamn it!"

Perry Cruz loves the yearning pitch of her voice. Since he can't mind-fuck anymore, he hopes someone hears.

I pull out and squeeze several solid streaks of Elmer's glue on those perfect ten-gallon orbs of her butt cheeks. Jeane slips forward hyperventilating, super-extended. Within moments, she is snoring, fast asleep.

With the tip of my index finger, I rub the stripes of semen along the purple-brown crack of her glistening butt-hole and the soft maroon tissue below her vagina, into her jet-black pubic hair — that's for you, Eddie boy.

And I did the entire scene without ever having to remove my trousers. I take a couple steps toward the tiny bathroom, but stop a moment. I stare at the chimerical scene; I would give ten grand to have my Camcorder with me. Biting my lip, I try to magnetize the image into the videotape of my memory. Looking around the room for a pencil, I consider sketching the vignette, this skyscraper of euphoria, this Mount Everest of erotica, which I plan revisiting time and again. There is a fresh pack of motel matches in an ashtray. I slip the matchbook into my jacket pocket and enter the bathroom.

Time to clean up the crime scene and dispose of the body. I wash myself, then dip one of the rough motel towels into hot water, squeeze it dry, and go back to the bed where Jeane is still lying on her belly, exhausted and intoxicated. I gently clean the semen and other DNA evidence off of the victim's beautiful back, only to realize that she's softly whimpering, delicately crying.

"Are you okay, hon?" I whisper.

She curls into a ball and falls asleep in my lap.

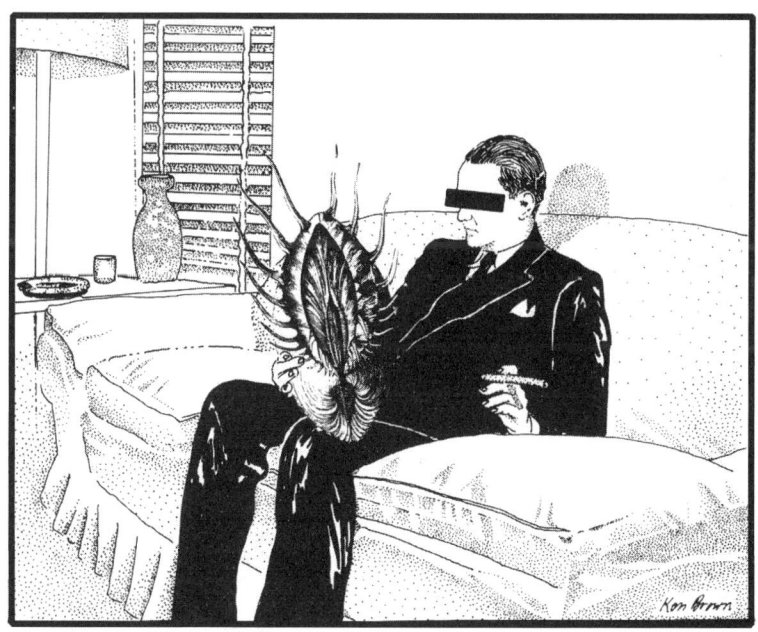

A MAN, A PLAN, A CLAM

DINOSAUR, IN
JOE MAYNARD

'm a Bible salesman. So what? So what if it's a silly job that keeps me constantly on the road and away from my wife? So what if I'm not really a true believer? I go to these Bible conventions, hang around evangelists, and even set up a booth once in a while near the end of a sermon when desperately poor believers here in the rust belt finish their altar calls and pledge their trust to the Lord.

It's the book. The big book. The one and only. The ethics of our culture are in there. The lessons. The arguments we go back to over and over, whether or not you're a believer: Sodom and Gamorah, Thou shalt not kill, It's easier for a camel to fit through the eye of a needle than a rich man to enter the kingdom of heaven. Some say it's the greatest collection of Jewish folklore. Some say it's the word of God.

For me, it's a $35 book, and $17.50 commission every time I sell one.

In Elkhart, Indiana, I was at Pastor Felix's show (yes, I'm such a cynic — I call them "shows," but only to myself), when I met someone from my home town of Elmhurst, Queens, you know, the borough of New York City. Yes, I'm a New Yorker. Born and raised.

"Ed."

I looked up from under the counter where I was trying to plug in my credit card machine. It was Tom Delaney, this grade A cynic who used to work for my dad, a furrier. Dad had a shop on 48th Street in Manhattan, back in the day. Tom had gotten kicked out of the Catholic school we both attended for allegedly telling a nun that he knew she masturbated. At least that's what he told me. He was about two years older than me. He was my dad's apprentice, and was constantly telling me stories like that. I hadn't seen him for at least twenty years.

"Lord Almighty!" I said using the language that would fit in this room, this dilapidated movie theatre with an organ to the side of the stage pumping and wheezing out the good music of the lord, while the preacher huffed, and puffed and blew the hopes and desires of hapless human scrapple until it ignited to become the flame of the lord, the body of the church, god's incarnation on this clueless earth. And here was a fetid hunk of sin staring at me as if we were on opposite sides of a mirror. Gray hair, crusty lips, each of us with a couple of well placed deep grooves at the sides of our mouths indicating the use of the famous sneer of disbelief that embellishes Jack Chick pamphlets whenever you see a well drawn sinner.

"Tom Delaney, thick as gravy," I said extending my arm for a handshake.

"So we both have memories, and in your case mamories," he said. "You sell these things? I mean, I heard they sell pretty well...."

"Yes, my friend, I'm a Bible salesman," I sighed.

"Well..." he paused, looking around the half-full room at all the desperate souls. People were walking up and down the isles trying to work themselves into a PTL frenzy. "...I guess I've seen it, so I have to believe it: Edward G. Monoghan, Bible Salesman." He leaned forward. "So, you hear the one about the traveling Bible salesman and the lady auto mechanic?"

"What are you doing here?" I asked.

"So his car breaks down and he..."

"Seriously, what are you..."

"I sell paper towels, paper cups, toilet paper. I used to run a theatre, but abused my privilege with a young female staffer. Now I work for the company that used to supply us with popcorn boxes."

"Sorry."

"It's OK. Movies are a dying business."

"Maybe you should move into Bibles."

"I think the Lord might spare me that tribulation. Hey, my car died so I gotta take a bus back to Chicago — can you give me a lift to the station?"

"I have to work here for another hour or so." I was hoping he'd be too impatient to wait for me and we could end this chance encounter. At that moment, a really grim looking young mother with a toddler asleep on her shoulder walked past. Two tattered looking urchins followed in her wake like a little duck family navigating their way out of a sewage pond. When I was younger, that would have been the bleakest, least sexy picture imaginable. But what she reminded me of was a one-time hot-blonde cheerleader whose luck took a horrible nose dive, and now that cheerleader, that I had so lusted after all those pubescent years, was within reach.

So just what had I become? A middle-aged guy with the beginnings of a paunch staring at miss-fortune as she walked by. Large, gray Irish eyes, large but pleasantly white teeth and full lips, large, plump bosom. Her ass still looked pretty good in a pair of mom-jeans as she made her way out the lobby door into the night.

Tom went on about his divorce, about how his kids were being raised as born-again Catholics: his wife had become what he could only describe as a religious nut job, even stopped having anal sex because…. Then he started the jokes. I acted like I was listening but I noticed out of the corner of my eye that grim woman with the kids looking back in our direction.

"…So the rabbi says, make it two, and don't forget the pastrami!" He laughed too loudly for the room. I stared blankly at him not having heard his joke, only the punch line. I didn't really want to hear it, didn't want to hang out with him. Christ, he couldn't even finish fucking high school.

"Maybe I'll close up," I said.

The crowd was thinning. I'd sold eight Bibles at $35 a piece, not a disaster, covered my expenses with about $40 profit. OK, not great. The sooner I got this prick to the bus station and out of my life the better. I had a $25 room in a motel on the edge of town that used to be a Holiday Inn. Shut eye. Glorious shut eye. Where I could dream about flying, sexy women and sports cars. That, or the recurring dream I have about trying to sell a Bible to a non-believer while trying to convince him of a belief I didn't even hold myself.

Tom watched me pack up, continuing his painfully dismal litany of high school memories: Bronwyn Giancano, the girl with the hugest breasts upon which all high school fantasies involving breasts were built upon; Dora McGuinness, the skinny chick from Rockaway who was famous for handjobs in detention (she had a car that was apparently a brothel on wheels); Fiona Applebee, who smelled like pee. She was always chewing gum and testing her breath in the palm of her hand. This is who Tom actually dated. Cute enough, but… the pee thing.

"Whatever happened to Fiona Applebee?" I asked while we were taking boxes to the car.

"She started seeing the gym teacher and became a lesbian."

Pastor Felix marched up to me in his black suit, skinny black tie and white shirt drenched in patches of sweat.

"How is the Lord's book doing, brother Ed?"

"The Lord is kindly providing just enough to catch your next revival in Lansing."

Pastor Felix laughed loudly, "Praise the Lord, and see you there!"

When he was out of ear range, Tom said, "What a moron."

"He's smarter than you."

Tom smirked like it was a joke, but I kind of meant it. We each carried a box to the car. I put them in the back seat behind me. The smell of my car hit me.

"Man, your car smells like a jail: menthol cigarettes!" Tom said.

"Not me — my wife smokes," I lied, not wanting to get into the whole whore story.

I had actually picked up a hooker a few nights previous, and the car still stunk like Parliament menthol cigarettes. I don't know why I picked her up. Maybe I was feeling my way out of this thing with Mary. I don't smoke. The smell makes me ill. Between her humid cum-soaked cigarette infused hooker breath and my tiny car, which is so small it prohibited any maneuverability, I had a tough time getting hard, even though I was hard when I saw her ass on the sidewalk. My dick: Another thing past its prime, suitable for a scrap pile. But really. She was fat under her arm pits. Like her tits started all the way over there. I mean, on a good night, she may have looked like Bette Midler, or that Ugly Betty, but once she got in my car, she just looked like a fat drag queen, only she was a real chick. Her skin felt like a plucked chicken rolled in olive oil. Her belly sagged over her pubes. All I could do was hold out $10 for her to get lost.

"So you don't mind if I smoke?" Tom asked. He lit up. "I didn't know you were married."

I told him about Mary. How she lives up in Royal Oak, just outside Detroit. We separated about three years ago, but just kept on seeing each other about once a week. Eventually, I stopped keeping an apartment and lived out of motels; I rented space in a garage adjacent Mary's house for my Bibles."

"How do you know she's not fucking every guy in town? he asked. "I mean, usually women who…"

"Knock it off," I interrupted. I didn't tell Tom about this, but Mary still looks good, and could probably fuck any guy in town. She's only slightly worse for wear. I didn't provide her with a great life, but we got along. Fights? Sure. They say it comes along with passion. Plus, it's in her blood. She's kind of a sassy half-Irish, half-Italian Catholic. Oh, but she has a nice tiny twat and can suck the chrome off a trailer hitch, to use an expression I learned from Tom back in high school. I mean, I love her, but I think our love peaked a few years back — but her tiny jaw, full lips, curvy little body, slightly tacky taste in jewelry — and her breasts that are so solid you could injure yourself if they caught you at the right angle; only medium melons, but tough little ones that I've been thinking about for years — thus the part-time thing we have.

I parked along the curb. The bus station wasn't very big. I almost missed it. As I got out of the car, I saw that woman with her three kids on the bench outside the bus station. We made eye contact and she kept looking at me as we approached.

"Could you spare some money for bus fare?" Her mouth stayed open after her plea, teeth almost resting on her lower lip, but beneath a crack of blackness. An unfortunate soul with a mouth like a black hole. Tom pulled out two bucks and gave it to her.

"Got a cigarette to spare?" she asked.

Tom poked one into her black hole and lit it for her.

"What are you doing with the kids out here?" he asked.

"Just trying to get back to Chicago."

The air was just starting to get nippy. It was mid-September. The thought occurred to me that the kids should be going to bed for school. Or maybe they weren't old enough.

"I'd give you money," Tom said, "but my pockets aren't that deep. Who knows with this guy, though. You know what they say about Bible salesmen?"

"No," she said taking a drag while staring blankly at Tom, "what do they say?"

"I'd better catch a bus," Tom said nudging me. As we walked towards the station, he added, "I might have been tempted if she'd just thrown me a bone."

I looked back at her and wondered why Tom hadn't tried harder to get in her pants. A guy like him would probably gladly miss his bus if he thought he had half a chance. But to look at her, where does one begin? Three kids, up way too late, destitute on a bench in a depressed Midwestern town. Perhaps if she'd been a hooker…. But, nah, hitting on that one was like poking at an injured duck with a stick. Just not right. Maybe that's why she turned me on.

Tom and I shook hands, wished each other luck. Took his wallet out and gave me his card. "Look me up if you're ever in Chicago."

He walked into the station and I back to my jail scented Ford Escort.

I turned the ignition, flicked on the headlights, and there she was again, big Irish eyes reflecting my beam. I clicked the high beams on and off, but she just stared blankly at me. I drove up to her bench. The kids were leaning against each other from either side, and it made me think that families were just so many houses of cards; they could be blown anywhere at any time. I don't know why that crossed my mind. I never think about cards — or families. I'm not sure how it relates to me and Mary, but maybe that's why I haven't gotten rich at the whole Bible salesman thing.

I rolled my window down. "Hey, come here, I want to talk to you."

She just looked over her shoulder at me. I wanted to fuck her black-holy face and make her kids cry. I also just wanted to do a good deed. I hated myself for both urges, one sick, one saccharine, then told myself I should just fill her hair with my cum, or fill her ass, mouth, cleavage... fuck. Sorry, Mary, but my dick is hard.

"Get in the car, let's go get a room." She didn't move. "Wouldn't you like that? I mean for the kids at least?" I turned the car off, turned the lights off and popped the trunk. The car made that bing-bong sound as I left the keys in the ignition while taking boxes of Bibles from the back seat and putting them in the trunk.

I opened the passenger door and gingerly placed her two older boys that I'd guess were ages five and four into the back seat. They were roused from slumber but made the effort to keep their eyes shut. When I turned around she was at the curbside with her youngest, who seemed to be about two. I shut the door after her, the two year old slumbering on her shoulder, chocolate stains ringing her mouth. We drove off. They stayed in the car while I negotiated a two-bedroom with the Hindu guy. He seemed disinterested in everything but getting ten extra dollars.

The room had a broken a/c unit, the tin cover lay belly

up on the floor, but it seemed otherwise clean. Agressively orange and gold decor. Kind of left over from the 70s or something. Shimmery wallpaper, peeling now and then at a seam. The two older boys were awake but docile. One grabbed the TV remote control and they sat on the edge of the bed closest to the door while the woman moistened a washcloth and washed their faces and hands.

It was a loving gesture, but I wondered if it was just instinct. Like a cat purring when you give it food. It doesn't mean it likes you. Maybe the mother doesn't even like her children. There's just a maternal instinct that makes her wash faces. I felt little respect for some reason. A disconnect. I began pinching the underside of my dick through my pocket. She went back and forth between the sink and her various kids. I walked to the back of the room by the sink and watched her conduct her motherly protocol in the mirror. The infant was on the free bed. It seemed I would be sleeping with her and her baby, which I thought sweet. At one pass she brushed my belly with her hand, a sort of brief, affectionate sweep.

The two older ones had found *SpongeBob SquarePants* on the tube. Why do they have *SpongeBob* on at eleven at night? Is that where we are in this culture? Toddlers staying up to eleven? She took off her jean jacket and was wearing a t-shirt. I noticed bruises on the back of her arm. She took out a toothbrush from the pocket of her jacket and bent over the sink, brushing her teeth, occasionally looking back at me.

My dick was hard. I walked over to her, put my hands around her biceps covering the bruises I had noticed. She continued to brush her teeth. My dick rested in her buttocks. She spit and began washing her face. I stood perfectly still. She tightened her buttocks around me. Kind of soft but firm at the same time. Perhaps she was a farm girl. Generally healthy, but down on her luck. Pragmatic and fearless. I imagined her running naked through a woods, jumping into a river, wet and slippery, while ever so slightly rubbing up and down with layers of fabric between us, fearing the kids would notice. She stood slowly, toweled her face and took my hand, pulling me into the bathroom a few feet away. We closed the door and began our embrace.

Inside she gingerly pressed me against the door, put her hands on my shoulders, and used one foot to wedge one sneaker off, then the other foot to kick off the other sneaker. Her mouth came up to my nipple. She inhaled against my armpit and fully wrapped her arms around me. I feared I smelled bad, but then, on the other hand, I didn't really care. I pulled her face to mine and kissed her. It was minty and primitive, like the farm girl I imagined she was. She bit at my neck and I slowly pulled her body downward until she was licking my dick through my pants. The restroom was so small that I was against the door and her ass against the opposite wall. She got on her knees, put her hands between my legs, pushed my balls outward and sucked at them through my trousers. My fingers were in her straight, wispy, dishwater blonde hair. I gently wrapped my fingers around her ears as her mouth slid back and forth over my dick.

I got down and straddled her, her head at the foot of the commode, her feet lying in the unused shower. I undid my trousers and my dick bobbed in front of her, she began jerking at it with one hand. I was starting to feel the pressure of orgasm coming on. I pulled her hand away, and laid down beside her, our heads to one side of the commode with the toilet paper roll above us. I thought of Tom, and it was a bit of a bummer. I got a little less hard, but the power I held in this arrangement made it easy enough to keep it up.

After a moment of kissing, I sat up and sat her on the commode. I stood and dropped my pants and boxers to the floor. I stood over her then slowly put my dick deeper, deeper in her mouth. She gagged, and though her hands pushed against my thigh, I pumped her throat a couple times before pulling back. She coughed and gasped for air when I released my hold. She didn't seem put off. I stood higher on my toes and she sucked at my balls while holding my dick. Her thumb made a circular motion on the underside of my shaft. She was no naive farm girl, even if she was a farm girl. I could see how she managed to be stuck with three kids.

Her breasts, though not huge, were ample enough, but they had no real form, no body. I squeezed them and they seemed to squish out the sides. I pinched her nipples and slightly twisted them through her t-shirt. She opened her lips around my dick and turned her head left and right. I let go of her nipples and grabbed her hair, pushed her face all the way down. I fucked her face hard and fast, coming deep in the back of her throat. I stopped while my dick spasmed away. She struggled to free herself, but I held her forehead tight against my pubes. She turned her head back and forth against me. Pulling her hair back with one hand I could see the red of her cheek continuing back around her neck. Fearing I was strangling her, I let her head go and she fell back against the tank of the commode, coughing up my cum and gasping for air.

She laid back, her bloodshot eyes rolling around. I stroked myself as the last bits of cum dribbled from my third eye, cum dribbled from her mouth. She was drenched in sweat, and looked like she was wearing rouge, though she was just naturally flushed. Her pixieish face slowly returned to its pale Irish color, her eyes tearing. I wiped her tears to the sides of her face with my thumbs. Her arms were limp. I pulled her face to my cock and she gently gave my dick small french kisses to its underside. She took my limp dick in her mouth a couple more times. After a moment I turned on the shower.

I gingerly took off her t-shirt, stood her up and escorted her towards the shower, kissing her forehead as she went around me. I watched her push down her jeans and turquoise panties that weren't in the least sexy. The flesh of her ass was smooth, but bore a couple dimples. The thought occurred to me that she was about thirty, as Miss Jean Brodie would have said, in her prime, but quickly losing it. I briefly wondered if she'd live to forty. It was a tough world, and perhaps her life after this encounter would entail child welfare officials removing her children, the solitude of soup kitchens, jobs programs, grim government housing in a quasi rural setting and eight hours a day at a bottle cap factory which would only hire her for the tax break. Grim. Sweet, meek and grim.

I washed her hair. She seemed to enjoy letting the water hit her face while I massaged her scalp. Once I rinsed her hair, I rubbed the tiny bar of soap over her body. She put the palms of her hands against the wall and pushed her ass into my semi-soft dick accompanied by an uninhibited gasp. She reached behind with one hand and laid my dick over the top of her ass crack. She continued lap-dancing me while I rubbed soap and fingers across her breasts, belly, back. I admired the look and feel of her skin. She had a nice creamy color and turned pink in spots where she had been touched, or the hot water had resided for too long. She was exactly my type. Reminded me briefly of how Mary looked when we were younger.

I tugged her mother's hips against me. She reached under and rubbed the underside of my dick through her crotch. Though I was only semi-hard, her vagina was loose as can be, and I slid in her gooey, hot, soft twat, though with slight trepidation, not wanting to get her pregnant again. I pulled out and tried to rub against her anus. It was a hard, little raspberry. She got the hint and bent lower, her elbows against the wall of the shower. She moaned, "Do it… do it."

I grabbed the shampoo again and washed her *derierre*. I poked her asshole with my thumb. I slid it back and forth easily with the lubrication of shampoo. I put my semi-hard dick to her raspberry. She slid her legs as far apart as they would and bent all the way over with one hand clasping an ankle. I slid into her like a squishy bar of butter. "Oooh!" she was nearly singing. I didn't go in and out, but the invisible thread of nerves in the center of my semi-hard dick seemed to swell and electrify. Shock waves seemed to go over me as her ass slapped against my pelvis. Somehow I managed the whole thing into her little raspberry, slowly but surely. Little pin-pricks began tingling my shoulder, thigh, calf, the onset of an orgasm, but somehow, the sensation past her sphincter was not optimal. I pulled out and a couple milk duds dropped to the floor of the shower. I turned her around and kissed her hard, aggressively, our teeth briefly slashing each other. I slowly licked and sucked at her neck, squeezing myself, then sucking at her flaccid mother breasts that had a mere rind of a string somewhere deep in the center that kept her nipples attached to her torso. I felt it coming on as I pushed against her belly. I stood, pulled her down and rubbed against her soap-slick cleavage. She was ribby, like a gristly piece of meat, too ribby, too hard, though her breasts were soft and formless against my thighs.

I ran my fingers through her wet hair and pushed her wagging tongue against my nuts. She shook her head while her lips and teeth created suction against my dick bringing forth that familiar tingle. Up and down she worked me. I grabbed her head and capped my cock, pushing my semi-hard butter easily to the back of her throat. I pumped, she moaned, it was less effort for her this time. I pulled out and a quick squirt of semen hit against the side of her nose and dribbled towards her eye. The rest of my second load simply drizzled over my fist, which she licked, then pulled away, so that my near flaccid dick was back in her mouth. While I ran my cummy fingers through her wet hair, she worked my melting butter in her mouth with her tongue and teeth for a moment, then unceremoniously stood, gargled into the water stream, and stepped out of the shower while I began washing myself. Before I was soaped up, she was out of the bathroom all together.

While toweling off, I could hear her putting her kids to sleep. I heard her answering a couple questions with reassurance. I toweled off in front of the sink, in view of her panty clad, topless torso, mistily moving about the dank, dark motel room, lit only by the bathroom light softly filtering through the steam out the partially closed bathroom door. I briskly dried my hair once more, felt the cooler air against my skin, then felt her arms slide around me and her naked torso pressing against mine, and her breath moistening my chest. My dick was once again yearning, though I didn't think I had it in me to give another go. I wrapped my towel around me, went out to the car to get my overnight bag from the trunk.

She was in bed with her baby while I brushed my teeth. I could see in the mirror that she was spooning around the child, her small feet rustling under the shiny, polyester bedspread. I turned out the bathroom light, felt my way to the bed, and slid in behind her, my content dick falling asleep within the embrace of her buttocks.

I awoke to the sound of the door opening and shutting. I heard her say something to the kids about breakfast. I went back to sleep. Then a knock at the door. I opened it. There she was. Over the top of her blonde head, the sun streamed in. I saw in the courtyard of the motel a grassy playground. The kids were happily swinging. The two-year-old was in a sandbox. The Indiana sky was big and blue, occasional cloud. No traffic. No other cars except mine in the lot.

"You should really put something on before you answer the door," she smiled, handing me a hot coffee.

"You seem life-like," I told her.

She pushed me back inside and stepped in after me. The reality of the evening before and the kids and all this morning hit me. She opened the drapes and the sun streamed in. She was in the same jeans, but in a linen shirt with a collar. The room was moist, revealing she had spent time with the kids in the shower. She opened a window to let in some air. I could almost see myself with her.

"I don't know your story," she said. "But the kids and I are grateful for the room and breakfast in the lobby, though I hope we didn't annoy the hindu guy too much."

"You're really a great fuck," I said, sliding the fingers of one hand between the buttons of her blouse and resting my morning wood against her ass. "You must have a story."

"You want me to start?"

I put my coffee on the table, and kissed her from behind just beneath her ear. "Yes," I said, groping her with one hand. "Let's start something."

She walked to the bed the boys had used and sat next to me with one hand on my boner while I sipped coffee.

"My husband disappeared after a camping trip a few years ago, my job as a key-punch operator at a potato combine was eliminated, and last week we lost our house. I had too much pride to apply for food stamps, but now I think I've swallowed more than pride."

She smiled. I finished my coffee and lay back while she continued to stroke me.

"You're an incredible cocksucker. You should be proud of that." I told her.

She kneeled down and, licking me, said, "I just need money for the kids."

"OK."

I lay still, she worked me with her mouth this way and that. That suction thing with her lips and teeth following a ribbon of saliva and nerves on the underside of my shaft. I came on myself, dabbed my finger in it and stroked her hair.

She kissed the inside of my thigh. "We need money."

I sat up, walked over to my pants and counted $74. I turned and gave her $52.

"Thanks," she said. "This will get us back to Chicago. My family is there." We stood in the morning light looking at each other. "What will you do today?"

I shrugged.

"You should probably jump in the shower."

When I got out, no one was in the room. I looked out the window and they were no longer in the playground. I imagined them shuffling back downtown to the station, the five-year-old dragging that pale blue diaper bag. I considered looking for them with the car, but instead fell back into bed feeling empty but serene. I dreamt of dinosaurs roaming about aimlessly, in flat, empty fields, occasionally copulating.

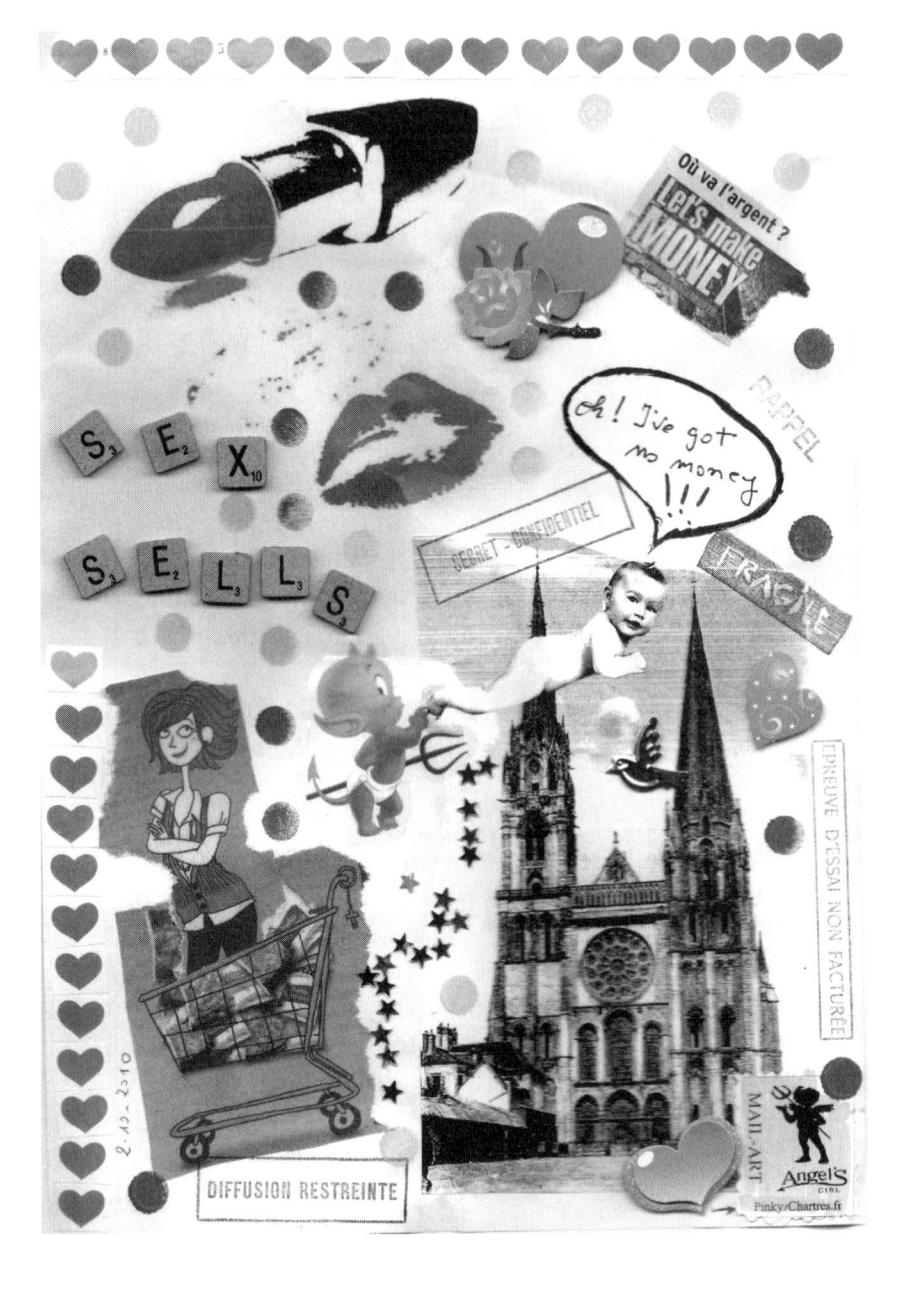

AN EASTER MEMORY
JOHN BAYLES

Today was Easter. It's the holiest day of the year for a lot of people, but not for me — I went out and got drunk and then had sex with a twenty-one-year-old. I'm thirty-one.

It used to have meaning, when I was younger, and when my cousins would come up to the city of Birmingham to swim in our pool and Peter would body slam me in the shallow end and hold me under water for what seemed like forever. (Back then, I never realized how much he resembled Cheech from Cheech and Chong and I never thought about him smoking weed and taking my father to a Steely Dan concert. I once took Peter to my pot dealer's house and saw him hit a big red plastic bong. That was a good Easter weekend.)

They would eat ham and turkey and cranberry sauce and go shopping at the mall. There was no mall where they were from. It was always special for them; to be able to go to one location and find all of the things they wanted under a single roof; there were over seventy stores in the Galleria in Hoover and each and every one of them posed a new shopping experience for my relatives from Eclectic, Alabama.

Easter. I think Easter was the last time I went to church, maybe twelve years ago — excluding Christmas Mass with Mary, which didn't really count because I'm not Catholic and I had no idea what I was listening to or what I was doing. Stand. Kneel. Stand. Sit. Kneel. Stand. And then there was communion — but I couldn't take part — I was a heathen in the Catholic Church's eyes. When communion was called, the entire pew got up and made their way to the pulpit and I was left sitting by myself. But when I turned my head I saw someone else sitting alone and we gave each other a nod as if to say, "Yep — I wouldn't be here if I didn't have to either."

I loved Mary. I loved her a lot. She was the first girl I tried to be a real boyfriend to; the first girl I honestly thought might end up being my bride — might end up taking my last name.

Who am I kidding, though. She would never have taken my last name. She was way too liberal for that. She would have insisted her last name remained to ensure her identity, to cement her role in the relationship as care taker, as mother. Well, really just to proclaim to the world that she didn't have to take a man's name.

She was from Massachusetts.

I used to hate fucking Mary. Well, not really the fucking part. That was fine and all, but it was the fact that she always had to cum. I mean, guys always have to cum. The ladies though, they should just be happy and thankful and that should be enough some of the time. Maybe they fake it every now and then, too, just to appease. But Mary was a different story. She would stay on top of me and press my finger to her clit and I would be forced to rub and rub until she came. At first, I didn't mind. It was fun. But after a year it got old as hell.

One night when I was feeling pretty good about my masculinity, I decided to just resist and pulled away and rolled over and muttered something about not being able to see straight and that I was dizzy. The next thing I knew she was no longer in bed and had retreated to the bathroom and I could hear her moaning, finishing the job herself without me. When she returned to bed I was appalled, and I made sure she knew it. She was all like, "I'm sorry, I just had to. I didn't think it would be a big deal."

Truth is, it wasn't. It wasn't at all.

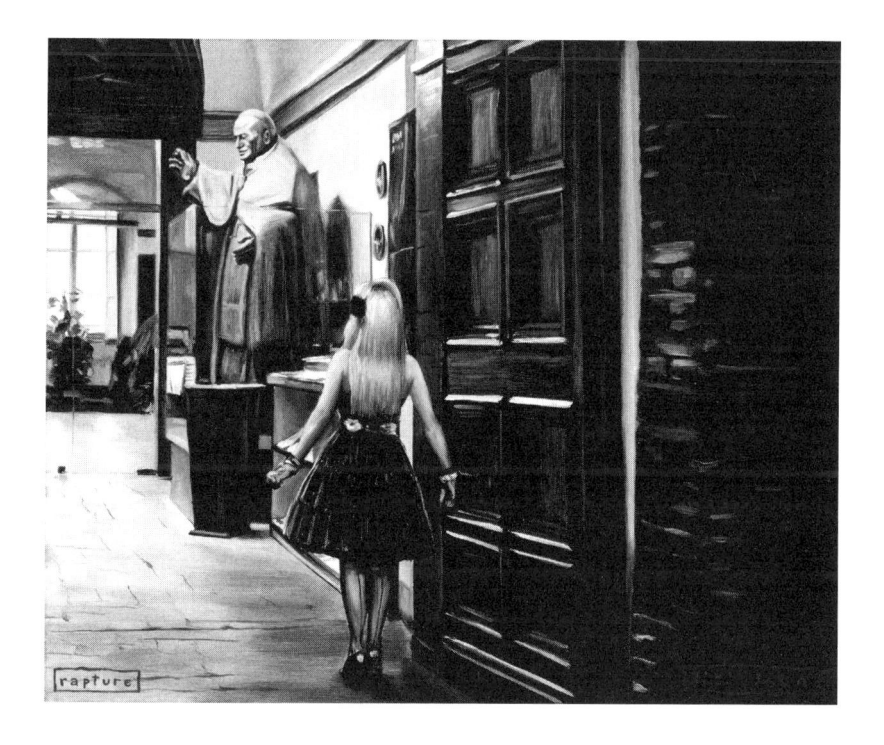

GIRL IN A BOX
ANNA MOCKLER

Helen sits on the stool by the windows full of sky, reading the *World Book* encyclopedia. She marks passages she doesn't understand with red pencil. Later Maurice, her lawyer, will explain them. Sometimes she crawls inside her sleeping bag, terrified by all the empty space. She doesn't want to get things wrong.

It's bad to get things wrong.

That's when you have to go inside the box.

Jesse petted her legs while he laid her in the box. Margaret folded Helen's arms. "Yes," she said, "you listen to Jesse. You're safe here. Anything could happen out there. Young girl like you? Want to be very very careful."

Couldn't be more careful than inside the box. That's where you can't do anything wrong. Long as you lie still inside the box, only knocking on the lid when you have to make water, you're not doing anything wrong. Can't be punished for what happens while you're inside. That's the rule. Longer you stay in, cleaner your record when you come out. Whole yards and cellars of bad deeds are wiped clean by long periods inside the box.

Now she was outside the box all day long. Memorizing heroes of the Revolution. Walking city streets, swinging her arms and laughing.

Opening her mouth and trying it. Before, it was, "My Lord is dead and how shall I laugh?" Now it was "He saith among the trumpets, Ha, ha."That was how Maurice laughed: he'd be talking along and suddenly end a sentence with Ha, ha. The boys who used to throw tomatoes at the fence ran off laughing like crows. Sometimes couples close together laughed under dusky skies, a sound that stirred the devil in his lodging.

Helen turns all this in her mind, walking. Maurice sent her to Claudia Bowdoin, the therapist, first thing. "Need to get your self-confidence up," he said. There was so much to relearn. How to walk without knocking people down; how to speak; how to do business — "Maurice will show you that," said Claudia with her lips inside her mouth. Claudia said there were living people everywhere who said there was no God. Said it right out loud and nothing struck them dead. Claudia said God helps them who help themselves. Maurice's secretary Marileen said God was in everything equally. Maurice said it was all a crock, a fairytale to keep the people quiet when their stomachs growled.

Everyone agrees that what Jesse and Margaret did to her was very bad, but: "They were just misguided," said Marileen.

"They took the Bible like a law book," said Maurice, "and, see, law bends to situations, you got to interpret it, which is just what most people don't understand."

"They thought their personal truth was the only truth," Claudia told her. Claudia said that people take what's inside them and imagine it's outside them — that way they're not responsible. Take their inner goodness and call it God; bundle their bad impulses and say it's all the Devil.

"Where does what's inside them come from in the first place?" Helen asked. If God and the Devil were just ways to look at things, what was the point of her life until now?

Maurice said people had been wasting their time asking that since forever; meanwhile time was going past and death sneaking up on you.

As she coffee-strode the streets, sanctity poured from an upstairs window: "Jesus Christ oh God oh Jesus!" The flat hand of the Lord pinned her against a wall, it always did, until the wailing ended. Listen, you miserable sinner. Here is the devil. Everywhere among you he walks.

Nobody in the new world seemed to know a thing about the devil. Marileen took her to lunch when Maurice was out of town: "The more you fear your shadow side the more visible it becomes," she assured her earnestly. "Maurice embraces and admits his own darkness. That's what makes him so free," she said.

Helen asked Claudia Bowdoin why no one knew Satan. "What does that mean to you?" she asked.

Helen burrowed in the wing chair set in the windowless corner of Claudia's office. "It's off balance," she said at last. "One time Zinnia had a calf born with only two legs."

"Okay, go with that! What happened to the calf?"

"Margaret chopped off its head and burned it."

Often Claudia urges her to visualize her severed past. Obedient Helen squinges her eyelids to make darkness but all she comes up with is wind in the pine branches. The office air chokes imagination. She hates the smell and feel of imprisoned air.

"That's good!" Claudia was all excited. "Feel strongly!"

Helen drew her legs back. Excited people were kittle-kattle. You never knew what they'd be up to next.

"What else do you care about?"

Helen thought. She sat upright, hands in her lap, legs crossed at the ankle as Marileen taught her: "Otherwise everyone can see what you had for breakfast." Helen marveled at the new world's ability to see through flesh. She couldn't even see through a shirt, herself. She was still sitting when Claudia leaned back in her chair, a chin-length strand of pale hair between her fingers. "That's it for today," she said. "For next time, I want you to remember, really remember, what happened between you and Jesse." Claudia believes the past must be recalled or it will sabotage the present.

Claudia the inexorable, her blunt fingers parting Helen's quiet, intent on rooting out the darkness in her and bringing it to light. Helen goes along with what's expected of her. She always has. Only the occasional afternoon, her head at the bottom of the sleeping bag, could betray her. And no one knew about those.

That afternoon, her head muffled in goosedown and the world dark around her, she remembered.

It was the first winter she was with them? The second? She came in early from evening milking, Zinnia and Chrysanthemum holding back for calves that grew inside them. She heard them talking in the parlor. She watched them through the pantry knothole.

Jesse said, "She could be the one. The one Christ's born through, this time. Be the right age."

"Hmmm," said Margaret. Spat on her darning hook. "Hand me those shears, Brother. Long as we keep her safe. Body's got a hundred doors on it, every one swung wide to the Devil. Only sure lock's the word of the Lord."

"Amen," said Jesse and sat silent, his socks against the woodstove.

Couldn't remember Jesse without remembering Margaret: standing in maple shade, arms across her breast, veins standing out on her ice-blue eyes like a scared cow's.

"Don't even think about it," Margaret said, though Helen hadn't even looked at the fence or the gate or the latch. "You are possessed, certainly," she said.

In the kitchen, feet planted either side of the stool, watching Helen rinse the breakfast things in hot vinegar and water. "What I don't see, the Lord does. You better take care," said Margaret, "lest death catch you in sin, the devil toss you over his shoulder and dump you in perdition."

Early mornings, Margaret scowling. Flames jumping in the woodstove, sour milk in the nostrils, chickens squawking on the doorstep, stink of manure from gumboots in the woodshed.

Once Helen tried to look over the fence—not climb even, just look. Margaret took her out back. "Stand there," she said. Laid four chickens, one after another, on the chopping log and clove their necks with a hatchet, one quick blow, four times. "I told you, keep away from that fence," she said.

Margaret's hands were flour and salt on Helen's naked body. Grunting. "Get into the box," shoving her. The box had just grown too small. Margaret shoved and folded. "In." At last Helen lay pinched in the box. Margaret outside, huffing.

Chronology. You list the things that happened one after another according to the day they happened on, which has a name and a number. This year has a number, and so did the one before, and so on and so on back until before Christ was born. (Things were very bad, then.)

Two houses before Jesse and Margaret, the woman locked Helen in a closet when she was bad. Before that, she remembered huddling on a concrete garage floor between a lawnmower and electric hedge shears. The metal teeth would come to life and grind her up, the blades would mow her down if she moved an inch, they said, and closed the door and locked it. That's how she learned to… not to wet the bed. It was so luxurious, lying in your own warm water, inside a world you'd made yourself, and warm for once. But no, not if they snatched her from the lovely sheets and put her under bright lights that showed the hedge trimmer inching up every time you closed your eyes, no. She learned to hold herself closed.

So much trouble from between her legs. Jesse hollered and prayed over her, trying to grab the Devil out. Helen lay on the tile bathroom floor the night the Devil started dripping out. Jesse and Margaret knelt in the parlor shouting, "Praise God! From whom all blessings flow!" Helen lapped blood from her thigh. Put the Devil inside her again. She lay on the cold floor, running her tongue against her teeth, until Margaret diapered her in rags.

No. Her life won't submit to chronology. The houses before Jesse and Margaret all run together. She hadn't remembered the day the Lord showed them to come and get her until Margaret sat her down in the kitchen with potatoes to peel, knowing what the Devil found for idle hands. Margaret said, "You didn't always live with us. We went into the town," she said. "You don't need to know its name, it's a place of vice — and found you trying to climb inside an icebox, nobody watching but a big yellow dog. Cardboard over half the windows anyhow, what could they have seen if they'd looked? Jesse grabbed you by your legs, you didn't say a word. We walked slowly down that street, case anybody thought we'd done something we shouldn't, but the angel of the Lord kept his wings over us, and no one appeared to bear witness for your people. Only the yellow dog whined after you from behind the fence."

But when did Margaret tell her all this? Helen can't remember.

Helen had been with them three winters? four? when the devil got so strong inside her Jesse girded up his loins to fight him where he lived. "Sister," he said, "go down the stream and get us some peppermint." Margaret scuttled out the door, her body rippling with the speed of her passage.

Helen and Jesse were alone in the bedroom they three shared every night. "Do I have to get in the box?" Helen asked.

Jesse shook his head. "You got the devil in you. I got to get him out."

"Where in me?"

"I'll show you," Jesse patted the bed. "First, you got to lie down here."

"Where you and Margaret sleep?"

"Here, I said." Jesse petted her ankles. "These bad legs keep trying to run away."

"It was only the kitten; I was afraid he might forget to come back and run against some people would hurt it; I just wanted to keep the kitten safe, Jesse."

Jesse stroked her calves, circled her scabby kneecaps with his thick fingers. "Bad, bad legs," he intoned. "Hush up now, Helen," his beard trickling down her neck, "you don't want me to do this because you're resisting the Good Lord, you're taken over by the Evil One."

Helen nodded. She clamped her lips shut.

It had been a long day, waking to do the milking, scrubbing the kitchen, tomato soup for lunch, sterilizing all the canning jars before they were carried down cellar and arranged on shelves with hundreds of years-past clean jars. Helen drifted off while Jesse rubbed her thighs, chanting under his breath: "Out bad devil, rise, rise from this body."

He pulled her dress up around her armpits. "Lord, reach down your hand and cast the devil from this naked body before you." Jesse's hands pushed her thighs apart: "Don't you resist the Lord or the devil will get a hold on you nothing can undo."

He stroked her wide-spread thighs until Helen was warm through. He prayed: "Anoint this body and possess its undying soul." His hands pressed her throat, once, briefly, the way he could strangle her with just one of those hands.

Jesse rubbed her thin chest like he worked over the calf was born too soon. He was making her strong against the devil. His right hand between her legs. "These're how I know the devil's getting strong in you. These hairs? Mark of the devil." He held her pelvis in his palm. He stroked holy healing into her so she squirmed with its power.

Jesse stood up. "Your body's trying to side with the devil." He doubled baling twine from a coil in his overall pocket; made her arms and legs fast to the four-poster that dripped with yellowed nightshirts.

The hands came upstream from her ankles like flood-water cresting, working with the lay of the hairs but always moving higher. Jesse put a calloused hand over her mouth: "Now Helen, you got to behave here." She nodded, peering between his fingers; she tried not to squirm as he rubbed her nipples that stood up the way they did in cold weather; she used everything she had to keep the devil from churning her around. It was much harder than Sundays, when she sat in a straight chair from sun-up to sundown while Jesse and Margaret took it in turns to read the Bible to her.

His hairy mustache, his long gray beard, tickling back and forth in the soft place under her arms; she held the devil still. He nibbled at her little breasts like he could get milk out of them. Her nipples were January, while the rest of her dripped sweat on sheets she'd have to wash, later, and wring them out and hang them up to dry. He hollered: "Out devil! Out!" and unbuttoned his overalls and out leaped what was huge, purple, hammer-headed. Jesse had the devil in him, too, she marveled.

But the devil in her twitched against the damp sheets, against the baling twine, against his moustache tickling her chest. Jesse pried between her legs with his thick blunt fingers, dirt under broken nails, until he found the place he had to get into. He stuck one finger inside a hole she'd never known she had. Moved it up and down. This was the pain the martyrs suffered.

He withdrew his finger and she lay gasping, not saying a word, mind, sweat cooling on her body. He made the sign of the cross above her and wiggled two fingers inside her: "You feel the devil now," he said. "You feel him spitting at me."

She got used to it after a while. Except his fingers pushed all the juice out of her body from where it was supposed to be, no place for it to go except out her skin.

The winter before, Jesse'd reached inside Zinnia and turned her baby calf so it came out right. His fingers far inside her, to grab that devil by the neck and turn him.

He put a knee either side of her hips and held his purple hammer and shoved it where the Devil spat. Screaming was the side door where the devil loved to enter unexpected. She lay still as still while he shoved that long hook into and out of her, over and over, devil-grabbing.

She didn't know how long it went on; the sweat pouring down her eyes, her muscles twitching, her tongue firm between her teeth; sunlight poured through his beard; he cried: "Out, devil, in, begone, out, God, in, Christ Jesus Christ oh Lord oh Christ oh my Lord!" and fell down on her. His beard scratched her throat. He lay there still as still while the sweat cooled on them.

After a while he stood up. He wiped himself dry with Margaret's nightshirt. "That's Devil's blood," he said. "I got him a mortal good one, that time. Almost yanked him out. You were good," he said, "there's no way he could have sneaked back in. You kept real still and didn't shout and that's the way to beat the devil at his own game." He untied her: "Wipe yourself. Then get in the box. You'll be safe there, likely the devil's sneaking around, trying to get back in while you're weak."

She rolled off the bed. She crawled into the box. He said, "I'm locking you in, case the devil tries to pry it open with his horny claws. You stay safe in there. Pray for your immortal soul. Good work we done today, getting the devil dislodged. Prayer's best now."

The door closed. The stairs creaked beneath his work-boots. Helen lay inside the wooden box and imagined there was room enough to fold her arms around her weak, cleansed body, but the box was tight now she was growing so fast. She lay on her back, arms at her sides, staring at the boards four inches from her face.

She fell asleep and dreamed the heavenly host descended and baptized her in the blood of the Lamb. Angels sang from the pine tree outside the window.

A few years later, Jesse lost interest in the project. He must have got the devil out? Holy days came around more often, found him and Margaret side by side on the plush sofa in the parlor, shouting and singing the afternoon long. Helen milked, she fed the chickens, she gathered eggs and berries and herbs for the teas that purified their blood. She barely turned her head when Jesse's voice rose among the dustballs in ecstatic praise: "Oh God oh Lord oh my God oh Jesus!" Often when Jesse summoned her to prayer, she fell asleep from sitting down, woke to find him lashing her thighs with a hazel switch. "Bad! Bad legs!" as he striped her, blue-black, white; blue-black, white. Margaret sat, the while, among cushions, shouting psalms so loudly the cows bellowed in response.

Wind and laughter came through the open windows, knocking the *World Book* to the floor. Helen wriggled from the sleeping bag. Darkness lay on the city; a thousand lights rose up in mute protest, striping the room blue-black and white.

She mashed her nose against the cold windowpane and breathed, fogging the whole world. It was the first time she could remember it, all of it; Jesse and Margaret didn't take her memory and put it in the box the police burned, she had it, she had it in her mind, she breathed and disappeared the world, inhaled and resurrected it.

She laughed in the empty room, the walls amazed at her loudness: "He saith among the trumpets, Ha Ha!"

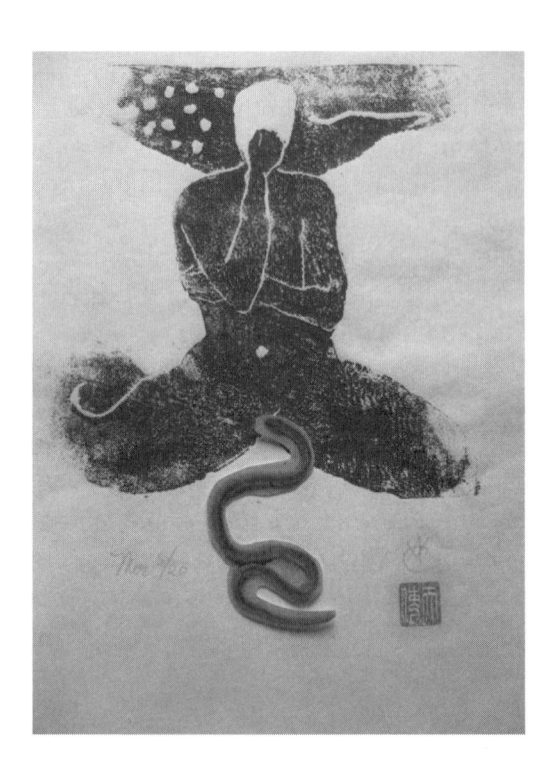

TRUST
JENNIFER HILL

The girl's thumbs pressed on the edge of the new bowl, petalling the edge. Her friend sat on a bench in the corner, elbows on knees, shoulders rounded. A radio corked out jazz from the local public broadcasting station. Pipes dripped above the boy, and their rain just missed his head and hunched form, splatting on the wood and peeling red paint of the bench. He wished he could smell her from this distance, but was too far away. She smelled of honeysuckle and lilacs, dry hair and the toffees she always ate. She was the sort of girl you wanted to put your arm around even if you weren't in love with her, just so you could borrow the trust in her bones. He ran his finger through the water on the bench and blended her initials with his. The girl had her hair pulled up, and he could see the hollows of her neck. He wanted to kiss her there, but he hadn't even gotten the courage to take her hand on the long walks they took after school. The girl turned and looked at him, held up a clay wadded thumb and waggled it at him, the song of her laughter ringing out in purples and blues, the rainy greens of a pigeon's feathers. He closed his eyes just to see it.

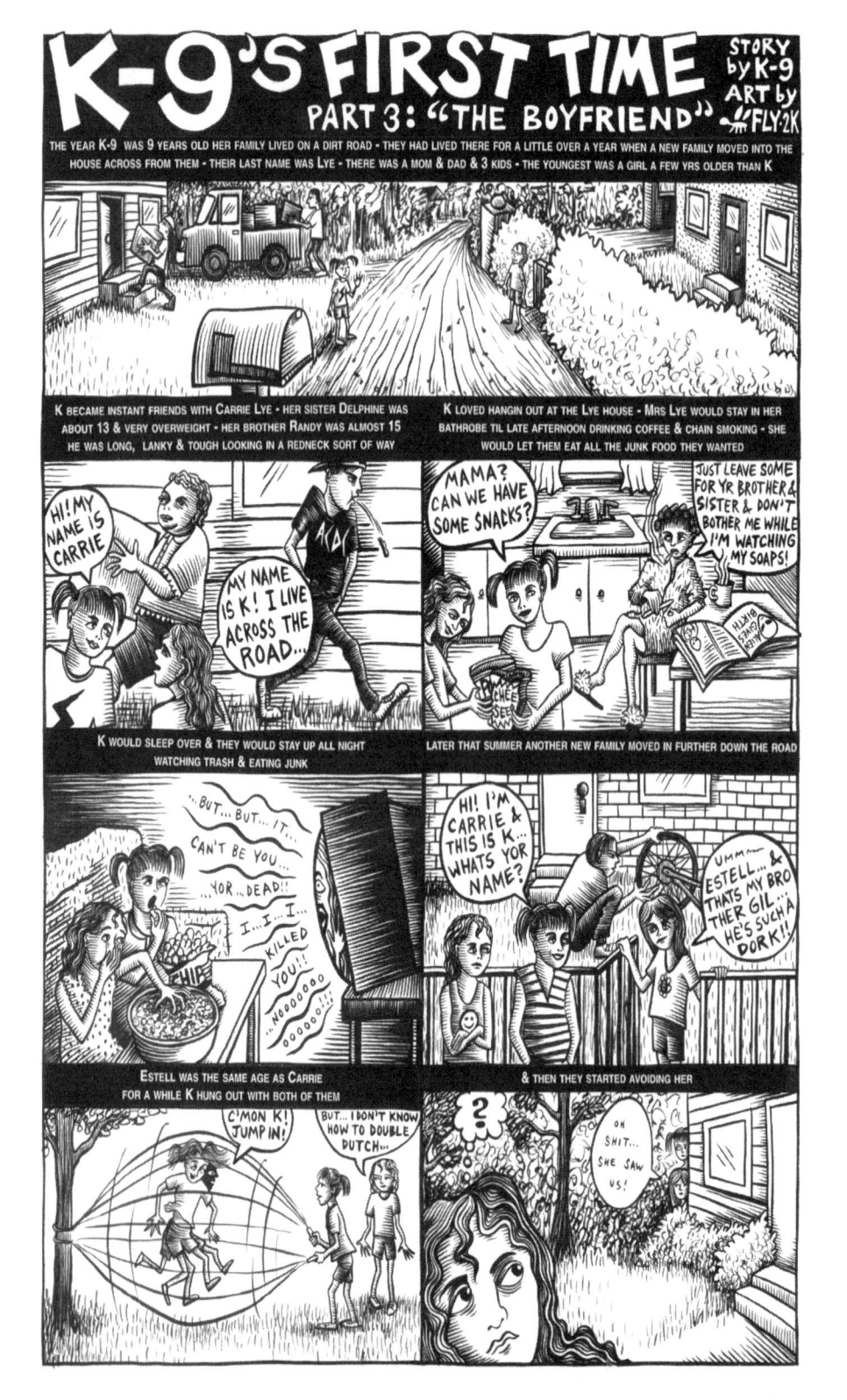

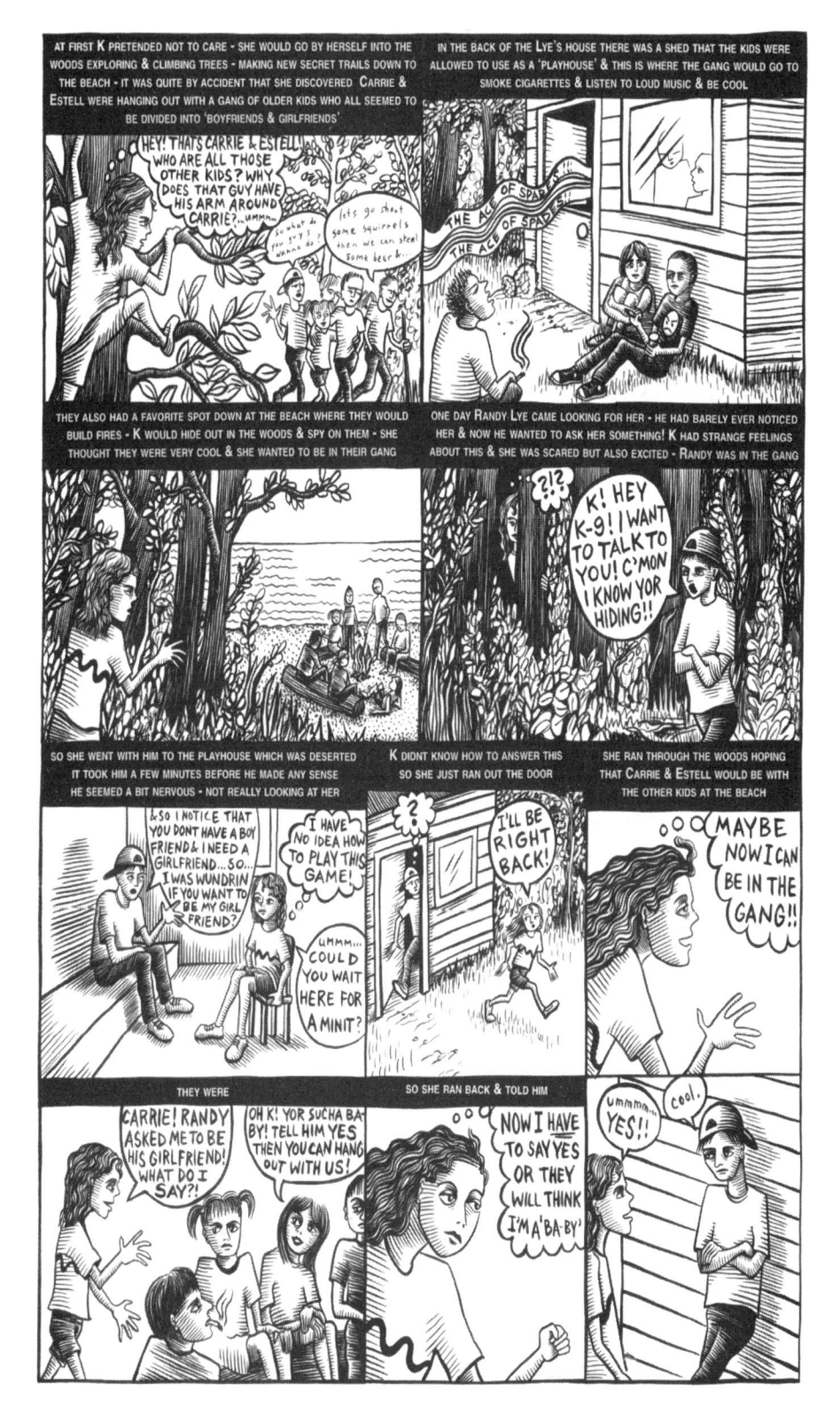

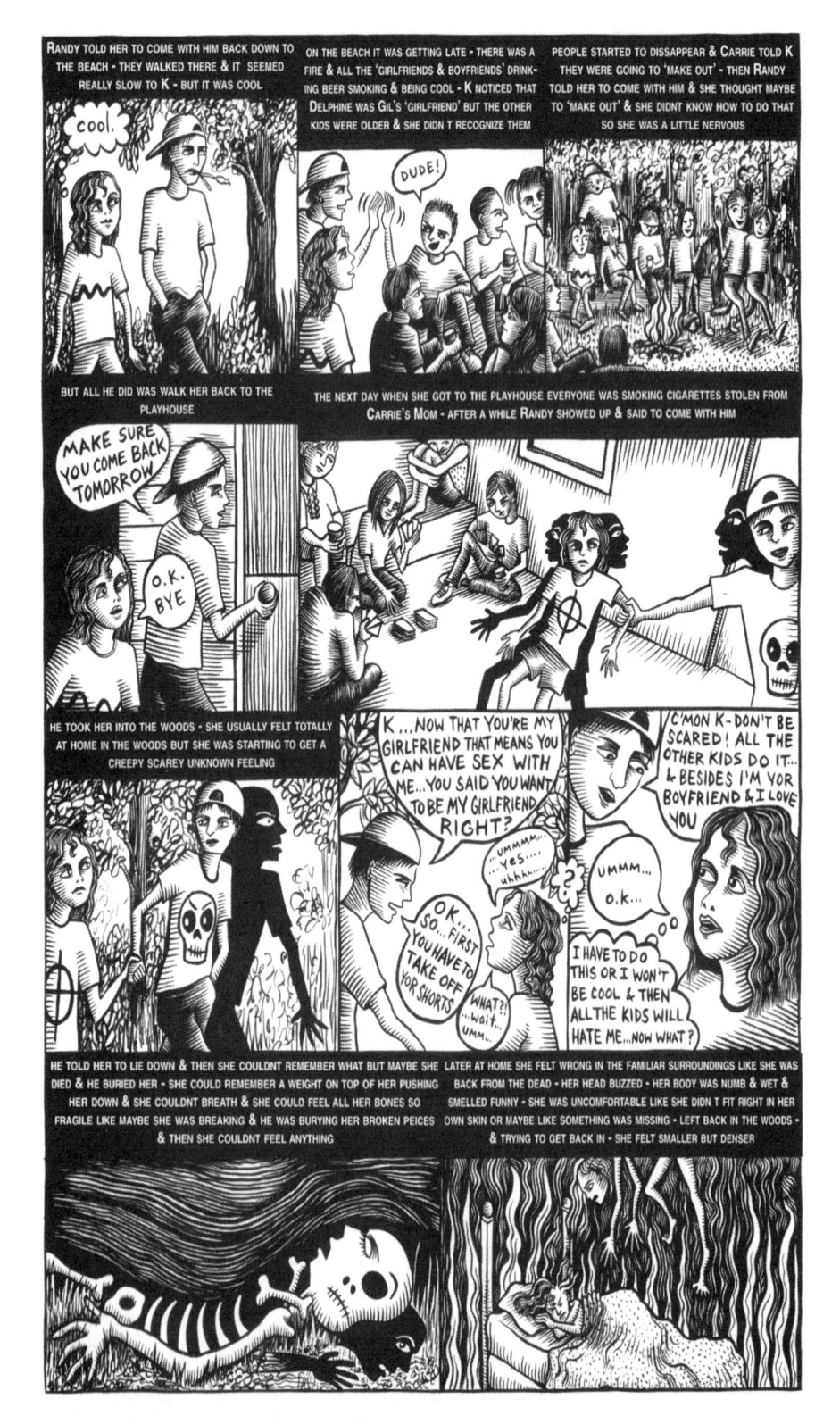

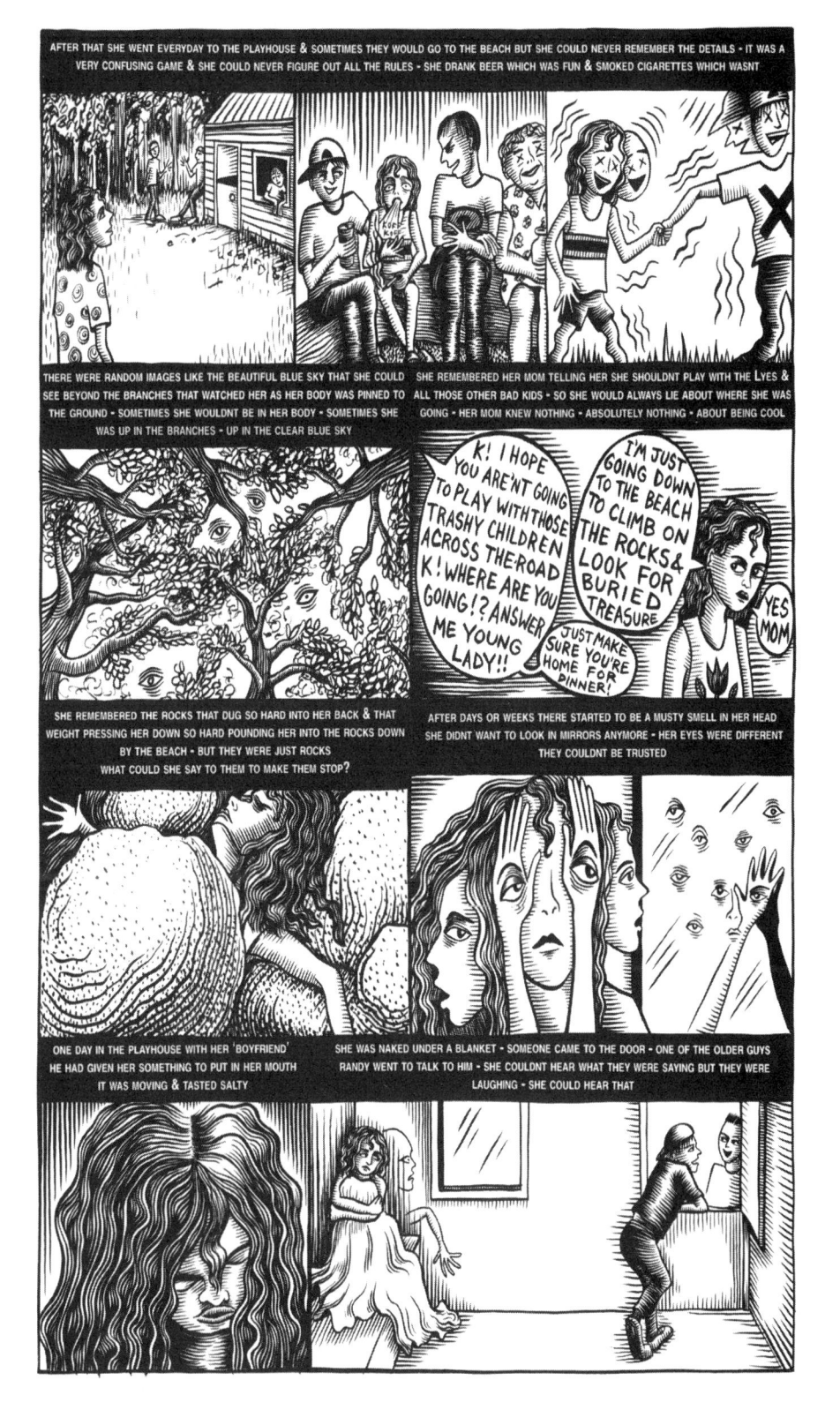

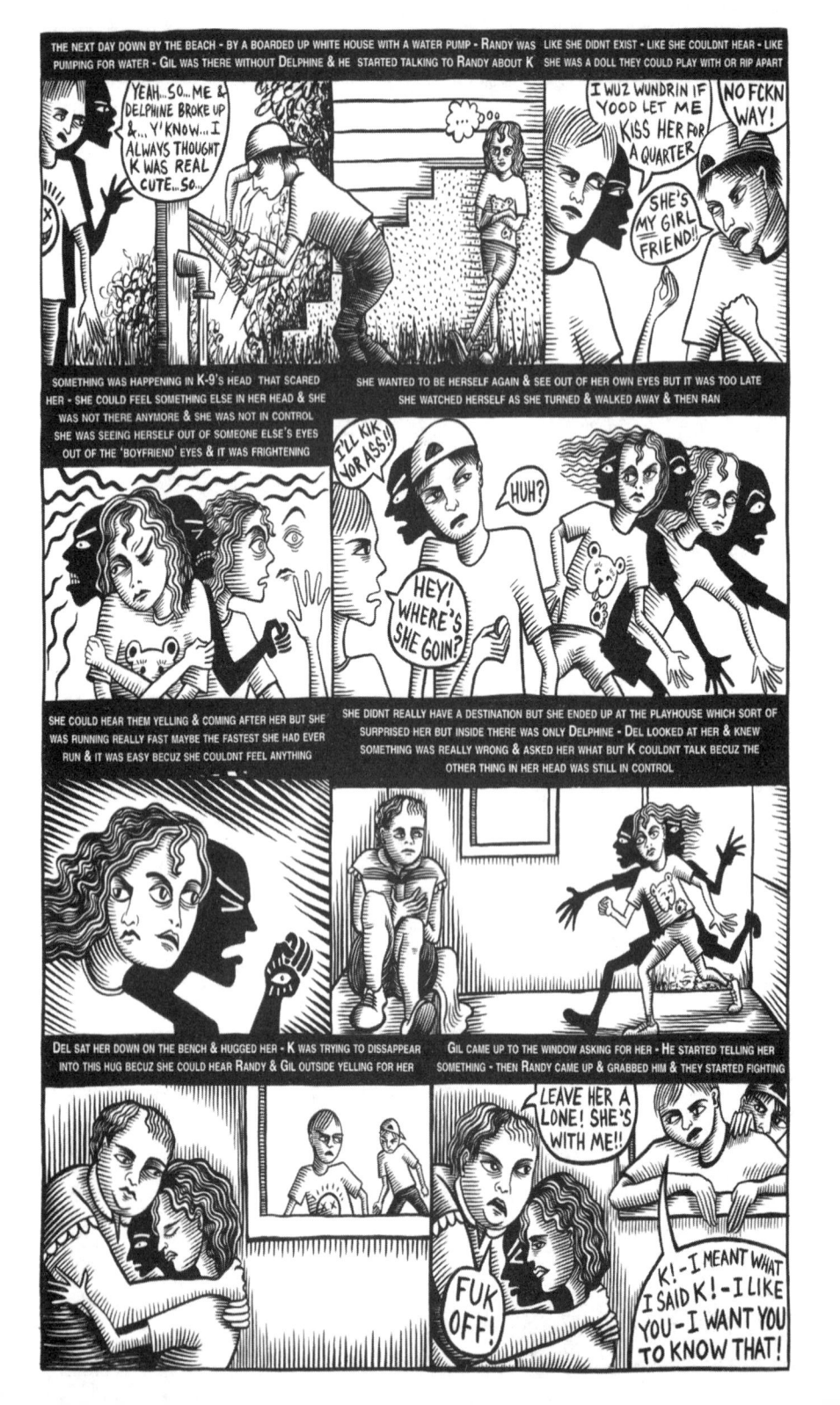

DELPHINE SAID SOMETHING ABOUT SHE SHOULD BE FLATTERED THAT THESE GUYS WERE FIGHTING OVER HER BUT K DIDNT FEEL ANYTHING · THEN THERE WAS THE DIFFICULT JOURNEY GETTING HER NUMB BODY ACROSS THE STREET TO HER HOUSE HOPING NOT TO SEE ANY OF THE OTHER KIDS

SHE STAYED AWAY FROM THE PLAYHOUSE FOR THE REST OF THE SUMMER WHICH WAS ALMOST OVER ANYWAY · SHE WAS CAREFUL WHEN SHE WENT INTO THE WOODS OR TO THE BEACH · ALTHOUGH THE REST OF THE GANG SEEMED TO BE BREAKING UP & SHE BARELY EVER SAW THEM

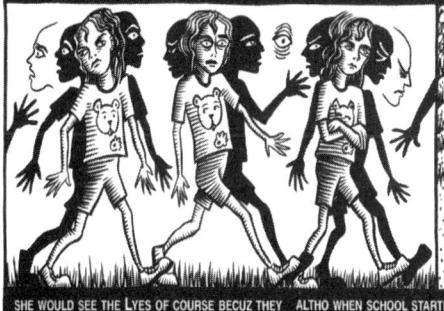

SHE WOULD SEE THE LYES OF COURSE BECUZ THEY LIVED ACROSS THE STREET BUT NO ONE MENTIONED ANYTHING THAT HAD HAPPENED THAT SUMMER AT LEAST NOT TO HER

ALTHO WHEN SCHOOL STARTED SHE STARTED TO HEAR RUMORS OF HER PROMISING CAREER AS A SLUT

THEN EVERYTHING CHANGED REALLY FAST WHEN HER DAD MADE THE ANNOUNCEMENT THAT ONCE AGAIN THEY WOULD BE MOVING

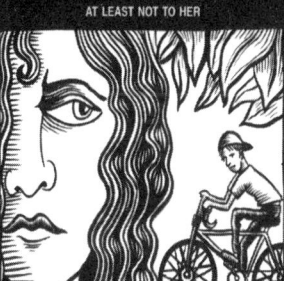

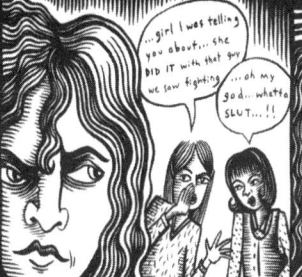

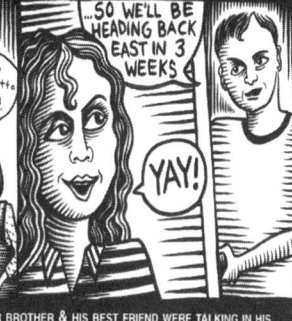

K-9 WAS SO HAPPY TO BE IN A NEW PLACE · SHE COULD FINALLY RELAX · IT SEEMED LIKE EVERYTHING WAS REALLY EASY AGAIN · SHE WAS BACK IN THE CITY LIVING BESIDE THE PROJECTS & FEELING MUCH SAFER · NOW SHE COULD JUST PLAY & FORGET THAT SHE HAD EVER BEEN A 'GIRLFRIEND'

BUT ONE DAY HER BROTHER & HIS BEST FRIEND WERE TALKING IN HIS ROOM & SHE OVERHEARD SOMETHING

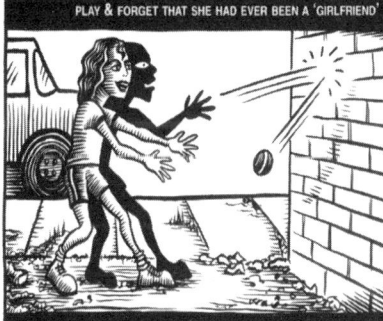

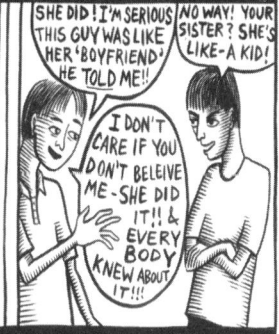

LATER SHE NOTICED HER BROTHER'S FRIEND LOOKING AT HER & SHE GOT THAT CREEPY SCAREY FEELING AGAIN ALTHOUGH BY NOW THIS FEELING WAS NOT UNKNOWN TO HER

SHE FELT THAT DARK EMPTY PRESSURE THAT MADE HER SMALL & DENSE THAT PRESSED INTO HER LIKE THAT ROCK PUSHING HER INTO SOMETHING SHE WANTED NO PART OF · SHE FELT THAT OTHER THING IN HER HEAD WANTING TO TAKE OVER

SO SHE BURIED THE FEELING SOMEWHERE IN HER MEMORIES BACKYARD & FIGURED THAT WAS THE END OF IT · NOT REALIZING THAT IT WOULD LATER GROW INTO SOMETHING BIGGER

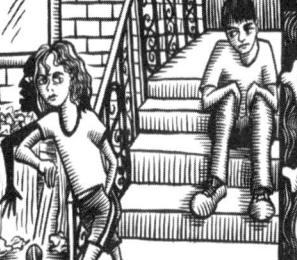

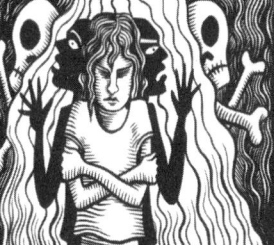

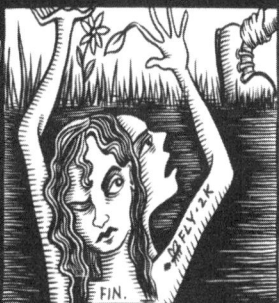

MY TVC15
JOSE PADUA

Leonard was not at all like me. Which, perhaps, was why he fascinated me so much. Because unlike me he was never able to lose his memory. No matter how far he traveled, his memory was with him. Lines from a popular song, a drop of liquid, a television program, a piece of furniture — the insignificant details and sentimental emotions always caught up with him in his universe.

To him the years he spent in the outside world were a blemish upon that universe. Every night he had gone to bed with Annalisa had darkened it. Every day when he hadn't used his imagination had diminished it. But as his universe collapsed, his memory expanded.

As for me, I learned to put my memories behind me. To build something with them, a monument which will speak of my heritage. And this history which I'm now writing, and with which I will soon be finished, will serve as my monument. A monument I can carry with me. A monument I can slip into the right hand drawer of a desk, or leave at the bottom of a duffel bag. A monument which will never harm me like the gun with which my great grandfather — and later my grandfather — killed themselves. And although I will know at all times where the monument is, I will never again think of what it says.

When Leonard got back home everything was the way he remembered it — the television, the stereo, the furniture.

The only difference being that although Lily and he were still married, it was Lemuel who was now, for lack of a better word, her lover. That and my four year old sister Marly.

Marly was a quiet child, and her eyes always seemed to follow you around the room like those of a suspicious cat. Still, Leonard saw that she was a beautiful little girl, looking exactly the way Lily did when she was that age. And though she would stare out into space when she wasn't staring at you, there were moments when she would abruptly run in the direction she was staring. As if there were something out there only she could see. When she'd get across the room she'd look around frantically — she was, in her own way, a very active child. Then rush back to where she'd been and once again stare across the room.

I was now seven years old and had gotten into the habit of watching television. I'd set myself in the middle of the living room, on my hands and knees, and gaze at the television for hours. What was on television didn't matter to me — Leonard could change channels in the middle of a program and I wouldn't even blink or show the slightest change in the expression on my face. Because although I was now aware of what was going on around me, I had no desire to take part in any of it.

Since the television was in the living room, which was now Leonard's room, he began watching it all the time. The show that interested him the most was *The Cosby Show*, because it presented what to him seemed the ideal situation for a young boy to grow up in.

Theo, the boy in the fictional Huxtable family, had parents who were both professionals. With his father being a doctor and his mother a lawyer, it was ensured that he would be well provided for. But what was more important was that Theo had not just one but four sisters. And so if things didn't work out with one of them, Leonard thought, Theo still had three others from which to choose, one of whom was bound to make a suitable mate. Though naturally he should sample each of them before making any kind of decision.

Leonard always thought that the perfect match in the family would be Theo and Denise. Although their personalities were rather different, Theo had a way of connecting with Denise that seemed more profound than with any of the other sisters. And although Leonard saw him getting his dick sucked by young Rudy, doing the six-pack with Sondra, and fucking Vanessa up the ass while playing with her ample breasts, Denise was the one he saw Theo going back to time and time again. She, of all his sisters, was the one Theo wanted the most. She was to him what Lily was to Leonard, the only difference being that Theo had alternatives, while Leonard did not.

After a time Leonard came to believe that it was his own fault that he lost Lily to Lemuel. When things had gotten difficult, he had failed to put the proper effort into their marriage and went so far as to completely abandon Lily for nearly five years. As he had been gone for such a long time, he couldn't blame either Lily or Lemuel for taking up with each other. Because, like Leonard, they had no alternatives. If only their parents had had more children, Leonard thought, things might have been different. And he wouldn't have to spend the rest of his days without a wife.

Shortly after Leonard returned to town Lily got a job as a waitress at a nightclub on Fort Myers Beach. Lemuel, who was still at the greyhound track, had decided not to go back to school, having taken an interest in dogs. He wanted to breed them, which was something he could learn about from being there at the track.

For Leonard it was enough to stay home and take care of the kids. He stayed home all the time now — he never left the apartment. He had concluded that in the last five years, from the time he set out west hitch-hiking to the end of that long bus ride, he had seen enough of the world. At any rate, all that he needed to experience first-hand.

He began living through Marly and me. He'd watch us all the time, hoping we'd begin to pay attention to each other. Which, to his disappointment, we never did. The closest we'd get to interacting was when somehow the same toy attracted our attention. This was a rare occurrence, since all our toys — the teddy bear, the fire truck, the Barbie doll — usually just lay on the floor unused.

Sometimes Leonard would put the teddy bear in my hand, then point to Marly, pulling at my sleeve in an attempt to get me to bring it to her. I'd look in her direction, usually towards her feet, but would never approach her. Other times Leonard would try to get us to roll the fire truck back and forth to each other, but he'd always end up rolling it back and forth himself as we wouldn't even look at the truck or at each other. And instead would merely gaze at the floor.

Leonard tried playing tapes or records. But music didn't affect us any more than silence. He'd play the old Tommy James and The Shondells tape. And when "I Think We're Alone Now" came on he'd look at my eyes, then at Marly's, hoping that somehow this song would inspire us. All he saw were our blank stares which to him revealed not a trace of recognition or understanding.

Things went on this way for a long time and he resigned himself to the idea that Marly and I would never take an interest in one another. But one day the following spring Lily came home with the news that she was pregnant. Leonard was happy for her, and for himself as well, as he believed that the presence of another child would be the catalyst that would finally bring Marly and I together.

Lily and Lemuel immediately left the apartment. Leonard thought they were going out to celebrate down by the river, but that wasn't the case at all.

As they shut the door behind them Leonard began to hear the sound of rain falling on the window, followed, in the distance, by the sound the thunder. He turned out the lights, lay back on the sofa and closed his eyes as the sounds grew louder. Despite all the flashing lights and noise, Marly and I, sitting by him on the floor, didn't cry, didn't even stir. This, he believed, was a good sign.

He clasped his hands together and dreamed of the day when Marly and I would make love for the first time just as Lily and he had some fourteen years ago.

He could see it all very clearly, and it wouldn't be long, he thought, before Marly and I saw it too: Rudy, in the sixty-nine position with Theo, sucking on his dick as if it were a popsicle; Sondra, the most conservative of the girls, lying beneath him and moaning, "Oh God, oh my dear dear God"; Vanessa, rubbing his cum over her breasts, then licking her fingers clean; and Denise, after having sucked him off, washing her mouth out with a steady stream of his urine. With the images of these fictional lovers in mind, he believed that Marly and I would create our own world and make our own way within it. Creating new legends, building new shrines, new monuments, and devising new ideas.

He believed that one day we would walk out into the storm to be by the river. That rolling around naked in the shallow water, caressing, kissing, we would spill our love over one another. That the day would come when our screams, the first sounds ever to leave our mouths, blend in with the clamor of thunder. When our bodies, in a fearless act of discovery, flash with each burst of light.

He believed that the day would come when Marly declares "I want you" as I push my middle finger in her ass —"I love you" as I slide my thumb inside her pussy. When gasping for air, she rises, then settles her young head between my legs to suck as if sucking and breathing were the same. When finally, with her mouth full of my cum, she brings her face up to mine.

He believed that the day would come soon, when in our perfect world we'd feel nothing but the gentle gift of rain in all its forms. That and the touch of skin upon skin.

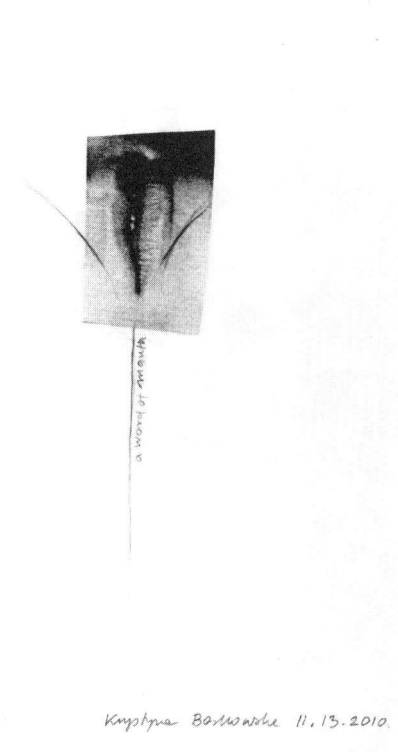

Krystyna Barkowske 11.13.2010.

PIN-UP
KEVIN RIORDAN

Hank LeBlanc missed his evening train and had an hour to kill, not that anyone would miss him. Even when he was married, his wife had been prone to start things without him — all kinds of things. From Aaron to Zachary and back.

Knocking around the moth-eaten fringe of the Loop, he was intrigued by a dimly lit doorway:

BOO
Novel

read the neon legend. Up close, he saw that the 'KS' of the word Books had been converted to squab roosts, and the 'ties' of Novelties had burned out, evidently in flames.

Inside, the few furtive patrons looked like try-outs for the Pink Panther. The racks of magazines seemed to be in a strange language that barely registered as erotic. *Modern Sunbather, Young Equestrian, Biter's Digest, Red Patent, Screw* and *Sexology* vied for space with *Dungeon Times.*

He grabbed a copy of *Playboy* without really looking at it, and approached the counter as if he were buying fish-skins or Zig-Zags at the local Rexall, feigning interest in the objects hanging behind the oily clerk. Maybe BOO was the right sign at that.

"You sell some interesting novelties here, I see," he muttered, in a hurry for the plain brown wrapper.

The clerk leered down at what was in fact the current issue of *Playpen* and said, "Oh yeah, we can float your boat all right," pushing a button that spun part of the pegboard partition to reveal another display of novelties, most prominent among them a big pair of leather diapers, along with saddles, harness, an inflated extended family, a mouth in a box, and what he recognized from the local confessional as a misericordia.

As he was about to express an interest only in the magazine interviews, a bell over the door rang and a statuesque brunette shimmied in, bearing a steaming Styrofoam cup.

"Montana, you're a sight for four eyes. You brought me coffee."

"Chicken soup, that's what you're getting, look at you, you don't look like you'll survive the week." At the appearance of a woman, all the men stiffened in one way or another. "Speaking of weak, what's with Casper Milquetoast here," she added discreetly.

"Special customer here, a regular little lost lamb."

Hank was speechless, in part because he'd never seen a woman who could carry the Grand Tetons around in her sweater with such aplomb. It was like watching the wombats waddle up Noah's gangplank.

"Aw, does baby want a binky? Show him the pacifiers, Lou."

Lewd Lou obliged with a drawer of paraphernalia, diaper pins like hypodermics, outsized pacifiers in a bewildering assortment of colors and shapes. My god, was that supposed to be a….

Hank hit the floor like it was a revolving door, the blackout whooshing him in.

He came to with a terrific sneeze, expanding the cloud of talcum powder he found himself in. His disorientation was complete for a moment until an elevated train rumbled past the window. Was he behind bars? He reached out then jumped back as he bumped a mobile with pink and blue plastic milkmen. He was in a room above the store lying in an oversized crib, complete with padded bumpers. The floor seemed a long way down. He needed to take a leak but realized that must be what the diaper was for; size 46. He felt like crying so he did, a loud bawl. The brunette with the frontispieces came in with a tangle of knitting in her hands. "Look what the stork brought me!"

Hank quickly ran through his options. His love life was literally in the toilet, adult life gave him a rash; what did he have to lose? Maybe the two of them could grow old together. Drooling ever so faintly, he gurgled out "MMMaaaaMMMaaaa?"

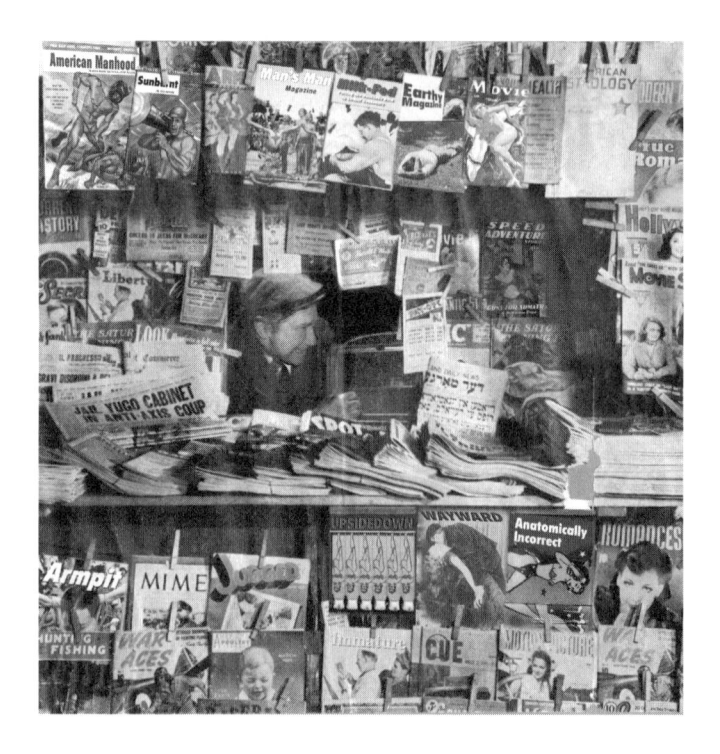

HELL'S ANGEL CIRCUMCISION
ALAN KAUFMAN

In 1968, at the age of 16, I worked as a floor sweep and general grease monkey in the Bronx Motorcycle Repair shop on Soundview Avenue. It was the main custom shop for the Hells Angels chapters of the Northeast, from NYC to Massachusetts, and was run by this guy named Eddie, a gearhead genius; who turned cherry red full dress Harleys into chopped hogs with extended forks and flaming Hells Angel death heads painted on the peanut gas tanks.

He paid me under the table in hard cash and kept me well-fed on take-out shrimp salad heroes, quarts of chocolate milk and cans of Schlitz beer. I think he retained my labor partly out of pity because I wasn't much with a wrench — couldn't tell a lug nut from a washer.

Tenement-poor sewer rat such as I was, the gig was an ultimate getaround boon that gave me bucks enough to take out my first real girlfriend, Kathy Gregorian, a short, hot 17 year old mixed Puerto Rican-Greek girl with long black hair down to her waist — she wore stiletto high heels, miniskirts and tight sweaters with uplift bras that turned her breasts into milk bottle torpedoes.

I belonged to a dead-end gang that had its own storefront clubhouse where we weight lifted, planned crimes and went down on Barry Gerber's mother, who whored to keep her son fed and would do us favors at two bucks a throw. But when I had Kathy in back, on the cot we kept there, she wouldn't let me go all the way. She'd moan "Keeese me, Alan! Keeeese me, my ba-by," and was great to make out with, rolling and sweating, grinding and thrusting those breasts into my face. But she wouldn't let me get further than a copped feel. To have the rest, I'd have to produce an engagement ring, which I had no intention of doing. All of which gave me blue balls so bad I limped.

One day at the motorcycle shop, I heard a ground-rumbling roar that sounded like a tank charge by Patton's 3rd Army and went outside to watch the endless ranks of the Massachusetts Hells Angels roll up in waves of chrome and fire.

They dismounted and Eddie, dressed in his usual ragged greasy jeans, black boots and ripped tee shirt stepped out to greet them, mopping his face with a sweat-soaked bandanna. He lead us into the cavernous shop and introduced me to everyone.

"This here kid's Alan," he said. "He's Jewish, right? So, his mother was hunted by Nazis in the war. And she survived. Ain't that right Alan?"

"That's right," I nodded shyly, avoiding eyes, hands jammed in pockets, shoulders slouched: a big proud strong kid planning to go out for varsity football that fall.

The Angels, fearsome, wild, studied me with interest. Then they parted ranks for an Angel with long black stringy hair, a grizzled face, and a certain familiar look of intense and torturous intelligence.

"My name is Jewish Bob," he said, "and that's my bike." He pointed at the armada of bikes parked in neat rows. "You see the sissy bar?" I followed his gaze to an iron Jewish star welded atop the sissy seat of the baddest chopped Roadster I'd ever seen. It had giant monkey handlebars and chrome everything; sat so low that cockroaches had to detour around it.

He pulled up the sleeve of his striped jersey and showed me a Jewish star tattoo. "You been circumcised, kid?" he asked.

"Yeah," I said.

"No, you ain't. You see this knife?" He slipped one out from an ivory scabbard slung on a black garrison belt with a grinning skull buckle. "Look at it. A genuine SS battle blade. My own father took it off a Nazi motherfucker in World War Two after he shoved a bayonet up his ass. See that Swastika on the handle?"

I saw it.

Balancing the knife in one hand, he took hold of the loose hanging tongue of my belt, sliced it off with a lightening stroke and held it up for all to see.

"Check out this fuckin' foreskin!" he shouted, and the Angels laughed and cheered. "Today he's just got a circumcision Angel style! Now he's really a man!" and shouted the Hebrew toast to life: "L'Chaim!"

All the grinning Angels pounded me on the back and jostled me around, making me feel like I belonged. I'd never seen a Jew like Jewish Bob. He seemed like the toughest, craziest Angel ever. As the day wore on he stripped off his shirt and colors and walked around bare-chested. He danced drunk, dropped some acid and careened laughing into doors. Back and front he was a rope muscle wall of black Gothic ink designs, including what I recognized as the Hebrew word for God.

From them on, I had friends among the Angels. One, a sergeant of arms for the New York chapter, drove a Dad's root beer truck to make ends meet and also worked the door as a bouncer for the Filmore East and every so often would pull up in the truck, drop off a few cases of root beer and hand me some guest passes to the Filmore.

One night I showed up at the concert hall with Kathy
and was greeted with a cheerful "Hey, Alan!" by the Angel
bouncer who let us in for free. She was so impressed that she
almost let me go all the way for once. Almost, but not quite.

Summer ended. I made varsity football at a sports pow-
erhouse, the biggest all-boys high school in NYC and
became first string offensive tackle and defensive end on a
team heading for the City Championship. But the coach
was this Italian guy who liked to shout at me: "What the
hell are you doing on the football team! Jews don't play no
football! You oughta be in synagogue, Kaufman!" and it was
getting to me so badly that I felt ready either to stab him to
death with my K-55 knife or else quit and kill myself. In
fairness, he insulted equally; Irish, Blacks, Puerto Ricans,
Asians and Italians too. Still, it bothered me to the point of
anguish. I wanted to make it stop, but how?

Next time I saw Jewish Bob, the Mass. Angels were in
for a big custom bike show at the NY Coliseum where
Eddie had a couple of flaming roadsters out on the floor
and I happened to mention to Bob about my problem with
the anti-Semitic coach.

Bob listened carefully and then said: "Where's this
school of yours?"

I gave the address.

"This coach," he said. "He around today?"

"Sure," I said. "He's probably out on the practice field right
now with the team. I took off to help Eddie with the show."

"You're a good kid," he said, and stood up. "This conversation?"

"Yeah?" I said.

"We never had it."

Heart pounding, I agreed: "We never had it."

I didn't ask what he meant or where he was going, but

next day at practice the assistant coach pulled me aside and asked: "You know the Angels?"

My heart jumped, but I kept chill, slumped my shoulders, nodded and said, "Yeah. What about it?"

"Well, a couple of them came here to visit, and there was this scary-looking guy called Jewish Bob. You know him?"

"Sort of. So?"

"Well, he scared the living shit out of the coach."

"Oh yeah? I thought nothing scares Coach. So, what'd Bob do that was so scary?"

The assistant coach proceeded to describe how Bob went up to Coach with the other Angels watching and stuck out a big, greasy paw, introduced himself as Jewish Bob and told Coach how proud he and all the Angels were that I'd made Varsity and how they all thought I was sure shot to make All-City and even some day maybe win a Heisman. And then he told Coach, looking him straight in the eye, that every Angel from here to Berdoo, Cali will be following my career real closely. And, dude, it better be a glad one. A very, very glad one.

"Coach almost shit his pants," said the assistant coach. "He said he's afraid to leave his house at night. Can you imagine that? Coach afraid?"

I shook my head in sympathy. "Yeah, well, you know, those guys, the Angels, like, man: you don't want to piss them off."

Coach never did reference my ancestry again. I never saw Jewish Bob again either, and I believe that he met with a really sad end somewhere out in Mass., because one day Eddie and the other Angels just stopped talking about him and if I mentioned his name they got all mournful-looking like they felt sorry for me for having lost such a good friend, which I guess I had. Now and then I think about him, even to this day.

And as for Kathy, I never bought her that ring.

And it goes without saying that she never let me get past her bra.

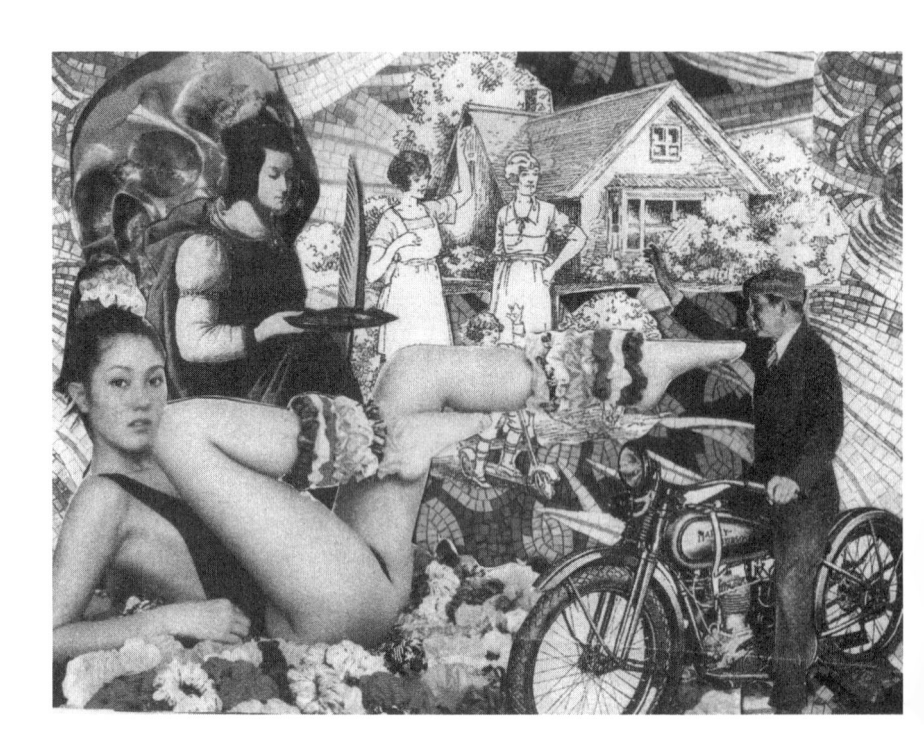

THREE GOLDEN RINGS
MICHAEL CARTER

Back in the queer-taunting Paki-bashing footballing days of my dissolute youth, my mates and I would gather round the perimeter of the field after work and attempt to project a higher degree of manhood and worldliness than was evidently the case, our circle-jerking games having become a cause to some for queer fear and overall to have lost their original savor of camaraderie and hormonal release. It was in such an uncertain querulous state that one our members — a stout red-headed lout given to boasting, then barfing come pub-time — suggested it was past time we'd had real experience of a woman, and said his older brother — a seaman (and who should know better?) — had told him of a swell little brothel near a big filthy incinerator in the East End. We drew lots and I picked the short match. At first I sought to maintain a visage of worldly knowledge and manly delight, a crooked smile stamped upon my watery mouth — then, as I turned towards the just-descending bloody red sun, small twinges of fear fought to overwhelm my smirky demeanor, for soon it would be nightfall and the deed must be done. But as a dusty moon appeared on the horizon to the west, my courage revived, a delicious fervor took over my entire being, my cock got hard and I was ready.

She was a fleshy young thing with curling red hair and skin like cream from a Jersey cow. Her hips were wide yet far from bovine, though her breasts were udderly magnificent; incredibly soft grapefruits whose large animated nipples looked pointedly in the general direction of my incredulous eyes. I think her name actually was Elsie. I lay myself upon her and as the log of my prick felt the bulge of her already well-lubed mons — a wild unconquered strawberry patch — oozing inside with ambrosial nectars the likes of which my youthful prod had obviously never tasted, I ripped my trousers completely off as my fingers stumbled through pockets in search of a protex, which the gentle ma'am kindly helped cover my now throbbing cock. So sensuous were her nimble fingers, I valiantly held off blowing my load right there and then. Soon, however, I was sheathed and, pressing my determined peach-fuzzed chin into her heaving bosom, plunged right in with all my newfound adolescent might. Oh it felt good in there as she let out a big groan; she began moving her hips around it and the ocean began to well; I could feel her tight muscles contracting holding it in, then letting it out, as I began to thrust and whump with sudden confidence, harder and harder. Suddenly I felt something like an iron-rod biting into the pleasure signals my cock was sending my brain. More whumping and I could feel yet another huge metallic thing and to the other side, another. Regardless, I could not stop whumping and thrusting until I was on the very point of losing my load, though whatever was in there felt like it was ripping into my cock. And in that moment a thought flashed through my delirious mind: If all women are so constituted, then god help our entire race — when, bloody hell, the damn lambskin ripped open just as great gobs of gleaming jizz spurted from my retreating member. She looked quite unhappy and exhaled a world-weary sigh accompanied by a pungent pussy-fart, then spread her legs revealing the font of my premature pleasure and subsequent woe… for there in that red and fertile crescent could be clearly seen three tiny golden rings, adorning the inner folds of her labial wings.

I had never heard of such a business, and I should certainly have something new to brag about at school; then again, on second thought, perhaps not.

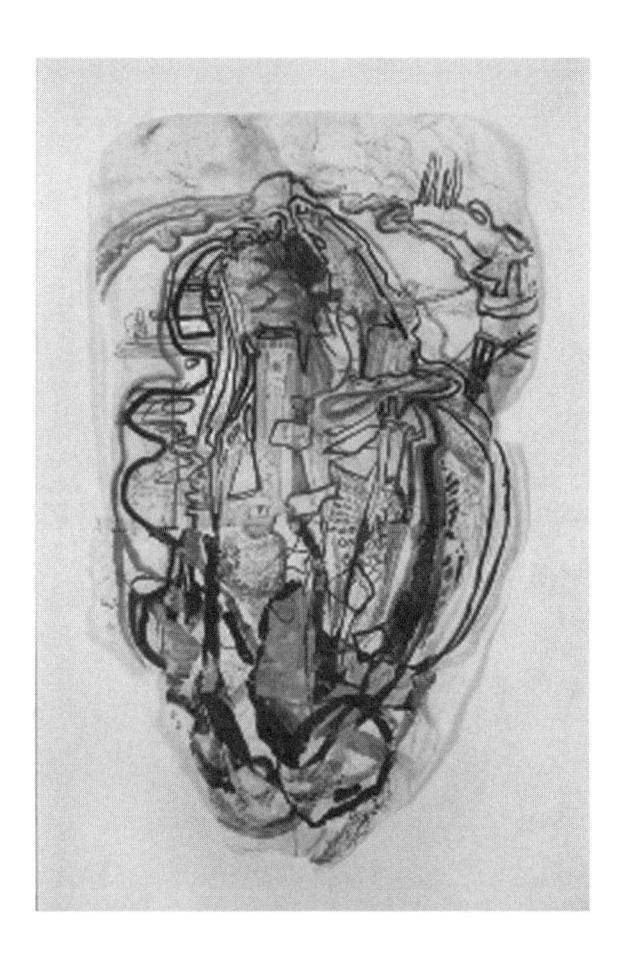

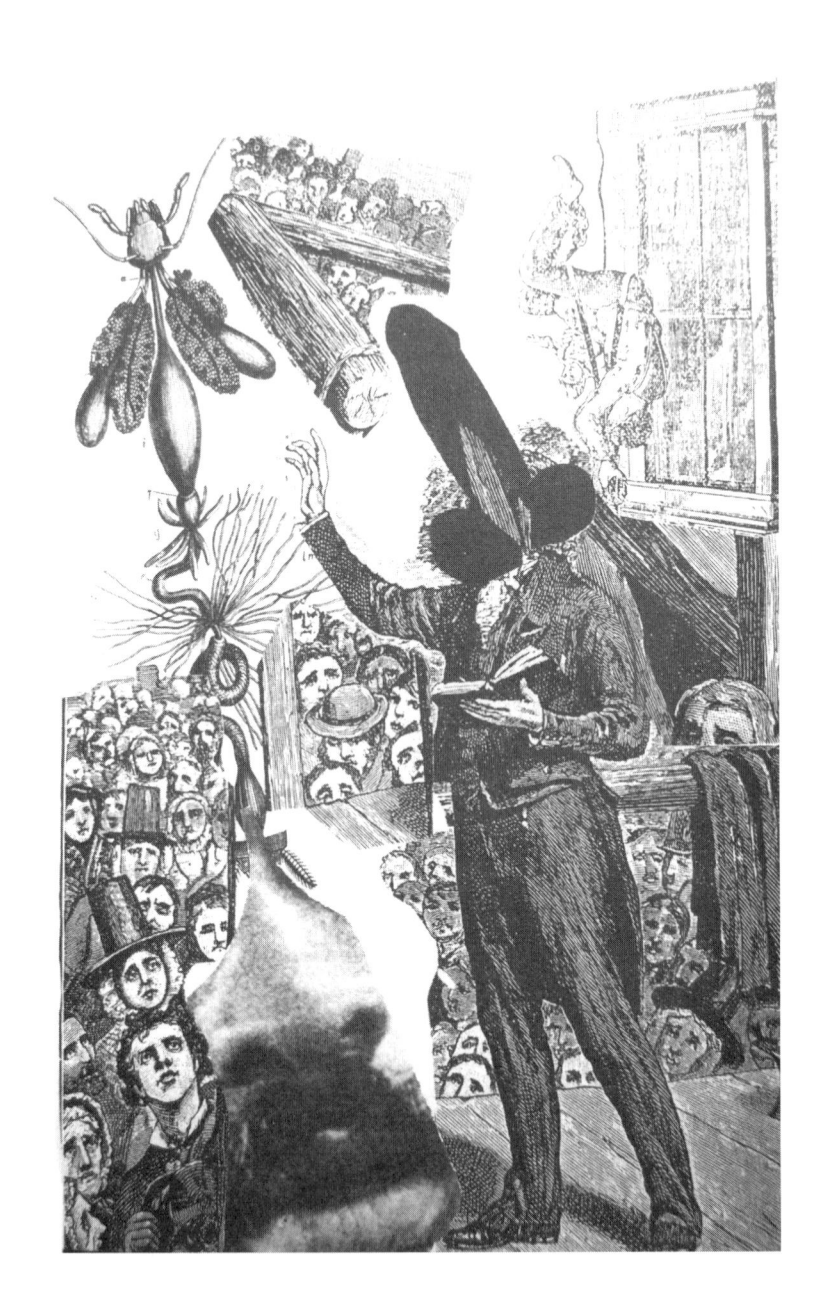

WHAT DOES TALKING TO THE ANIMALS HAVE TO DO WITH SEX?
DARIUS JAMES

I don't think I ever really recovered from the trauma of reading Hugh Lofting's *The Story of Doctor Doolittle* — wherein a cannibal the color of coal, armored in a suit of rusty mop buckets, is bleached by the titular hero (famed for yakking with the animals) to aid said cannibal in his quest for the heart of a silken-tressed fairyland lass.

"*Boo hoo hoo!*" cried Prince Bumpo with sooty tears rolling down his chunky charcoal cheeks, splashing the delicate watercolor of the golden-haired princess pictured in his fairybook.

"*Boo hoo hoo!* Woe is me! Damn this *damnable* darkie skin! If I were white, with blood in the face, I would mount my noble steed, and charge to her rescue, gleaming as brilliant as the sun in my shining armour! I would slay the dragon with my trusty spear, and get down on bended knee, asking for m'lady's fair hand!"

Prince Bumpo paused in mid soliloquy, his shifty eyes betraying the black intent of his devil's heart!

"*And tap dat ass with som' o' dis' big black jungle dick!*"

WET WIGGLE WALTZ
ART RAVESON

Soda jerks, sand hogs, day laborers, correction officers, foot messengers, fight promoters, bail bondsmen, postal clerks, arc welders, dish washers, house dicks, longshoremen, stumblebums, brewers, bookies, pool sharks, shills, touts, johns, marks, saps, chumps, panhandlers, hobos, bums, jailbirds, out-of-work burlesque comics, degenerate gamblers, pederast priests, scapegoats, suckers and patsies, typesetters, sign painters, fish mongers, draft dodgers, deviants, racketeers, blackmailers, Bible thumpers, atheists, stool pigeons, arsonists, strike breakers, idiot savants, ex-cons, swindlers, chiselers, crumbs, crooks, cranks, crackpots, second bananas, grease monkeys, goofs and gimps, all belly up to the bar, belch and stammer, "Whu-whu-whu-whu-whu-whiskey."

They gasp, whimper, whisper, wheeze, hem and haw, spit it out fast and catch their breath, trying hard to play the innocent. Lot of water under the bridge since the bartender, a morose, emaciated, old geezer answers to the name Lawler, has heard anything that's given him pause.

"Sumpthin' t' drink an' sumpthin' t' eat, mister. Hol' on, will ya? I know what I want, jus' can't remember what in hell they call it, nowadays…"

Whiskey, bourbon, gin, boilermaker, shot of rye, beer chaser, hard boiled egg, pickled pigs foot, beef jerky, stale bag a' peanuts….

Lacking any discernible social graces or particular gift of gab, he mumbles and stammers, recites stale jokes, yaks it up and spews it out; all manner of piddling, daft hooey, ever so slowly sidling up; edging closer, moving in for the kill, with an uncharacteristic, delicate touch; "Take y' down t'Voinon Boulevard, lady, c'mon. No trouble, 's' on my way."

Squat, flea-bitten, down at the heels, old gal, putting on a good wrestling match with her coat, shuffling out through the warped, sagging front hallway, dizzy, hopeful mug in tow, gives her the once-over, in the light; "Decent enough sort. Pretty good egg, really. Solid reputation as a dedicated adultress. Keester like a Sherman tank and hard, pudgy gams, like steamship pistons."

Standing in doorways, empty lots, alleyways, under bridges, the dark, deserted periphery of a vast industrial zone, in loose, frayed, rolled-up, soiled workpants, ankle deep in icy, stagnant, shallow puddles. Shoes saturated, waterlogged and overflowing, laces undone, socks sucking up oozing, acrid, dense batter of bubbling, oil-slicked sludge and chemical-laced groundwater.

Shivering, knock-kneed, cold blooded and queasy, sluggishly burrowing beneath heavy horsehair coat, unbuttoning, pulling, tugging and hauling, attempting to sneak past an undefended, easily penetrated, flimsy outer layer of cheap, threadbare, dime store, hand-me-down duds.

The soothing, intoxicating, familiar smell of warm female flesh, emanating from beneath tattered, disintegrating fabric, sparking foolish, romantic, schoolboy longings. Sliding into a light hypnotic, sexual trance, only to be instantaneously slammed back into shocking, hard reality. Stunned and flummoxed, by the sudden appearance of an ingenious line of defense; outlandish, confounded, cursed, female contraptions of an unknown vintage; heavy, rubberized, suspender-hung, double wire-ribbed, reinforced, obsolete, roll-on foundation girdle, and bizarre, jerry-rigged, molting, mule-hide utility-brassiere, thin and balding in patches; a present, no doubt, from some grateful, smitten sodbuster. Stymied by an impressive array of old-fashioned, impenetrable defenses, and morosely contemplating humiliating unilateral surrender; his obstinate, mule headed, contrarian nature kicks in, and battle plans are quickly redrawn for a hopeless, last-ditch, all-out storming of strategic, well-defended, fortified, primary bastion; a clumsy, worn out, immobile, stiffly starched, iron-clad pair of home-made, tattered, patched and resewn, reinforced, button and hook secured, front panel, rough cotton-canvas bloomers, Houdini'd have a hard time breaking into.

Joyless, bleary-eyed, silent and wheezing, grim-as-death, gurgling foul, deadly oaths under his sour breath, with a determined, sardonic, cold rigor mortis grimace plastered over his grotesque, unshaved mug, he proceeds ever-so-cautiously. Vexed but unbowed, struggling in the dark with no assistance whatsoever, from our good-natured, woozy, hapless, reluctant, lumbering battle-ax, who, for all the good she was doing, might as well be waiting for a trolley.

"Kinda dismal 'round here, if ya want my two cents," she quips. "No chance mistakin' this for the Onyx Club! The hell is that, anyway? Wildgrass, dead skunk an' sumphin' else I can't put my finger on," she blurts out loud, taking in the local air. "Smells like some rotten corpse has had hisself a substantial bowel movement, hereabouts. Howdya ever settle on this godforsaken' spot, anyway? You weren't actually searching for the place dead guys come to shit, were you?" she asks.

Bony, calloused mitts, skating underneath her trampled, twisted up skirt, now hauled up above her beer barrel torso, draping her behemoth shoulders, offering no easier access to her vaulted and secured nether parts.

In knee-jerk response to his primitive, boisterous pawing, and a sudden, accidental elbow to the bread basket, she involuntarily jerks her hips backwards, nearly tipping him headlong into the freezing, poisonous Newtown Creek.

"As reluctant as I might be to broach the subject, Minnie," he wheezes in a weak, gasping, emphysemic drawl, "but is there any remote possibility of you takin' a slightly more active interest in these here proceedin's?"

"What proceedings might you possibly be referring to, yew half-dead tramp? Not your last court hearing for public indecency, is it, yew scabrous, stunted, walking cadaver? It's still fairly unclear to a lady what in hell you're even up to," she replies.

"Just an innocent bystander — that it?" he prods. "I guess no one ever gave ya that little talk about the birds and the bees!"

In one ear and out the other. She pipes up again, raising the flood gates higher, "Much longer's this honeymoon sposed ta take, ya guess? Gotta shove off sometime, ya know. A woman needs her beauty rest! Prob'ly missed *Life With Luigi,* by now. By gawd, I hope yer happy!" Rattling on, unabated, her croaking, sledgehammer voice, known to dislodge boulders, initiate landslides, trigger earthquakes and set tidal waves in motion, bores through thick skullbone, dense brain matter, viscera and nerve endings, alike.

"Despite this uncertain, dubious outing, I'm no damn night bird, pally. Get that through yer waterlogged noggin, once an' fer all. If that old man o' mine ain't started off on his regular Friday night bender, already, he'll be wond'rin where in the hell I'm off ta, pretty soon, you bet." She blubbers on, unabated, conversing in turn to her recently

deceased, fat uncle Leonard, her imagined childhood play-
mate, Gertrud, and other vaguely-perceived spirits, with an
occasional aside to the man in the moon. "Still not done by
a longshot, are ya? Had the feelin' this was another bad
government job, yew glimpsy, miserable, dilapidated mug!"

The unrelenting, battering-ram, blunt, raw power of her
fearsome, bellowing voice and incoherent, mindless, unconscious prattling has finally started to take its toll. Eyes bug-
ging out from the prodigious strain, puffing like a tubercu-
lar case, punch drunk and ready to throw in the towel, he
summons up his last ounce of human strength.

"I've played the gent an' I've held my piece, but
enough's enough, dearie!" he growls. "Cursed undergarments be damned!" Bunching up and violently tearing
through damp, stiff, ancient, threadbare, damaged goods,
discarding wide, uneven, scattered, curled-up shards along
the already littered, soggy, fetid, waterlogged ground.

Worn out, discolored, cheap fabric gives way, leaving a
raggedy-edged, wide band of yellowed, stretched, worn out
elastic-rubber, loosely encircling her now heaving, considerable girth, like some fat, three dimensional, unhinged
equator, slowly sliding off its globe.

"I guess we're entering the tropical regions now,
Minnie," he demonically cackles, as a battered, sweating
paw slides down an immense mountain of undulating
flesh, searching blindly for her warm, hidden mons pubis.
His hard-won victory punctuated by the sudden, horrific,
savage, ear-splitting, yelp-like war cry of "Pay dirt!" temporarily deafening his stunned, dazed partner, nearly
bursting her eardrums.

Slowly regaining her equilibrium, she responds in
kind, initiating a renewed series of extemporaneous, bel-
licose oaths.

"Yew vandalous, no account criminal! Yew uncivilized, heathen Mongolian horde!!!! Them's a perfectly good pair of ladies undergarments!" she wails, heaving her massive, herculean hindquarters, wriggling under his grizzled, skeletal frame.

"There's no denyin' them drawers was headed for the heap," he attempts to assure her. "I'll stand ya to a new pair, come payday! For fuck's sake, listen to reason, sister. This here's the twentieth century, aint it? We're practically livin' in the future, far as I can see! I hope you'll excuse my bluntness, Minnie, but despite yer mounting bar tab an' the ol' mans paltry paycheck, it just might be time for a change of undies!"

The word "undies" gives her a surprising start. The sound of it has a strange, erotic effect on her, calming her raging tantrum and lulling her gently into a more romantic mood. Practically swooning, she clings helplessly to the scruffy, bouncing bag of bones wrapped around her.

Calloused hand gripping chain link fence, fighting for leverage, off-balance and clumsy. Amazon laundress shoulders and behemoth, musclebound, elephantine ass, pushed up hard against half-submerged, salvaged, galvanized bulkhead, leaving dime-sized white spots, where frosty-cold steel rivet-heads imprint pink, squishy flesh.

Slammy, bouncing, hot-headed and punctual, veins flowing with sweet, old nonna's Bensonhurst marinara, deranged, slap-happy hips beating out rhythm like Oscar Pettiford.

Up to his old shenanigans; rubber legged and spastic; the wet wiggle waltz.

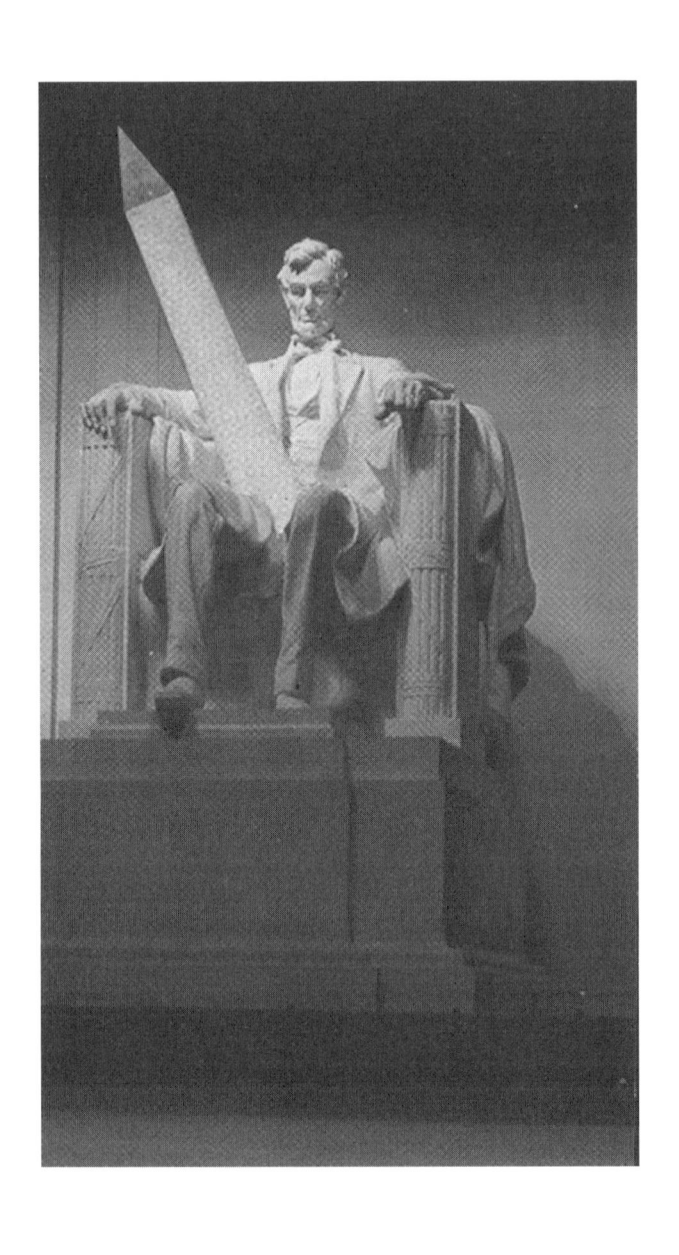

HUNG JURY:
A SECRET HISTORY OF THE O.J. TRIAL
JIM FEAST

all me Jason, Jason Argonaut. Some of you may have heard of me. From day one, I caused trouble as a juror on the celebrated O.J. Simpson trial. As those who closely followed the trial back in the day may remember, I was removed from the case by Judge Ito, just as were Michael Knox, Jeanette Harris, Tracy Kennedy and others. However, while the reasons these jurors were booted out of the courtroom were soon made public, the rationale behind my dismissal is shrouded in mystery, unfounded rumor and bad mythology. I personally signed a document in which I agreed to not reveal any of the circumstances for a certain number of years in order to avoid prosecution. That time limit is passed and the truth can finally be known.

As you'll remember, the Simpson trial brought to the surface the tensions between blacks and whites, which, even with the election of a black president, still mar American life. Perhaps I alone, among all the jury members, am qualified to understand prejudice.

You see, as a child coming up, I had it hard, being of mixed parentage. My father was white: a high-priced, high-octane corporate lawyer at one of the most prominent firms in the country, my mother was black: a ghetto drug dealer. Their marriage didn't sit well with the posh suburban community of Ioclus where we lived. People would point at us, often making insulting comments, as we strolled past them along the malled streets. I guess they weren't used to interracial couples. It didn't help that, due to a unique genetic condition, I had a stripe down the center of my body, neatly dividing my Afro-American left side from my Caucasian right side.

I think that makes me, not Jeanette Harris, who broke the news of the sheriffs' prejudiced attitudes, the jury's resident expert on racism. I had seen it from both ends.

Too often I faced scenes like the one I experienced on my first day at Lemnos U. I had gotten to my biology lecture early and seated myself in the last row. Pretty coeds sat down on either side. There was a black girl to my left and a white one to my right. We got on well during the class: exchanging little notes, gazing at the professor's slides of jelly worms, shuffling around the syllabi. I thought I had made two new friends. But when I stood up and was no longer in profile, the women shrunk back in distrust and horror, realizing I was neither an Afro-American blood nor a Caucasian WASP, but both.

I'm afraid that multiple experiences like that diminished my self esteem and made me feel like a contemptible loser. It was this baggage I lugged straight into the jury box.

Anyone who digs up an old copy of Michael Knox's *The Private Diary of an O.J. Juror* will learn that, as a sequestered, isolated group, we jurors felt we were being put through a sensory deprivation experiment. We couldn't listen to the radio or watch TV. Newspapers were censored. Only occasionally could we see relatives and this under heavy surveillance. Since the jurors were not allowed to talk over the case until the prosecution and defense rested, interaction among us was carefully monitored. We couldn't visit others' rooms though we could talk on the phone, listened in to on both ends by hovering sheriffs. If you didn't want to call another juror who had retired for the night, then, as Knox explains, "Jurors were told, 'You can approach the [other] juror's room, knock, then step back and stand at a minimum distance of three feet from the door. When the juror comes to the door, you may have a brief conversation. If you wish to have social contact, you can invite the juror to join you in one of the common areas.'"

All this led to our shared sense of being coerced. Knox put it like this: "There was a subtle change in our behavior when we realized the deputies were always positioning themselves so they could eavesdrop."

Think about it. Here we were doing a public service and we were being treated like cons. Even Knox, the most generous-spirited of the jurors, got hot under the collar, letting go with this comment: "It's strange and unnatural for human beings to be isolated and not allowed to talk about things weighing heavily on their minds." It's also as if we were at war with the judicial system.

I personally came to see jurors as spoilers. I mean, after all, any large institution will act to maximize its influence. No one has even accused lawyers of being shy of grabbing power, and judges (usually former lawyers) have the same instincts. These people and other court functionaries resent juries, who grasp a little of the power they would much rather monopolize for themselves. All judicial employees prefer backroom deals, agreements worked out in the judge's chambers by the parties' lawyers, those parties themselves kept outside and in the dark. Again, the jury process represents a crimp in this action. No wonder trial by jury is disliked if grudgingly tolerated by legal professionals.

However, few of these professionals so dislike the jury that they would play the dangerous game indulged in by

Judge Ito, who encouraged the lawyers to pack the jury box with a combination of Black nationalists, former Panthers or still active Black Muslims, and white supremacists, including many vocal Kluxxers, hoping for an explosion that would discredit the idea of allowing average citizens to participate in the judicial system.

I daresay these jury bashers got more that they bargained for. For it was as if the different antagonisms within our little camp, as we were fused by the outer pressure from the restrictive rules and pettifogging guards, became the imperfections that temper the hardest steel, making a sword that would eventually not politely ask for but take what is every American's god-given right to booze, guns and the occasional hijink.

It was this rebellion by the majority of our jury that got my dismissal officially hushed up, unmentioned in the press or other memoirs. You see, my simple if lusty action was the spark that catapulted our humble group into creating a temporary autonomous zone.

1. From Little Acorns

In the poisoned and oppressive atmosphere that reigned in the hotel, cafeteria and box, even the smallest infraction, if it was carried off with aplomb, would be a cause for jubilation in our ranks. Now one thing that had really ticked everyone off was the booklet we were handed on our first day of impaneling, *Judicial Briefs: A Dress Code for Celebrity Trial Jurors.* How demeaning and humiliating to be told, for example, to wear argyle socks and penny loafers. One day I couldn't take it any more and decided to test the limits of the system.

That morning as we were waiting for our ride in the underground parking garage, a husky white guard singled me out. "Argonaut."

"Yes, sir," I responded.

"Where's your right shoe?"

Everyone was staring at my bare, light-skinned foot.

"Oh, that."

The guard moved menacingly forward, unholstering his .45 magnum.

At just that point, Hercules (like Knox I'm using fake names to protect identities) strode between us. He was a former NFL linebacker and card-carrying Bircher, who one might have thought would side with the police. Instead, he said in his guttural Irish voice, "Nuttin in the book says you got to wear two shoes."

The guard backed off. "I guess you're right."

A victory, small but sweet, for all of us.

2. HOTSIE WATER

At first I thought the high spirits evident among all the jurors that evening when we returned to the hotel were due to a belated savoring of my triumph over the guard earlier in the day, but then I remembered that it was the night of conjugal visits. Knox talks sensitively about how lonely such nights were for individuals like Tracy Hampton, who had no partner. As he puts it, "One sad note. Poor Tracy Hampton looked very upset. She'd be alone on this conjugal night… what a shame that such a fine young woman is destined to be alone on this night of all nights."

Needless to say, I was in the same boat as Tracy. I, also, was too shy to have made any conquest of the opposite sex. And yet, uncharacteristically enough, on that charmed evening, emboldened by how I had stood up to the authorities, I had the courage to approach the jury's other outcast, Medea, who was, like me, a racial outcast, being an Afro-American albino.

Shy as I was, I was not about to pitch woo in the hearing of the guards, but there was one avenue open for semi-unrestricted talk. For exercise, both men and women were allowed to jog down the long corridor of the men's floor. As our overweight guards were not about to jog beside us, this was the one place a minimal privacy was possible.

In the hothouse atmosphere of the jury box, emotions develop quickly, and in no time we had each confessed our love and desire, to the point of figuring out whose apartment we would go to in order to consummate our relationship once the trial was over. Our relief at being able to reveal our long smothered feelings was balanced by the frustration of not being able to take action more immediately. Suddenly, noting that we were both wearing baggy sweat pants, I had an idea.

"You know," I said, "we could look at each other's…"

"You first," was her game reply.

To tell the truth, I was more afraid she would reject me when she saw my peculiar equipment than that we would be apprehended. I gritted my teeth, pulled my sweatband open and displayed all — revealing one small, shriveled white ball and one bulging, throbbing black one. In the center was my staff, looking like a barber pole with a white line zebra-striping up the brown shaft.

Without comment, she opened her pants, and I glanced down to see something I'd been searching for my whole life. Her kinky black pubic patch had a circle of gold at the center through which her clitoris could be discerned. It was like a donut with the sun glimpsed through its center.

I was so mesmerized, I crashed into a guard.

3. REDEEMING MYSELF

The guards were furious that night, but we didn't really

grasp the magnitude of our offense till the next morning when we found military personnel pulling up the carpeting on the men's floor.

"What's going on?" I asked.

"We're forbidding jogging and," he added, "to make sure people don't try to break the rules, we're laying in electronic land mines."

Everyone blamed Medea and me, rightly I guess, for this new restriction. It wasn't the jogging — you could jog around your bedroom if you were really that gung ho — but that tonight we were expecting a shipment of guns and ammunition. Don't get the wrong idea. We weren't planning to blast our way out of the courtroom. It was just that Judge Ito had ignored our reasonable request (and Fourth Amendment right, I may add) to carry small arms. Many of us felt understandably nervous with so many trigger-happy sheriffs around and needed a "rod" as a security blanket. And that's not all. Accompanying the weaponry was our bi-weekly shipment of bootleg liquor.

I realized that if I didn't come up with a solution, I would irremediably damage the growing unity of our group — blacks and whites had come together in planning and executing the smuggling operation — and it would start my romance off on the wrong foot.

Ignoring whatever was going on in the courtroom, I thought long and hard about our problem. That night, I whispered to all those involved in the operation, to open their doors at midnight. No danger of the guards noticing anything since, given a false sense of assurance by the presence of the electronically controlled mines, which they switched on at 9 pm, they had all retired for the night.

"Everyone," I called out, "put on those x-ray specs I distributed earlier."

"But those don't work," Hercules objected.

"They may not help you see under girls' skirts, Herc, but they can detect ultraviolet rays," I told him.

Then, surprising everyone who could see from their doorways, I took three mice from my pockets, ones I'd caught in my room and whose feet I'd swabbed with UV paint. I let them loose in the hall. "Genius," someone muttered. He realized, as I did, that a mouse will instinctively avoid a land mine. Once they had scurried away, and we donned our x-ray specs, we could safely navigate the floor, following their little paw prints.

To protect our outside contacts, I won't reveal any more about our shipment, but let me mention what happened after all the guys got together in Herc's room after the mission was accomplished. After downing three shots of straight "corn," Orpheus started singing my praises, and ended by asking, "Is there anything me and the boys can do for you?"

"I'm really horny and I've got the hots for a girl you all know…" I gave him some background on the budding romance between Medea and myself, "but we have no place to be alone together."

Orpheus, after a moment's thought, turned to me with a twinkle in his eye. "There is one place where you and Medea can get real tight, with our help…."

4. Last

The next day I was kicked off the jury. I think it was the worst/best day of the whole trial. ("Worst" as viewed from the authorities' point of view, "best" from ours.) It was the day that goings-on in the courtroom totally degenerated/ elevated and the unruliness/free-spiritedness of the bad jurors/true patriots was fully exposed/allowed to flourish. It let the world know that all the jurors were at heart near anarchists/anarchists.

Remember that Judge Ito occasionally relaxed the seating rules in the jury box and that day he allowed us to choose our own chairs. The six men sat in back, the six ladies in front. So, I had Hercules to my right, Orpheus to my left; with in front of the three of us: Calypso, Medea, and Persephone. By coincidence, I had whites to my right and blacks to my left. The pattern was this:

Hercules moi Orpheus
Calypso Medea Persephone
_____ railing

Security had gotten tighter since the jogging foul-up, and conversations were more strictly monitored than ever, but, getting onto the transport bus, I had managed to whisper to Medea to ditch her panties.

There were a lot of reporters present that day because Johnny Cochran, O.J.'s lawyer, was scheduled to re-enact the crime. Not that anyone on the jury was much interested in the case by that point, not with my relation to Medea occupying everyone's minds, but we hoped the lawyer's actions would provide a useful smokescreen for our activities.

We bided our time until all eyes, human and camera, were on Cochran. He had chalked crosses on the floor where Nicole (the victim), Ron Goldman (the other victim) and Mr. X (the man the defense claimed was the real killer) stood. Suddenly, with a dramatic flourish, Cochran set inflatable doll pellets on each marking. They gave off dreadful wheezing noises as they filled with air. Everyone was straining to see the face on the Mr. X puppet.

Meanwhile, I had slipped my rock-hard organ out of my pants, signaling the men on either side to move in. Disguising their actions under the pretense of inspecting the inflatables more closely, they leaned close. Now the layout was like this:

Hercules moi Orphesus
_ _ _Calypso Medea Persephone_ _ _ _ railing

The close reader will note that the group had moved nearer the railing, which had begun to bend slightly forward — indicated by the dotted line — as we pushed against it. Medea had raised up a little from her seat and braced her legs against the rail. Her skirt rode up to exhibit her bare underneath.

No longer able to hold back, I plunged my erection into her creamy wedge.

My co-conspirators were doing their best to cover me, drawing ever tighter to hide my quaking limbs. Hercules grabbed my collar to prevent me from lunging out of my seat. Thank god for the wheezing of the Nicole doll which hid Medea's appreciative whimpering.

The greatest danger was posed by the rail. Medea had her whole body's weight on it now, and as each of my thrusts went deeper, I could hear the wood groan. Apparently, it hadn't been built to endure this kind of punishment.

My pants had dropped to my ankles, exposing one black and one white leg. Out of the corner of my eyes, I caught sight of the men in the back row, who, without telling me, had decided on a daring maneuver. They all began unbuckling and dropping their trousers. This way, if anything went wrong, we would all hang together. As they eased down their pants and drawers, I heard multiple clunks as pistols and hip flasks fell out of back pockets. Miraculously, the female jurors, not all of whom were privy to our plans, quickly figured out what was going on, and joined in. Although being in the front row, they had to be ultra discreet, they began stripping off their panties and lifting the back of their skirts in a beautiful gesture of solidarity. Drunk with erotic ecstasy, plugging away, I realized that for the first time my mongrel birth was being ignored. Glancing to either side, I saw black and white dicks, white and black pussies, all equally displayed as shields to my romance. This was the high point of the Simpson trial for me. Who cared about judicial niceties and lurid details when one could experience real racial harmony beyond all barriers? (Let me not exaggerate the selflessness of this moment since, in fact, many of the jurors, both male and female, with exposed genitals and sex in the vicinity, couldn't help but begin vigorously stroking themselves.)

Suddenly there was a shout as the mystery doll was fully inflated. The timing was perfect. Medea reached orgasm at just that instant. The waves of pressure flowing through her vagina were tickling my cock so deliciously that I threw caution to the wind and pumped like mad, disregarding the splintering of the railing which gave way, sending the twelve of us cascading out of the box.

There was panic in the room. It must have seemed like a dike bursting and the muddy Mississippi, its brown water cut by golden currents of foam, pouring through.

Personally, locked as I was to my honey, and in the throes of a mammoth orgasm, I kept my eyes closed. Knowing and not caring that I would be removed from the jury, I disregarded minor bruises as I hit the floor, knocking over a table.

I was later told that Johnny Cochran, Marcia Clarke and even O.J. Simpson himself jumped onto their desks, seeking higher ground to escape being drawn under by that torrent of booze, vaginal fluid, gunpowder, sperm, blood and illicit fire.

PAIN
MIKE GOLDEN

Naturally just when I couldn't imagine things getting any worse, they did. My friend Otto called. The closest thing in the world I had to an older brother, Otto was right there for me in this the most critical point of my life. "Hey, I'm really sorry about what happened between you and Jesse."

"Who?"

"I take it you haven't heard from her."

"For all I know she's dead."

"No," Otto said, "she's doing fine. In fact, that's the reason I'm calling. Jesse wants to sleep with me. But, and I want to emphasize this to you, bro, I'm in your corner, I'm your friend, and I won't sleep with her if you don't want me to."

Well what could I say? "I don't give… a fuck… who she sleeps with!"

Since I was emotionally incapable of taking that solid healthy middle ground and admitting *this hurts too much for me to talk about right now,* it might have been easier for me to have said, "If you lay a fucking hand on her, I'll kill you, you swine Nazi pig fucker!" But I had seen too many Belmondo films, and was too cool for my own good. And not exactly capable of admitting what my heart felt at the time either. I was in too much pain. Filled with too much rejection. Too much pride. Too much anger. And oh yes, guilt was there too…. For me to finally lose it, it took Andre, buried in the bowels of my poor carburetor in the garage next door, to send me over the edge by suddenly pulling his head out from under the hood when I started cursing about how long it was taking to fix the piece of shit car, and saying, "I know what you are thinking, mon, but I want you to know I did not do the nasty with your wife. I admit, she wanted to, but you and I are friends, mon — "

"No we're not!" I snapped. "You're my fucking mechanic, man!"

"That is an even stronger bond."

Winky ducked in the garage then. "How's it going?"

"We're almost there." Andre smiled at the brain dead shrink, then quickly ducked his head back under the hood.

I looked at Winky, stared into his eyes, and suddenly I admired David Berkowitz. I had an overwhelming urge to pursue a second career as a mass murderer. Pure rage filled me like the joy of Nitrous Oxide, before the pain kicked in again. I don't think I'd ever felt anything that overwhelming in my life. It started like a vibrating electric current in the arms. That was the fear, and I could barely breathe once it started. Which is why running helped. Yoga helped. Punching the bag helped. Everything physical helped, because the energy you got from the physical broke up the vampire emotions of despair sucking the lifeblood out of you. Sitting and smoking and drinking and singing the blues, on the other hand, was like turning the heart valve into an electric accordion being played by Edith Piaf while her mournful wail romanticized fucking the monkey demon on your back to death before you could talk it into blowing you.

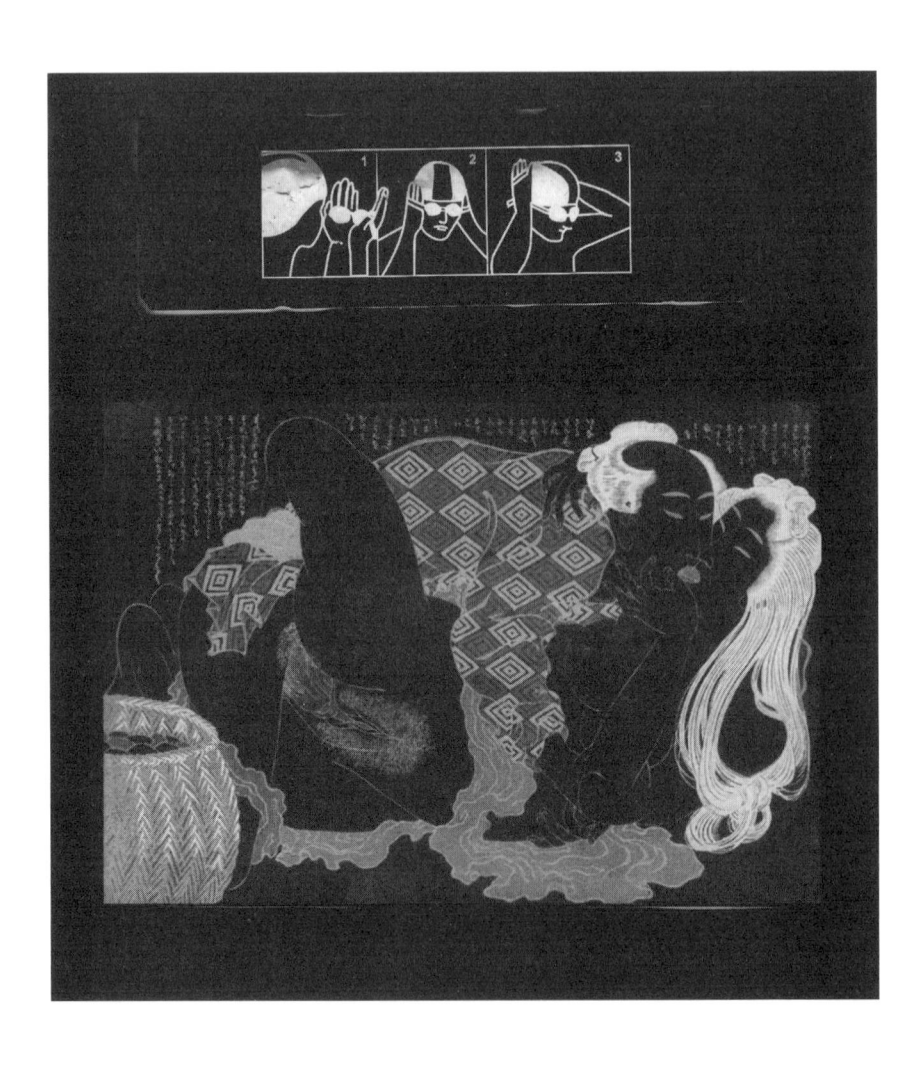

MY FATHER'S LAST CONCUBINE
NHI CHUNG

1) An-Dong Market, Saigon, May 1965

My mother was always flanked by two servants when she went food shopping. You might say we were rich since my father, Thanh Chung, owned a noodle factory with 200 workers, but mother still shopped, cooked and cleaned with our five maids, four of whom ran our in-house shop. But that day, the maids stayed home and as she examined kitchen utensils she was alone.

The An-Dong Market was a gigantic, partially shaded oval. The outdoor part sold sweets, vegetables and fast food while inside, under a vast dome, were innumerable stalls retailing meat, bowls, clothes, dead people's money, incense; just about everything.

Mother had paused to examine some fancy chopsticks when she overheard a fish merchant remark, "There's Mrs. Chung. Her husband is very rich. He owns a noodle factory."

Mother looked up pleased, then displeased: pleased to be recognized, displeased when she saw the merchant was not talking about her but a jauntily dressed, 19-year-old girl, who was passing by, dragging what appeared to be her daughter.

It wasn't until mother got home that she noticed six red-lacquered chopsticks clenched in her fist. They were unpaid for.

2) Saigon, 1960s

One thing about the Cholon (Chinatown) district of Saigon in the 1960s through the early '70s was that it lacked men. A war was going on so young males were continually being drafted. As soon as a boy reached fourteen, he was put in the army. No one could escape.

Or almost no one. One of my brothers was born very weak and could barely do any chores. He was too weak to be sent out of the country, so we found a place for him to hide in the attic. South Vietnamese soldiers would show up unexpectedly at 1 a.m. and search the house looking for young men but my brother was so well hidden he escaped detection.

My three healthy brothers went to Hong Kong as stowaways on military transport vessels when they reached the age of twelve. It cost one million in Vietnamese money to bribe the army for passage on a ship. Given that a white-collar wage at that time was $48,000 a year, you can imagine how much that cost. We borrowed money from our rich uncle to help cover part of the price.

Because of this scarcity of men, women had very little chance of finding a husband or boyfriend, so it was normal for any man left to collect one, two, three wives and even a few mistresses. In Vietnam, polygamy was legal and a man could legally marry ten times. Even a man pulling a *sik lo* (rickshaw), the type who would eat a morning meal of a slice of bread and a banana and whose clothes were full of patches, would have two or three wives, all with kids. He didn't have to take care of his women. A woman would go to work in a factory or sell fish in the market to provide for her kids. It was ingrained in Chinese culture that it was our obligation as women to carry on the family name. As these women saw it, having a husband was a nicety that could be dispensed with if necessary as long as they had children.

Perhaps the most notorious example of a man having many women was the so-called King of Binh Tay. Here's how I met him: When I graduated high school, I began to work with my father at the factory, which was a ninety-minute drive from our house. (Remember all my able-bodied brothers had departed to Hong Kong.) I had to deliver noodles to various places, including to the king. He had acquired the name because he had seven wives. He was about fifty, and owned a big business and a large mansion. I found out that each wife was in charge of one thing. One did the cooking, one the cleaning, one the bookkeeping and so on. Each had a bedroom and every night of the week he would stay with a different one.

The chauffeur would drive the van to bring the noodles, accompanied by me and one worker who would unload them. I asked the chauffeur if those ladies fought. He told me, "If one fights, he will kick her out and get a new one. That's how he got the latest one." She was an eighteen-year-old girl who had just graduated high school.

In those days, a man was considered the master of the household. The Vietnamese men were very violent. More than once, I saw one chase a woman and beat her with a stick in the open street. No police or passerby would interfere. Of course, the man would not beat the woman to death but just to the point of injury so she would be taught a lesson. Chinese men never beat their wives, but they still maintained strict control.

My father was not as blatant as the king, who kept a whole harem, but he couldn't resist the overtures of attractive women. Because he was very successful, and had power and money, and because he was tall, good-looking and good-natured, he had many opportunities to meet women. Holding a high position as a factory owner, he had to go out almost every night to socialize with other businessmen, such as engineers from Taiwan, contractors from Hong Kong and Vietnamese military men. Not only did he go out to dinner frequently, but he had to make trips to Japan, Taiwan and other places. On his trips he was bound to meet women, women of all sorts. Years later, my mother showed me pictures of my father with a Japanese woman and one from Hong Kong.

At that time, middle class women were not independent. They stayed home to raise the children (our family had seven), cook and clean. So, though my mother knew her husband had many women, she didn't have much to say, because he was the breadwinner and made all the decisions.

When my mother encountered father's mistress Hoa (flower), who was shamelessly masquerading as the legitimate Mrs. Chung in the market, she didn't take any action. At the time, I was eight years old, but if I'd been older I would have told mama to act like Mrs. Chu.

Mr. Chu was my father's chauffeur, and like my father, he stayed all week at the factory. He must have been lonely. At the time there was a Vietnamese woman, Nam, who cooked and supervised the cooking of the meals for the workers who ate in the canteen. She was younger and prettier than Chu's wife and had a small house right outside the factory gates. And don't forget, Vietnamese women liked to get Chinese men because they had more money and didn't beat their wives. So, Nam and Chu had an affair.

This happened before I was living at the factory, so I scarcely would have known anything about it except that one afternoon Mrs. Chu came to our house to talk to my mother. She said she'd found out that her husband had another women with whom he'd had two children whom he kept hidden in the factory compound. She was angry and wanted to know what my mother had to say about it. Why, she wanted to know, did my father allow such things to happen. Mother, lying, protested innocence, saying she knew nothing about it.

That answer, as you can imagine, was not satisfactory to Mrs. Chu. She took the recourse that many other Chinese wives had chosen. The next week, father told us, she suddenly appeared at Nam's front door, screaming like a mad ghost, cursing Nam for stealing someone else's husband and shaming her in front of her neighbors.

I thought my mother should do the same thing, but I couldn't advise her. In Chinese culture, an eight-year-old girl can't tell her mother to attack her father.

3) Thu-Doc, July 1972

One hot afternoon when I was sitting in the factory office, our van came putt-putting over the pebbles that formed the factory compound's street that ran between the workplace and the workers' dorm.

This struck me as odd since father didn't allow anyone but me, himself, the foreman or the chauffeur to drive the vehicle and all three of these men were sitting in front of me.

I ran outside, closely followed by my father, who was fluttering along like an agitated butterfly. A smartly dressed, slightly chubby young woman climbed out of the van, then dragged out two young kids, five or six years old.

My father, right behind me, said to the young girl, as if trying to introduce us, "Hoa, call her auntie."

I couldn't speak. I was so angry.

I had heard about this woman many times; this was the one who had stolen his love from my mother.

I walked away to the other side of the compound and went into the shower room, becoming more and more furious. I had heard my father had another woman, but I couldn't imagine that she'd have the nerve to show up in front of me.

I was thinking, "How dare you come onto my territory."

Yet, I couldn't confront her in front of my father. It had been drilled into me never to attack seniors. So, instead, I walked into a shower stall and stopped, looking up at the nozzle, like a dummy, as if it was that which was putting the water on my face.

4) SAIGON, 1970S

Among all these women my father had, the only one I met was Hoa. She was the last woman my father had before he died. She was younger than my older sister. Hoa was a waitress in the restaurant where my father dined with other businessmen. She was sixteen when they began their affair; back when I was eight years old.

My mother didn't uncover this affair until after Hoa had a few children by father. She found out Hoa was living in our neighborhood and that father had even bought her a house. We didn't have a house! We rented.

I suppose you think my mother was very stupid, that she didn't know her husband had a mistress till she had five or six children. You see, she did know he fooled around, but not that he had anything long-term. At first my mother kept her mouth closed, but then she'd had too much.

One day two little girls came to our house, looking for "papa." They were Hoa's kids. Father ran out and took them home. When he got back to our "rented" home, mother yelled at him, furiously, "Doesn't this woman have any shame?"

Father tried to explain — I was eavesdropping —"It was an accident." He said he was drunk when they'd started their affair. Then they had children and now it was too late. How could he break up with her now, he asked. Could they kill the children?

My father was getting more and more upset. He was not like the King of Binh Tay, who could control multiple women. Confucius says that all one's relationships have to be in harmony for the family and nation to prosper. Those children coming to our house created an imbalance. Father said, lamely, that he'd told Hoa never to do that, never to send her children to our house, but she hadn't listened.

Who can say, but perhaps this contributed its small part to the breakdown of everything else in South Vietnam. The economy collapsed and the communists took over the country.

After the war, the government seized the factory, shut it down and did an inventory. The soldiers came and recorded everything, every desk, every machine. They told us that if anything was lost, we would be responsible so we had to live in the factory and keep an eye on things. Father had to attend nightly self-criticism sessions. A young secretary from our factory, Hue, who never got the promotion father promised her, now accused him of being a reactionary and of having hidden gold. They kept this up for weeks, hounding him to reveal where the gold was hidden. Finally, he had a heart attack and entered the hospital. After that, they left him alone.

5) Thu-Duc, August 1976

I wish I could make a pilgrimage to that great, broad-flanked tree that stood, bigger than anything, on our factory grounds.

I have never returned to Vietnam since escaping (as one of the boat people) in 1978, but that tree with its heavy, thick greenery in the depth of summer and its thousand parasols of shade has often been in my thoughts.

After a leisurely dinner, served by Nam, in the empty expanse of the dining hall, clad in a thin veneer of sweat that covered our dark skin like red lacquer, father and I would retire outside to sit on our striped beach chairs under the tree, each of us holding a big gray fan, made from a large palm-like leaf.

We'd talk over the past, which, though recent, seemed separated from us by a great reef, a barrier reef, because the Communist takeover had totally altered everything. Many of our friends had been put in jail or been sent to re-education camps in the countryside. Others had fled the country, or like us, been labeled reactionaries.

Everything in the past, even a few years back, seemed so far away. When I tried to remember, it was like looking through water. Things were losing contours, details and dimensions. I say this because I want to emphasize that even the moral code by which I had lived so diligently now seemed to unfurl. Or maybe it was because, with father half-incapacitated, I was running things and became bolder.

I brought myself to broach the subject, there under the tree. I asked my father, "Why did you marry my mother if you didn't love her?"

"I never loved her," he said simply. He told me his story then. When he came to Vietnam from China as a young man, he met her grandmother. She kept urging him to marry her daughter. My mother was too unsophisticated, father said, but her relatives were rich. Besides, he said, he had a terrible weakness. He wasted money. He needed a woman who was good financially. My mother operated a fruit store. My grandmother proposed to him in mother's stead, as it were. He accepted. He wanted to continue his line, connect to a rich family, and have a good money manager. It was an arranged marriage.

"But why," I prodded, "did you have to take up with so many women?

"Listen, Manh Nhi," he said, "in business circles *Ö yun joy gang wu, sun but yow gay*." That's a Cantonese expression that means, "When you are in the water, the current pushes you along." That's like saying, when you are in society, there is nothing you can control. There is a protocol and you have to follow that protocol to survive. So, he had to go out to business parties where he met young women, and that's how sex is created. In the business circles, he said, he drank, he smoked, he had women, in other words, almost everything needed to be a bad man, he did.

I continued stubbornly, "It's still too many, too many women."

"But in that environment," he told me, "it's like when butterflies see a flower, they flutter to it. I have many juices like a big flower." I frowned. "Bok oy," he said, "I am like a god. I have a lot of love to give whoever wants."

Sometimes I hated my father. But this time, I couldn't help laughing. I couldn't get mad. I looked at him and saw he was dying. Now he was dying, I thought, and where are all the women. Even Hoa didn't come to see him. Only my mother was serving him loyally till he died.

I guess by this time he was feeling guilty. He kept

repeating, "You are too young. You may not understand."

That was our ending and soon after father died.

I had no pictures of him when I came to America and, come to think of it, none of the tree. Then in 2009, thirty-one years after I left, my one remaining relative in Saigon sent a black and white photo of our whole circle, sitting and standing on some steps in the park.

I'm on the top step, ten years old, smiling, beside my twenty-year-old sister. Mother holds the baby, next to older brother. Three younger kids sit behind father, who with hands folded, sits looking forward seriously, a touch disappointed, and all along the side of the steps, behind and above us, were the luxurious, lush bushes of Saigon, still willing to cradle us or, at least, our memory of happiness.

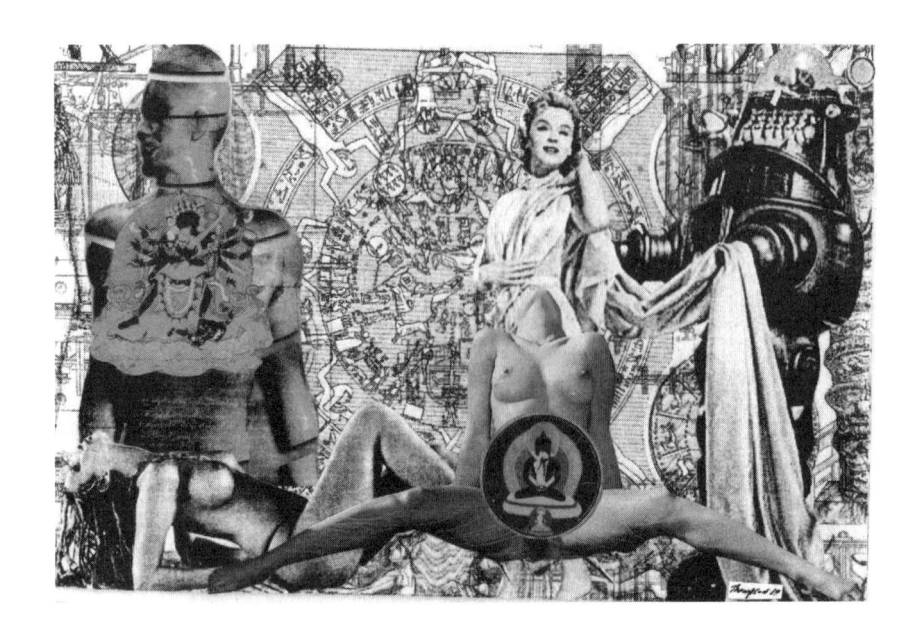

THE ROYOMA'S CHOICE
S.A. DERN

It was time for the Royoma to take a consort. As always, there was an overabundance of choice; handsome trinkets had been sent by countries far and wide, each of them vying for the honor of providing the Royoma's bedmate. And as always, these males were well built; a fine dusting of powder had been applied to accentuate their musculature. Though in general they were innocent of court ways, they carried within them great potential as national assets via their ruler's personal bed chamber.

Though her country's future did not depend upon her decision, it was an important choice nonetheless. The Royoma could not be stuck with a man who was as ill suited for the bedroom as he was for making decisions.

So she had watched them all perform 'The Dance.' This was not a delicate performance, but pure male sensual seduction. A relic of the time when men carried swords on the battlefield, it had become the way men showed their bodies to those meant to appreciate them.

Finally, she narrowed her choice down to two final candidates. Lucius was accomplished, very talkative, olive skinned and came from a nation where it was said that feminine power taught men the best way to please a woman. Ren was intense, silent, and ivory skinned with long hair as black at night. He came from a nation of honor where female swordswomen still practiced with ancient skill and men were able to perform intricate ceremonies with great ease.

"Come forward," she ordered Ren, not wishing to waste time with idle ceremony. "Disrobe."

With a flick of a pale wrist, the crimson garment fell to the floor, revealing simple perfection below; light tufts of hair surrounding a sufficiently large cock. His hair whipped forward as he bent his knees in a low bow, a sign of his submission.

Satisfied, she turned to watch as Lucius' olive skinned hands grasped the waistband of a pair of tight leather pants. A quick motion and they were unfastened, dropping to the ground in a heap. He bent down to pick them up; his long legs, delectably firm ass and beautiful abs were power and symmetry in motion. She made a mental note that his cock was also large enough to please her.

She moved towards Ren, stopping once she stood atop his silken robe. Then she reached down to grasp the folds of her own robe, opening it without removing it. "Please me," she commanded. "Use your tongue and bring me to climax."

His black eyes seared her as he tilted his head, his tongue penetrating the exposed folds of her flesh. He moved slowly at first, then steadily increased the tempo. She liked that he did not slow down once she felt the tightening. It was as if he fought for every moment of her enjoyment. And she took it all, wrapping herself in the pleasure, in the orgasm that wracked her body. "I want you inside me," she said, breathless.

She knelt down and spread her legs to meet his member as he thrust his hips upward, his legs giving him the leverage he needed to enter her. Rocking on her knees, she moved forwards and backwards, using his full and ready cock as a fulcrum. Faster and faster she swayed, thrusting downwards to get as much of him inside of her as she could.

And then the glorious moment of release; the thrill of the orgasm overtook her as she struggled to hold her balance. Bended knees turned to jelly and she reached to grab his ass, squeezing tightly as the afterglow washed over her.

She pointed to the other candidate. "Your arm," she commanded, in a voice that threatened to tremble. "Help me up."

He gave her a deep bow before crossing the room to obey her. He reached his olive skinned arm out to steady her, and then waited patiently as she found her footing.

Once she had balanced herself, she led him to the wall on the other side of her bed chamber. She pressed her hands against his shoulders, seeing and appreciating the hungry look in her eyes. "Your turn. Inside me now."

She braced herself against his body, before lifting one leg, then the other, and wrapping them around his waist. She captured his cock inside of her, and rode it up and down, slowly, losing herself in the rhythm. In the feel of his body. It seemed that he was giving everything he had; she could see the determination to maintain control in his sky blue eyes, as his strong arms lifted her lithe body up and down. He seemed tireless; powering her past the sweet and glorious point of release, moving her at full force into orgasm.

How was she to choose?

"Take me to the bed."

He obeyed, and with powerful strides brought her, still clinging to his body, to the soft bed in center of the chamber. She dismounted, moving to kneel on the mattress. "I must choose," she said, looking at both men, one moving towards the footboard, one standing next to her. "Come to me."

The men stood side by side in front of her. A study in contrast, but she had to choose. It was how things were done.

"Kiss me," she said, looking into unfathomably dark eyes. And the mouth that had pleased her so well met hers, their tongues dancing in unison. The kiss showed her intensity, devotion and dedication. This man would serve her not because he had been offered, but because he wished it. She allowed her fingers to run through his silky hair, and she knew she could not decide against him.

She pulled back, breaking the kiss and smiled at him before turning towards his counterpart. He did not need instructions, his mouth finding hers as if it were starving, Their tongues met, but they fought, dueling for space, and power. The kiss showed her that this man would fight for her, even against his own wishes. He would be hers. Her hands ran through the coarseness of his shorn hair. She could not decide against him either.

She was the Royoma. Who said she had to follow the rules? On the next day, she sent a proclamation. In short, it said:

> *I choose them both for my consort, and any other man who I deem acceptable can find a home with me in the palace as well.*

In time, she would be known as the first Royoma who had a great and honorable harem. But for now, she had Ren and Lucius to fulfill her every desire, and every need.

CLITORAL, OR THE NINTH ORGASM
LORRAINE SCHEIN

The society of Gyna II is centered around women's pleasure and the exploration of alternate realities. Its rites take place monthly in the inner sanctum of a large triangular temple.

The room is large, very large. It is dark, save for bluish lights shining faintly from below. On the floor, on their backs, lie the new female supplicants aspiring to the farthest reaches. Naked, their legs parted eagerly, raised and placed in the velvet-covered steel stirrups embedded in the floor.

All breathe in time as the humming polyskin vibrators lower from the ceiling and are placed slowly and accurately on their genitalia, starting to move with broad light strokes across the whole vulval area.

The clitori of the supplicants are tinted — the hoods in contrasting or matching colors, as can be clearly seen in the close focus control room monitor. Some of them are average size, but most of them are so long they can be sucked on like a nipple. Their pubic hair has been completely shaved off, so that all parts can be seen clearly protruding at acceleration, like pistils in a flower.

The trainees are taught to push back the hood over the clitoris so that the overhead machine may more easily stroke its center, as they kneel over the supplicants and their hands wander over their bodies. They know how to make it grow and shudder, draw back under its hood from the intense stimulation, yet wanting more.

Soon, the room is filled with the sound of heavy breathing. Each orgasm corresponds to another dimension and another altered state of consciousness.

The first orgasm takes you nowhere, but makes you feel energized, complete and ready — the second takes you to Alpha State Two. One by one the supplicants, those courtesans of time and space, are masturbated into the higher dimensions of space described by modern physics, unreachable any other way. The room resounds with moans and screams now, as the vibrators are placed more accurately and precisely on the inner vaginal wall of each, locating the individual pleasure spot and stimulating it in a special pattern of withdrawal, rest and arousal, until the ultimate reality is reached.

One by one, the supplicants reach the ninth orgasm — at last penetrate to the ultimate dimension of reality, convulsing uncontrollably in their pleasure at its beauty.

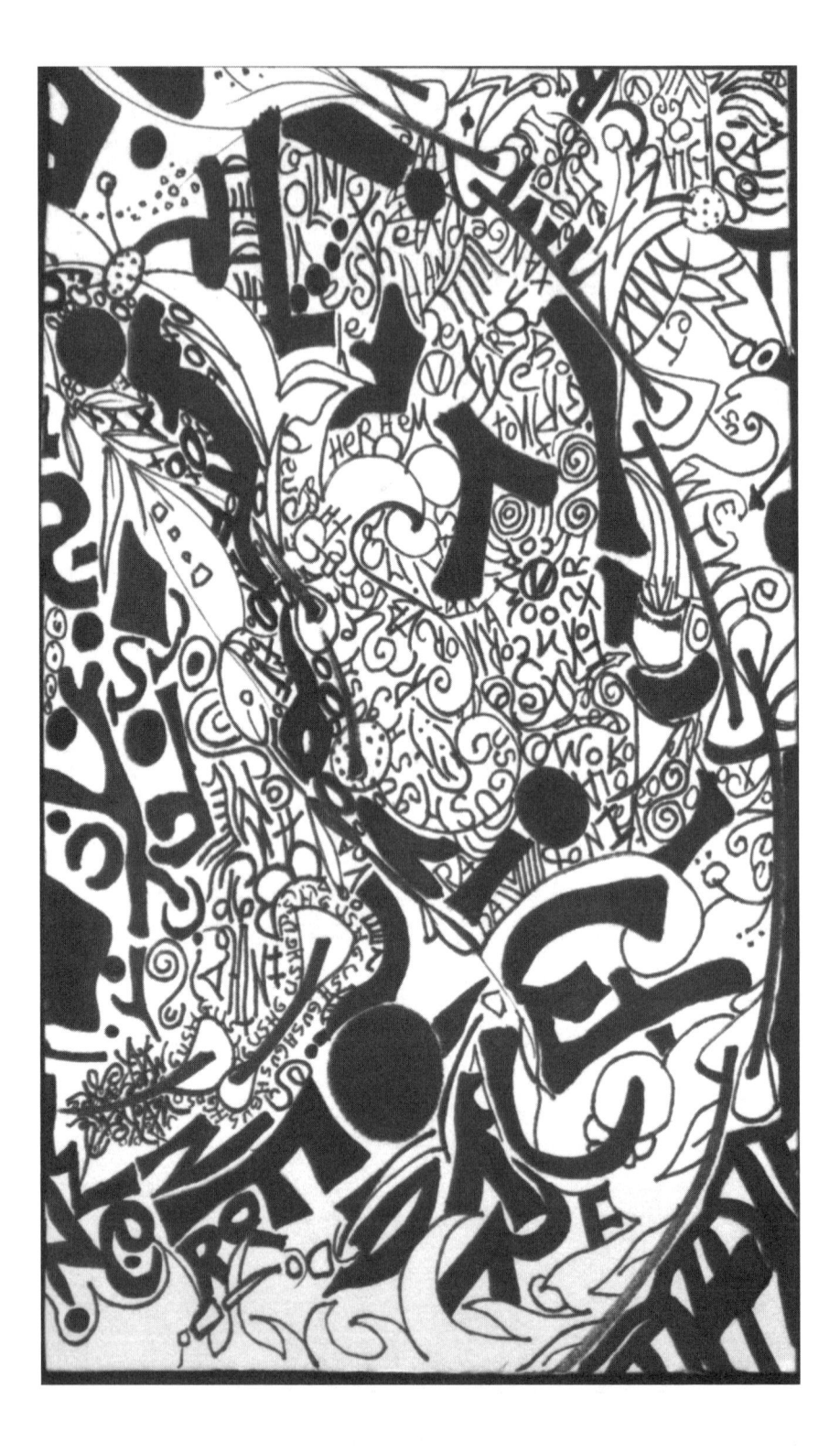

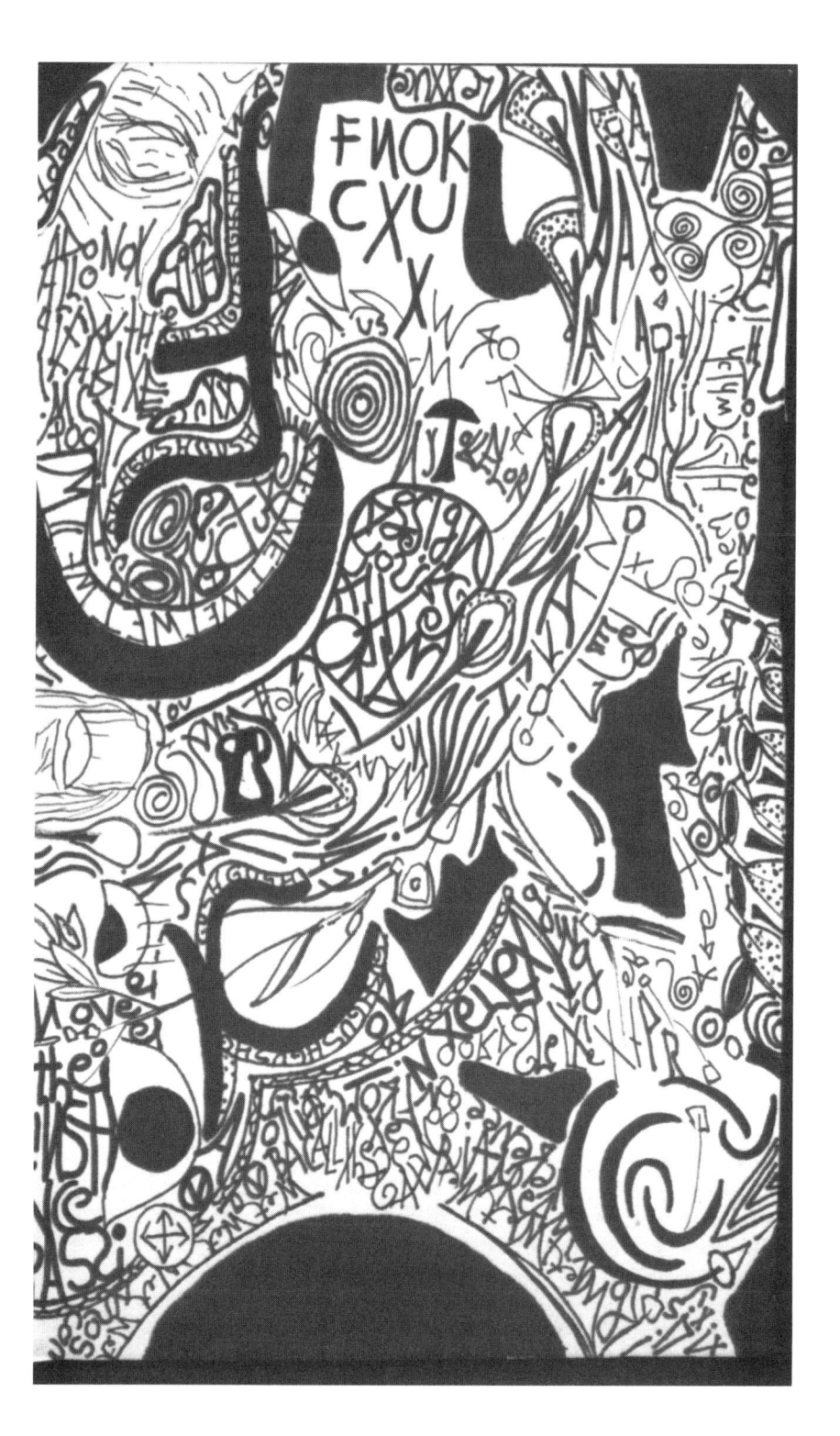

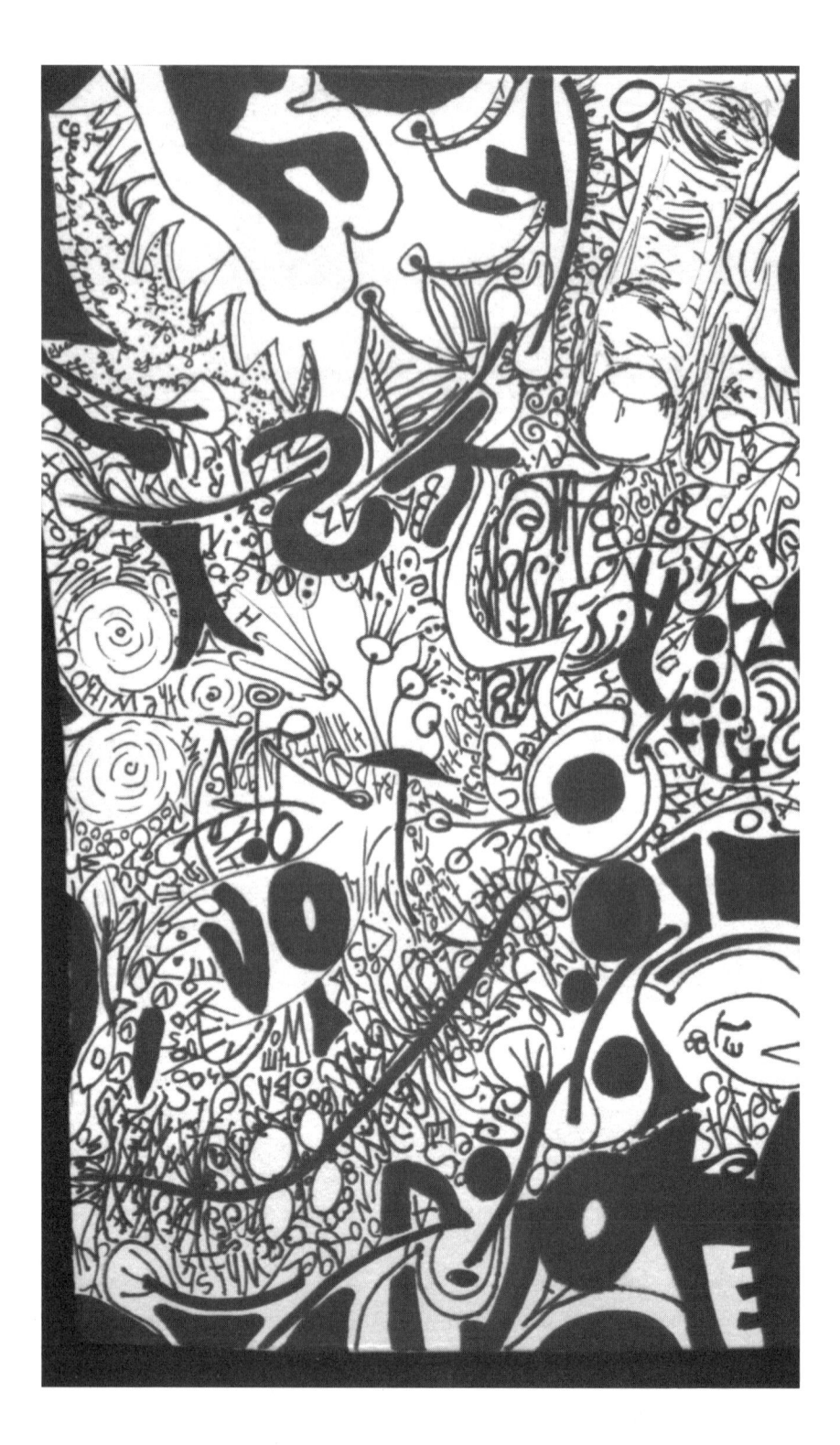

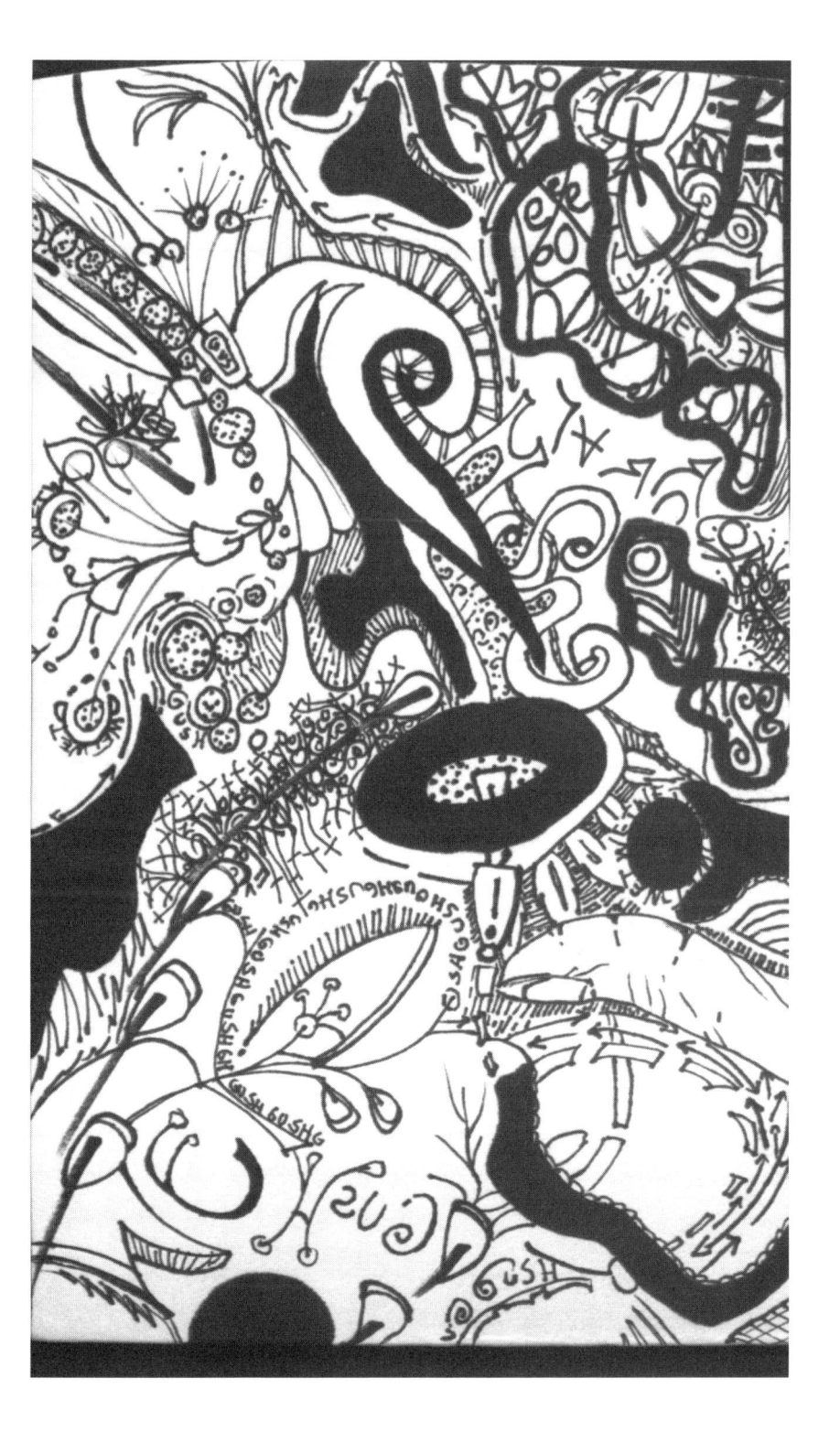

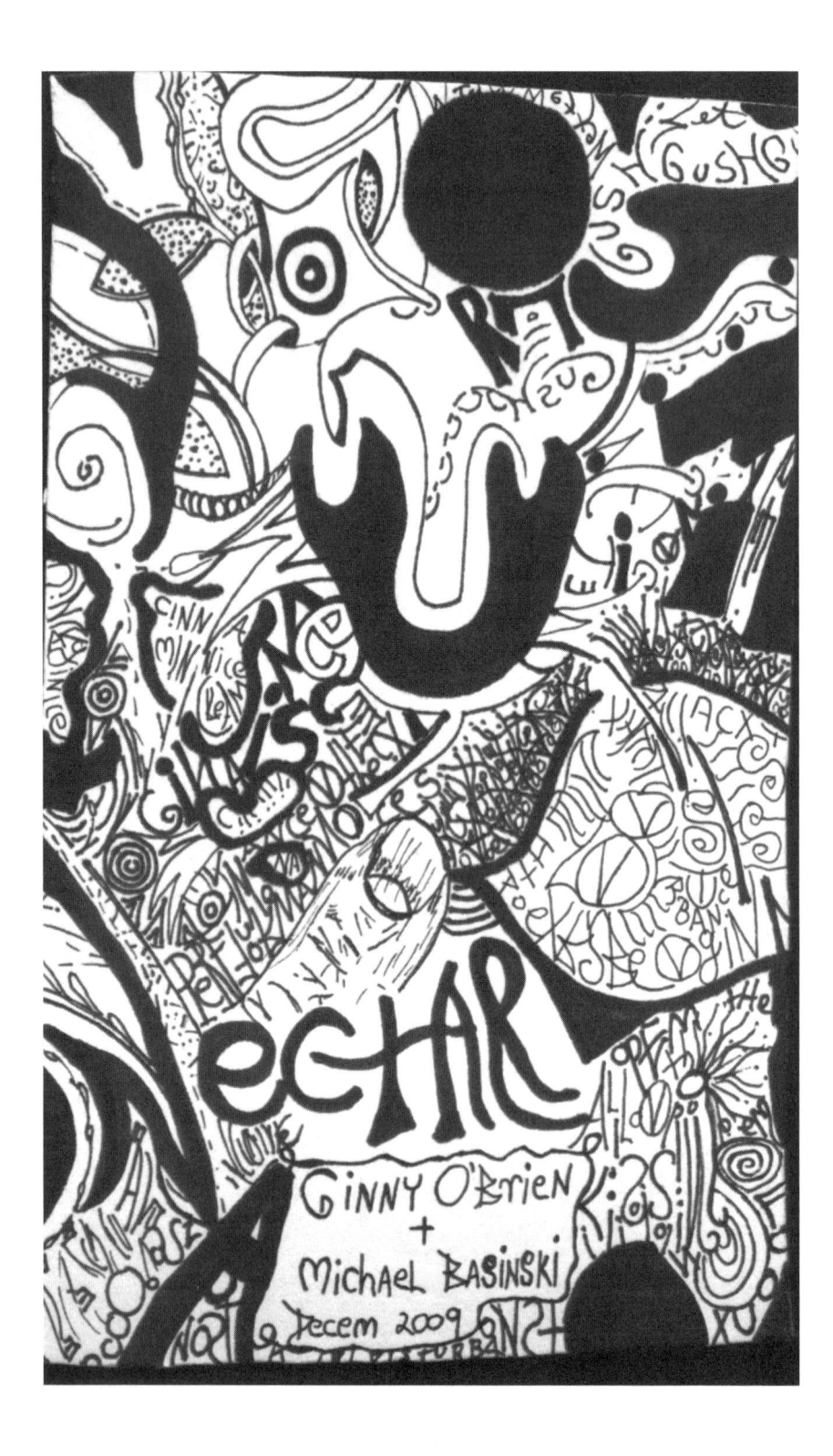

OMO GETS LUCKY
DOUG NUFER

mo was put back in place for study of him as prime boy specimen. Lab men did tests on him, as he, in some way, did on them.

Nobody was up on his true lab identity, as if no trace of his former cv remained. But Omo knew this could be only his take on reality. Mom and Pop, as if shut away in some bin, eluded him as he took his off time, as often as he was given, to seek that duo that science had set in a memory bank for him to cherish.

A loner kid, Omo lived as one put aside by isolation. He also tried, as one may in such a fix, to befriend a fellow chum. Now this proved way difficult, as every chum to be had for a fellow chum was, more than Omo even, a prime lab specimen. For a full decade, most lab specimens had been prod subjects. Any child so put in a study role was bound, really, to be off his nut: i.e., many resembled gaga juju zombies. Drug injections, a lobotomy creed in a common use, and regimes to feed only PEZ candy for meals did abet or always contributed a lot here to having boys emulate spooks.

But here too were a few girl subjects. Among the boys, the girls had some trick ways to defy walking corpse kid cult modes. A hormone buzz made girls of age to desire a boy rage in a frenzied lust for pud. Locomotive fad puberty anima pushed any girls onto a lubricious jag to be sadly unmet by catatonic juju males of a dud membership. And yet, as puberty was to waylay Omo presently, Omo had some tactical edge v. his would-be xy cum spew rival boys, in that drugs, etc., had yet no time for taking much vital body effect on him. No gaga juju zombie, stud Omo was like a monopoly tsar in a harem of lusty female cunning, a pin-up boy girls could wank for as if he put on a new lurid male rut mojo standard of beauty.

Virgin to all erotic ya-yas, Omo was in a nice spot, demanding lusty femme calls of every gal here, in a sex toy mêlée auction by rank-a-hunk bid.

"Seven," a bid went in shorthand quickly, as "hundred" was of a well-understood affix or suffix.

"Ten," a horny up bid overcame it, by and by.

"Twelve."

"Six thousand."

Well, that ended all bidding.

As it came to be, a teen girl band of gangsters bid a tidy ransom they did amass by shake down thuggery, as five or six would threaten guys or gals who dared to be solo in the dour halls of the lab when it was before dawn or even at high noon. This gang ruled so well, not even adult science work technicians of muscular body suit armor upended a reign by Teenage Pussy Vixen Molls.

But in vulgar definitions by diction, a "moll" is attached by sexual fit as dependent fix to a butch gal or man type gang member. In all, nobody here in the lab terrorist gang could be put down, as in slotted by some habit or classified by appearance, to be a butch or male consort. If Omo were to qualify them by making the rank of Buck, they could name this group by the brand of Teenage Pussy Vixen Molls.

Unique as Omo was, in odd upbringing as well as bio freak myth of a genesis by scientific aha!, it amazed his ward men to envy (or, in a non-prejudiced way, to express it here) to duly observe a boy reach up to a level of puberty as one fit on a destiny for sexual work as one buck of a stud in a pussy gang posse with molls. Every man here in a niche to view or study him was from a more staid cub development way of learning to be a sexy adult. Nips and bites — no fully savaged potluck grab of a gulped orgy — had been how any of them found the way to be carnally fed. Masturbation fed most, if not all, of them.

And so here was Omo, a boy deprived of a prime boyhood rite, by virtue of being a sex god in a slot ahead of a puberty mood funk that would set him on a binge to have it all. Some did resent how it was for the boy stud. However, many were of a curious mental powwow nature. If a boy raised by females to be a buck of a fully sexed maturity of a virile man could exist or adjust in a love digs to dig a dug captivity, he would generate bucks in the dynamo ripples of news to demand for a movie.

As luck (or designs by guess work) had it, a system of surveillance put cameras in each nook here, so every last move was to be put on film.

But an oops lurked, as one staff member had some juridical know-how in matters of sex law to share: Omo, even if capable of randy coitus a willing temptress of shy age would egg on, was verily a minor, by some gap. Even if he was too big for his age, Omo, any film had to define, was too far this end of sixteen for a public vent of sexual romping. A much older mating coupler was open as well to charges, but even if a girl of a likewise youth were to be caught on film as willing rut accomplice by dint of desire, any who made such a film was guilty of a third level extortion by rape.

"Hmmm," lab director Bull Whip Mason put on a show, deliberately, of care to seem to be an upright man, devoted in awe to human body ethics. A scientist had to be so pledged in duty, even a scientist who trafficked wholly in tube kid meta-humans.

"I have it," he said, once a decent pall rose in a lifted ah. "We put a young crew in charge of any film. Underage by acting, by directing, by filming to final cut, a dummy corporation ekes by. Sales might be tricky, as well. Distribution we can do later. Now, let's work up deniability."

"How can we slip by channels of regular show biz moguls? By going east. Who cares if Burmese TV plays it all week? China bootlegs, India buys: a mod triangular set of tradewind co-ops. And, for a good cause. I mean, it'll fund research of science! Our vital work," said Cy, the boss's head flunky. He, Cy, knew almost zip about science, but many here did non-tech gigs.

None did object in theory. Bull Whip took a vote by a huff, and it was done.

"Put cameras on, cue my sexed up action!"

By the dim glare of a very institutional cheer, Omo learned to fuck, on film by lights no eye could fix to see how any figure was defined. Blobs they did resemble, in a groping mad gesture of a body stretching awfully to quell an itch by scratching bloody pus in traces of painless but dreary mojo ecstasy. Goo evidence shots were a trope, as if a film auteur in a silly mood were to be known by signature of spent goo in close-ups. A spewed cum wad into fresh condom gave its only aftermath in a picture of realism by release: not by faked or substituted proof.

"We can't do this jack-off shit," came to be a vetted quasi-unanimous expert conclusion. "Amoeba shots in a mitosis hubbub are hot fucks by comparison."

Yet, a dull minority was content, as film to film ground pelvises to have Omo spew amok gleefully his pearly goo.

Nevertheless, a suspicious many were of a view that Omo's gang of teenage moll vixens had purposely hid the goods a porno lay might reproduce. By such deliberate muck-ups, the gang triumphed. A dissenting rumor had another fuck phase foot in the door by focus: were molls having sex fun, i.e., orgasms? In that, nobody was in place to verify.

But lack of ability for making truth known had no effect on the draw sex had, for sex truly was like that, webbed in mystery. Analogical hubby spider Omo plied among web strands of a love myth as he took his fly wives for a ride as they said one classic quote, if revised a bit: "Please! Oh my, help! Oh! Please!"

Rooting by rote in rut yowling made it all seem flatly insincere, but a rhythmic swap conquered all need to link a felt ahh of a sigh to real hug emotion. As every nook had its camera, no sex act did occur in secret, in a kind of way; but, as no light was lit enough, it (sex) could remain put in a physics of a modest nun shade. Moll nuns of an order in a vixen rut of rhythmic swap yowl had powers faith supposedly fit as fixed as if by fucking howdy fact.

So a solution came to any who pined to cash in by making the spunky Omo a porno Duke of Earl: by sonic tape — no hack video fuck drama loop — the Omo experience would rise to be a hit on the mojo circuit (as well as with an esoteric yap dog tweeter and woofer bunch of rare music folk). With so many tech savvy nerd boy fans here, panning some hi-fi nugget was jiffily done by flipping a switch. A cousin related by marriage to Bull Whip used rap music hall connections, a quick deal got inked for a tip jar sum, and Omo Gets Lucky was in play for all.

OBJECT LESSON
ROB HARDIN

PORTLAND, OREGON
MATRICIDE CENTER FOR CHILDREN (THE "MARTI CENTER")

Chills insinuated themselves like strangers' recriminations, like eczema after a night in a bum's hotel. Window light grayed and the hallway lights switched on, making the glass appear darker still. As the space around Shoner cooled, the whistle of a cartoon ghost rose and fell. *Inhospitable wind. A reason to tolerate confinement.*

She hadn't realized she was cold until she shivered. Was it too late for a visit? She didn't know because they'd confiscated her watch. No alarms buzzed in private rooms, no grandfathers' clocks chimed anywhere. Patients weren't supposed to revert to their Circadian ruts.

Shoner disliked being manipulated, so she counted improvised sundials: The chills and the lights in the hall. The Roman formations of crows outside the window. That *shlemp* sound just now, which meant it was time for dinner: The slimy kid, Viscid, had just dropped feces on an intern's head.

Shoner stuck her head into the hall to find their "treatment specialist," a Reedie in her 20s, rigid outside Viscid's room: Pensive from the back, hair still wet after a hasty toweling. Appalled but dull-eyed, as if she'd been evicted before morning coffee.

An idiot savant of timing, Viscid had gotten her during last rounds at six. He lingered like an infestation, eyes drawn to her pinched ponytail. She hadn't restrained him for some reason. He seemed happy about that: His frown of incomprehension softened.

He gazed without giggling because it wasn't a joke to soil her. All he wanted was for her to stand in front of him so that he could savor a long look: Sloppy and gangly but provoking to him for some reason. The need was more visible in his body language than his slack expression. In his erection, specifically, which shouldn't have been visible at all. It wouldn't have been if they'd lived among civilians.

His clothes had been adjusted from the outside, half-fixed by aides and volunteers who always paused just long enough to correct the obvious. They tucked ends back into place, tied his drawstrings or fastened a single button. As soon as they focused on someone else, he squirmed his way back to blithe exposure.

Shoner turned away, annoyed she was stuck with Viscid. It was Christmas Fucking Eve, for the love of god. Other inmates got to visit their families, but she and Viscid were still in here with the kickers dosed and strapped into place. Prone as roaches and trapped in a roach motel.

From her window, the ice looked half-melted and then frozen over. Holes had swallowed most of it; what remained on the grass was a stippled glittering gradient. Somehow, she'd missed the waft of white falling feathers. Now there were only leftover smears, botched flourishes in leprous frosting.

No one was picking her up, but that didn't stop her from imagining what to expect: Rich and compulsively attentive parents who tried to visit so often she had to ban them from coming more than twice a day.

Only five presents per visit, she insisted. She conveyed this by means of coded gestures to her ever-attentive staff: Owl-faced seraphs, their patience made infinite by their life-spans, who'd flown there from Carrion Heaven on a trip that began three centuries before she was born. Their message: She was the most important person on earth, her life at the Marti Center, a necessary cover. Incognito Birds of Minerva, who traveled through Eastern Europe making deals — any one of which could pay for a lifetime's indulgences — needed her to convince billionaires of the necessity of their projects. Eastern Europeans, it was said, found Shoner irresistible. She was to clinch each sale by making mystical gestures while whirling around the room. A powerful art critic and *Athena noctua*, who'd established and destroyed international careers while grooming himself, came to inspect her drawings after being told of her incredible promise. A man with a key to its cage invited her to evaluate unclassifiable owlet works — each more plumose and Gordian than the last.

She told herself these stories periodically while arranging the objects in her room: A book she'd found in the campus library, for example, with menacing illustrations of the Kirkbride Plan. She liked the book because it proved her life could have been worse. She envied those objects. She'd have liked very much to be one of them.

When she tried to fathom what it meant to be sent to this place, she couldn't. The idea seemed distant and frustrating, an itch she couldn't even reach without growing spindly mile-long nails. It was fun to think about that: Calcite tracers that nearly grazed the pate of the far gray road that led her here.

Isolation was, as people in group used to say, "triggering." Thinking about it could lead to the dismantling of a watch or a person, ending with a rubber tube taped to her arm for days. She didn't like that — being forced to sleep. She believed that people should allowed to choose their own oblivion.

Still, she preferred being fed quetiapine to staying up nights worrying that someone had hidden an embryo behind the soda machine. It was better than being afraid to ask for cereal. Better, for sure, than having to listen to the Voice of the Disapproving Elder, which always told her she was stupid, selfish and ugly, and that everyone hated her. She'd repeated that to herself so often that the sentence now played in the background of her thoughts like muzak.

She didn't think these things because she was weak. It seemed to her that self-hatred was more brutal than machismo. Grown men couldn't survive doubting themselves, let alone believing the kinds of things she thought routinely.

She suffers because she's was a genius, her mom used to say to her irritable father — another reason that mom had had to die. The word *genius,* as mom knew, was an instrument of torture. A way for witch-hunters to refer to outsiders and narcissists to refer to themselves.

Slivers of blankness had insinuated themselves between Shoner's thoughts. Lately, they'd expanded, obliterating her powers of invention. She couldn't make new observations but only repeat the old ones. Casting for insights led to clichés about holidays and the weather, banalities that didn't express her fear she was doomed to relive the same insufferable evening.

Thought-loss, blankness, flatness. It happened throughout people's lives until, like her mother, they could hardly say anything at all. They could only struggle with the idea of the present and fail to overtake it.

No one "should have to live like that." She's "better off this way." Her death was "a tragedy," but "I guess it was her time."

Shoner pushed her chair away from the desk. It was that feeling exactly, of cheesy sayings cheapening grief, that made her want to swallow a gun barrel and shut them all out.

She tried to read a book but the words only made her feel worse. Cogent language and perfectly expressed thoughts were beyond her. They whispered that the conscious life of the ordinary was worthless. Dead language and hackneyed sentiments trivialized all pain. They whispered that life was numbing because experience was repetitive.

"'How's everything over here?" the Reedie asked out of nowhere, startling Shoner by tapping her on the shoulder. "Are you OK? Are you getting worked up again?"

She turned away so the Reedie couldn't see her face. She needed a way to stop crying when she didn't want the intern to see.

There was only one way.

Places from her old house flickered into being around her, resurrected incongruously. The dusty living room filled with anguished carved shapes. The "string family" on the mantle. The chairs with talons for feet. She could feel her mother behind her in the kitchen making deviled eggs and singing to herself.

Release for a moment, then the tired truth. Shoner couldn't keep up the trick of pretending she had company. She was choking for no reason and trying to make it sound like careful swallowing. "Like picking at a scar."

Shoner glanced at her doorway: *Oh, shit, it's Viscid.* He wasn't watching her so much as sensing her proximity.

Being stalked was repulsive without being interesting — it was tediously repulsive — yet this was her social life. On this Night of all Nights, her peer group was a single spellbound waterhead. No conversation for her. Only penises and feces.

But what if she was wrong? Maybe everything she'd gone through was leading to one defining act: Using an idiot's urges to defy mass indifference. Maybe idiot semen was the key to a special puzzle, and led to a precious heirloom concealed in a hollow wall.

Or maybe his grunting is the only interaction I get, she thought. *If that's it, then that's it.* She lifted herself from the mattress and looked Viscid in the face to get used to him. He appeared especially confused, so she flicked him on the back of the skull. "We're going to the living room," she said.

He emitted a nasal yell, reached over to hit her and missed. "My head!"

"It's OK," she told him, fingers grasping his arm. "You like me. You do. So come on and I'll let you do something about it."

She led him out of the hallway to the stairwell into the dark. Viscid looked aimless and angry, a damaged horse waking from tranqs.

With the first turn of the stairs, they were out of the harsh light's range. The second submerged them in shadow, which felt good. *Fuck you, Santa.* The bookshelves massed together in semi-silhouette, physical entities that would soon be gone, reduced by tech to discorporate scrolls of paperless binary. For now, they were familiar to her as banalities: Pep talks for suicides disguised as stories, bland textbooks ditched by interns after mandatory courses. *Mainstreaming Emotionally Disturbed Children:* useful for anticipating people's strategies for controlling you. *Straight Talk about Psychiatric Medications for Kids:* a list of their rationalizations for doling out doses. Nothing about sex, of course, since therapists were oblivious to the good reasons for teens to have it. To gain entrance to a place with alchemical properties, for instance.

Next to the grandfather clock without a pendulum and just below the couch: A five-foot-seven area of space in which anyone who was young enough became invisible. It existed beyond the habits of perception of adults, who could no longer absorb the minutiae of experience. Shoner was still part-child, at least — enough to sense boundaries beyond which the interns couldn't find her.

Even when they were looking right at you, your parents could never see you once you climbed inside. They couldn't even figure out which part of the room you were in. It worked the same way with medicos in a mental institution. It even worked on her:

Chiaroscuro of little girl falling just behind distant car, her brown dress, hooped with gold, settling and flattening until she lies still. Little legs unbend amid fabric and falling dust. She remains there until, slyly, Angerona, goddess of secrecy and impatience, makes you look away, and the girl vanishes as suddenly as the childhood you must have dreamed.

They stood there until Shoner remembered what she was doing. "Here we are," she announced, pushing him into the space. He got in, moving with a luxuriant passivity. He was tingling from being touched and didn't want to do anything that might make it stop.

She got in after him. It smelled of cats and moldy fabric in there. He was still tense in places even though he'd relaxed. She unfisted his hand and put it on her shoulder. She expected it would stay there happily, but the claw soon descended to her chest. Just as quickly, the other one was on himself. Boys his age were like that, weren't they? "Bib boobs," he chanted. "Bib boobs." Repulsive and obvious, just like any other boy.

He rubbed himself sleepily before suddenly tensing and gripping her breast like a suitcase handle. She suppressed a yell, then studied his face: a confused expression, even for him. He stared at her cautiously, removed his hand, raised it to his face, and sniffed it. Then he was twitching and struggling to speak.

"What is it? What?"

He began to cry, hitting himself with the fisted hand that had hurt her.

"Hate me," he said, swinging and crying. "Hate me. Have a bad head."

"I can't hate you," she whispered, amused at the idea he'd understand. "That's a feeling I keep for myself."

She was getting used to his awkwardness. It was more interesting to explore his body than waste time recoiling; more efficient, to distract him from tears than expect him to stop. Braced for pain, she replaced his hand on her chest, then lowered her own onto him mechanically, lips buzzing in a puckered embouchure to imitate a toy crane's claw. She was almost confident about how she looked to him. As for him, he looked better to her from above. She decided to keep that vantage.

The two of them traded spidery touches in their five-seven hideout. Hers was a delicate *nesticus reclusus* taking it all in; his, a wandering slippery-limbed *atypus,* woozy after feeding on the prey it stabbed through silk.

Shoner pretended they'd holed up in a mile-long crawlspace bordered by Thailand and three other neighboring countries: A place without laws that was relegated to no nation. Only criminals lived there, all safe from extradition for as long as they stayed. She and Viscid belonged in that category. They were illegal idiots perpetrating crimes against themselves. She used him without his realizing it, just as he used her without his realizing it either.

She thought of herself as precociously corrupt but had only touched a penis twice before, when she escaped from the Marti and had had to share flophouse rooms with bums. Their appendages had been leathery in her hand, porous and cured in nicotine. This penis was different. It felt cloying, crusted over, as tender as baby flesh impaled on broken cartilage.

It made sense that Viscid's was viscous, but perhaps all the young ones were like that: Hard and malleable simultaneously, bent and breakable. Distressing little things.

It was also smaller than she'd imagined, since people were always making them out to be so important. Another secret you didn't share with males: Scariness had little to do with being big. It was more that men were switchblades wanting to stab you. Anger, not size, was the part you couldn't control.

She slid her palm back and forth across the tip, enjoying the idea she could frustrate him. She stopped moving entirely and then it became more insistent, pushing against her and trying to force her to move. Hands emerged to move her back and forth.

She wasn't having it. She stopped completely and moved away until he yelled and groped for her. To him, she was an object whose job was to provide necessary friction. Normally, that would piss her off, but she didn't mind being understood that way by an idiot who was actually institutionalized for being an idiot.

But she still hadn't warmed to him sexually — he didn't have that effect. Maybe if she wiped the tip, some of the stickiness would come off.

Some of it did, but the roughness made him twitch and yell. "Shut up," she told him, then slapped him for emphasis. "Shut up or I'll leave." He began to cry again, so she stroked his hair as if he were a little dog. That seemed to calm him (though his tears weren't exactly erotic).

She was about to try another experiment when his penis twitched against her arm. It seemed to explode and leak at the same time Abrupt, uncoordinated, drenching. She reached up and wiped her arm on the side of the sofa, flicking the goo as far away from her as possible. Some of it was spreading under her, too.

She slid away from him and tried to clean herself, but there was too much dust. *Dinner theater's over,* she thought. But then she had an idea.

He'll probably last longer now, she realized. *And I can always make it hard again because he's that young.*

I can do anything, but what do I want exactly? She knew she didn't want it inside her because the thing felt strange enough in her hand. She didn't want to find out how it tasted.

He's had enough thrills in life. It's my turn now.

She massaged him until it was hard again, then moved herself lower and pressed it against the hollow of her pelvis. It felt better than she'd thought. She slid it lower and then along the edges of her lips, teasing herself with it. She positioned herself so that it made contact with her clitoris only through the folds. Direct contact was too much.

He emitted the syllable *eh-h-h-h.* What she was doing felt so good, apparently, that his self-expression was confined to single vowels. Good for him. She could move more slowly because he was happy and if he wanted to stay happy, he'd have to keep still.

She sped up ever so slightly until the back-and-forth felt pneumatic. No need to worry that Viscid would try to put it in because he didn't know where "in" was. Now that she could relax, she found the perfect place to press herself with him. She hit on an ideal rhythm and stayed with it just long enough before changing. He tried to stay still but it was frustrating for him. A hand grabbed her neck and, for a second, she didn't exhale.

His hand relaxed slightly but stayed where it was. *Go ahead and kill me,* she thought. She focused on the part of him she was sliding against, which might have belonged to anyone. To an owl seraph, perhaps, glaring down at her with its reflexively severe expression that always seemed so serious and lost. A creature like that would feel too lost to stop. Contact mattered too much to such a being.

As everyone knew, Carrion Heaven was filled with angels who fucked each other in innocence. No Adam and Eve, no Ten Commandments for predatory beings. Only the animal in front of you, rubbing against you. Friction. Right there. There... there....

She registered how disgusting the appendage felt, but, for some reason, that helped her. A freak-show penis, such as you might find in a circus tent. Even the barker was yelling about how disgusting it was. *This is what you deserve what you deserve what you deserve kill yourself kill yourself kill him —*

And then it happened, though much slowly than it had with Viscid. She leaked on him for a change while his tip slid up and down mechanically. The feeling was incredible, almost worth the awkwardness. Sex worked best for her when others moved like robots. Just as her little sister had when she commanded, then other little girls in the neighborhood and now this idiot. Just like that. Like that, like that —

The tingling got more intense and then a huge hand obliterated her thoughts. She went blank with joy, thought nothing and was nothing. And this was pleasure.

She and Viscid lay in darkness for several decades as

she imagined the ticking sound of faraway timepieces in a death house grown calm.

She felt herself running on a treadmill in the expanding darkness as wet remains chased her and revenants from the last cave marked her with luminous chalk. It felt good, or distracting, at least, until someone called for her and she became aware of the narrow space around her; of Viscid and the couch and the dust and the bones in her hands.

The must of old fabric and cobwebs; soiled intricacies of uncoiled springs, frayed cloth and leaked stuffing — all existed where others couldn't see. These details became clearer as claustrophobia returned. She'd felt frightened like this before: In her mom's house, watching once-cherished things accumulate like bacteria. Mom had loved them too much to throw them away, too little to allow them any room. Little animals everywhere, stuffed, ruffled, glassblown, mechanical; tiny and misplaced, awaiting Shoner beneath the furniture and now in here with this thing next to her. Sickly-cute, Shoner had decided, though the creatures always seemed strange and carnivorous. Densely packed, preoccupied, cheery, obsequious, scowling. They watched as she sat in the corner with a mouthful of shaving cream, where her father liked to force her to sit for hours.

She sat there needing to escape the tiny figures and ravenous flowers around her, even though she knew she'd miss them once she had. Flee them like Viscid, only to crave them later. And this was company.

The intern was yelling. She thought that Shoner and Viscid had gotten lost. The yelling stopped for a moment and Shoner became aware of a nauseating sound.

Viscid was snoring, it seemed, but it wasn't the sound of a person. The noise was immense and imposing. It tore down all sense of separation, submerging her in the mucoid workings of his throat, then lower still. A human chest slopped open to reveal an escapement with pallets of slime. The wheeze of apoplexy. The bellows of corrugated caves.

She woke him as quietly as she could and tried to push him out. He kicked her in the eye viciously before realizing where he was. She bit his thigh, then held him by the leg and crawled out herself. Then reached down and slid him, struggling, into view. She even righted him. She made him stand.

He crinkled his eyes, pushing a snot-wet hand across her belly. She waited for him to stop gasping and heaving, then led him back upstairs. The moment of territorial fear passed and then he seemed loose and groggy, falling back into barren contentment.

They passed the intern first, who was braced as if for an onslaught. He peered at her sleepily, smiled open-mouthed and kept walking.

Shoner made sure Viscid got to his room and then returned to her own at last. She slid into bed knowing it was still an empty Christmas night. She tried to read, but every page looked like a transcription of Viscid's fistic monosyllables. Growls and vowels.

No one understood her, she knew. But now she couldn't understand them.

A pencil lay beneath the covers, pricking and chafing her. She found it and picked it up. She tried to draw but couldn't. Horrible, always to end up drawing by herself.

She pressed the graphite point against her wrist until it broke the skin. That made her smile like antic perfume: Overtones of sawdust and blood, then bassnotes of a slaughterhouse floor.

Usually, she liked to think about murder but couldn't find any comfort in it because she was caught in a different rhythm — the rhythm of her interlude with the idiot.

She hated being a person who thought about time and timing, who always rotted and thought. *I want to feel like an object.*

She reached down to trace the scar-line she'd carved on the side of her arm. She hadn't meant it to when she made it, but the scar reminded her of the place on a doll where you can feel the ends of the plastic molds. The border where the edges don't quite meet.

She might have found comfort in being a doll tossed into the back of a crowded car, a staring plaything that provided amusement and served some purpose.

She missed the intimacy of the things the nurse had taken. Her little picture watch, for instance. It had been orange and brown and didn't go with anything. It was perfect.

When the nurse carried it off, the little owl on the display goggled at her with its set expression of alarm, wings inching toward future time. The limbs of a crucified Metropolis worker.

Now, months later, the watch had probably stopped working, but it still called to her. It still had that little face.

She was feeling drowsy at last, drowsy to the point of drifting, and perhaps a little sad. It was only when her eyes closed that she heard the Disapproving Elder.

"You looked stupid," it said. "Stupid on the floor under the couch posing and trying to control him. What kind of place was that to bring a retarded boy? 'Secret world,' my ass. And he didn't like it there.

"You think people don't know the reason you lower yourself, why you try to force people to stay? It's not self-hatred or anything so dramatic. Simple loneliness, that's all: No boyfriend, no friends, so you seduce an idiot, and all he does is let you. *You* saw his face. You felt him in your hand: Half-interested. Bored. He didn't even want you."

No more.

"He wanted the Reedie. He's always wanted the Reedie. You think he hates you? He wouldn't bother. You think other people hate you? They can't even see you."

Please, no more.

"They only know someone's in your way. You should get out of their way."

Maybe they were in my way first, bitch, and maybe I want them dead. All of you, dead in a circle with your heads in a bag.

There was only one way.

She rose to turn on her little music player, selecting "Nostromo" by SleepResearch_Facility. The nurse let her have that sound because it wasn't overt: Glacial and forbidding, but quietly so. And they couldn't see the cover.

No words in her head, no thoughts but the ones she shut out. No rhythms but that of machinery on automatic, functions suspended. The periodic rhythms of instruments. Drifting instruments breathing.

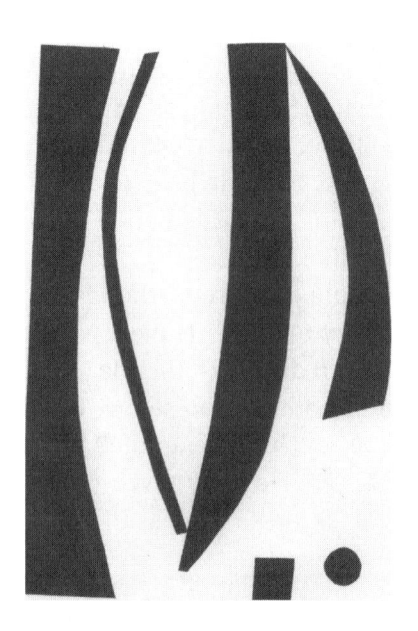

TRYSTS
RUSSELL HOOVER

River Wind arrives at Penn Station his cell phone is dead he immediately goes to a phone booth to call Tongue for instructions after a brief exchange he is told by a woman at Tongue to cross the lobby go to the last phone booth on the far wall she says then call Idlewild two quadruple zero that's Idlewild two quadruple zero ask for Noble Dancer. River Wind crosses the room sits down in the phone booth closes the door and calls. Idlewild two quadruple zero Hello may I speak to Noble Dancer please can you see me. What? Can you see me I am wearing a red silk tie and a fedora straight ahead no the other way yes that's it now look away. I am going to walk by your phone booth I will drop a black racing glove as I pass if I don't drop it the first time wait until I do this may take several minutes. When I drop the glove wait until I have passed completely out of sight then pick it up and go to the news stand give it to the man with the cashmere scarf and the cigarette holder ask him if he dropped it. He will go into the ice cream shop another man with mirrored shades will come out of the ice cream shop with two packages wrapped in green cellophane the man with the shades will give the green cellophane packages to the man with the mutton-chops who is waiting at the north escalator the man with the muttonchops will pass them along to a small boy with purple sneakers who in turn will give them to a man wearing a straw boater. This man will put them in a locker while you wait at the news stand wait for three minutes after three minutes go to the cigarette machine beneath the clock the man with the straw boater will then walk over and stand beside you ask him for change of a dollar when he unfolds his hand take the key to the locker along with the coins buy a pack of cigarettes and go to the coffee shop. At the coffee shop there will be a woman with long blonde hair wearing a silver dress her name is Crest of the Wave she will give you further instructions good luck.

River Wind waits in the phone booth Noble Dancer drops the glove and disappears into the crowd River Wind picks it up and takes it to the news stand he sees the man with the cashmere scarf and the cigarette holder ah pardon me did you drop this why yes I did thank you very much. The man with the cashmere scarf and the cigarette holder goes into the ice cream shop River Wind picks up a magazine and pretends to read it the man with the mirror shades comes out with the green cellophane packages he takes them to the man with the mutton chops who passes them on to the small boy with the purple sneakers who delivers them to the man with the straw boater. All this takes place quietly and smoothly almost too smoothly River Wind thinks something is going to go wrong. The man in the straw boater puts the green cellophane packages in the locker three minutes have passed River Wind heads over to the cigarette machine he sees the man with the straw boater heading in the same direction they arrive simultaneously. Excuse me would you happen to have change for a dollar I believe I do yes mm-hmm here you are. River Wind takes the key with the coins gives the man a dollar bill thank you very much you're welcome buys a pack of cigarettes and goes to the coffee shop.

He sees Crest of the Wave in the silver dress waiting in a booth you must be River Wind. He sits down across from her for several minutes they exchange information about what is to happen with the green cellophane packages in the locker during the course of this it emerges that before her affiliation with Tongue Crest of the Wave was with the Children of God. Like I just got so tired of that pious bullshit I mean those religious twits were trying to ball me every hour on the hour before that she was a receptionist at a Bic Pen factory. He notices her nails are painted green she seems breezy as if not a care in the world he decides that she is definitely hostile by the way I love your shirt where did you get it. It was made for me by a friend she shows him her pet waterbug I call him Dark Night because of his big dark wings but I'm worried about him he's not doing so well I think he might die. They continue to exchange information about what is to happen with the green cellophane packages she tells him that the green cellophane packages each contain the two halves of a manuscript entitled The Starry Skies author unknown it turns out they both have several hours to kill before fulfilling further obligations for Tongue in fact nothing can be done with the green cellophane packages until the following afternoon. They decide to take a taxi to a Cuban place she knows you'll love this place he agrees he is interested in the nature of her arrangement with Tongue he is unable to determine what it is. At the last minute before grabbing a cab they agree it's better to have the green cellophane packages in their possession River Wind takes them from the locker they grab a cab oh wow there're some really together apartments in these buildings along here she says look at those windows no but really I'd prefer a tree house all things considered barring that though I think people should have names for their apartments don't you for example I call my loft the Great Outdoors because there's so much raw space I mean it just reminds me almost of being in the great outdoors sometimes but like I have to have that space to be in mentally and physically so it's a thing with me. I know what you mean he says space is a really important thing you don't want anyone invading it. They arrive at the Cuban place and sit at the bar Crest of the Wave drinks anisette he drinks drambuie the guy who owns this place is really an asshole she says oh yeah? yeah but he's a good asshole I was getting it on with him for awhile basically he's very insecure even more insecure than my boyfriend I find most men are like that no but you seem OK. She touches his arm as she talks anyway I don't have time for relationships anymore she says I mean hey let's face it they're not worth the hassle. By the way says Crest of the Wave have you noticed that so far in this story I've been portrayed as an utterly one-dimensional cartoon-like bimbo bird-brain hey don't look at me says River Wind I didn't write this thing I'm only a character in it like you besides I haven't exactly been portrayed as Einstein.

In fact Crest of the Wave is not a one-dimensional cartoon-like bird-brain. She scored sixteen-hundred on her college boards and her LSATs finishing both tests in twenty minutes flat. She apprenticed as a metallurgist in Fuji and has an encyclopedic knowledge of the sharpening and finishing techniques of Japanese and ancient Samoan sword making. She composes award-winning scores for orchestra and tape codes the trading software for market-makers on the Tokyo commodities exchange punches meddlesome grizzly bears square on the nose sending them running in holy terror plays a mean prepared piano and though deaf in one ear has been feted in international audiophile circles for her contri-

butions to the Direct Stream Digital specification for Super
Audio CD. During her frequent swims in coastal waters
adoring groups of manatees porpoises and sea turtles form
concentric protective circles around her. She has designed
aquifer filtration systems for entire lakes and rivers she was
the only person to win the Indy 500 by completing an extra
twenty-five miles she was scouted by the Mets in 2007 for
pitching six consecutive no-hitter games after having ingest-
ed a half-gallon of ayahuasca. Her research involving the
production of stable micro black holes has effected a thou-
sand-fold increase in the safety of particle collisions at the
Large Hadron Collider. She led the Zapatistas alongside
Subcomandante Marcos in Chiapas once saving an entire
village from a horde of malevolent Burmese pythons using
only toothpicks and a fishing line she played Lady Macbeth
at the Old Vic to nightly standing ovations she developed an
award-winning line of Bavarian lederhosen she appears on a
postage stamp in Kurdistan. On New Year's Eve she broke
the blackjack table at Monte Carlo after which they had to
shut the place down and apply to the French government
and the European Central Bank for emergency funds under
the CRAP financial assistance relief program for casinos.

Crest of the Wave tells River Wind that in collaboration
with Tongue she has invented and patented a unique form
of erotic stimulation of the ear get out of town says River
Wind. No it's true here is a demonstration this is an urgent
communication from Tongue she licks his ear I can't do this
tonight says River Wind what about the green cellophane
packages he asks I'm the only package you need this is an
important message from Tongue you must listen we've got
to get back to the Great Outdoors she licks his ear. From
the back of the cab they give each other further instruc-

tions from Tongue riding in circles endlessly going nowhere seemingly though winding up finally at her apartment he puts the green cellophane packages on a shelf above the bed she puts her waterbug on the bedroom floor. And there in the Great Outdoors under the Starry Skies the Dark Night passed with the River Wind riding the Crest of the Wave.

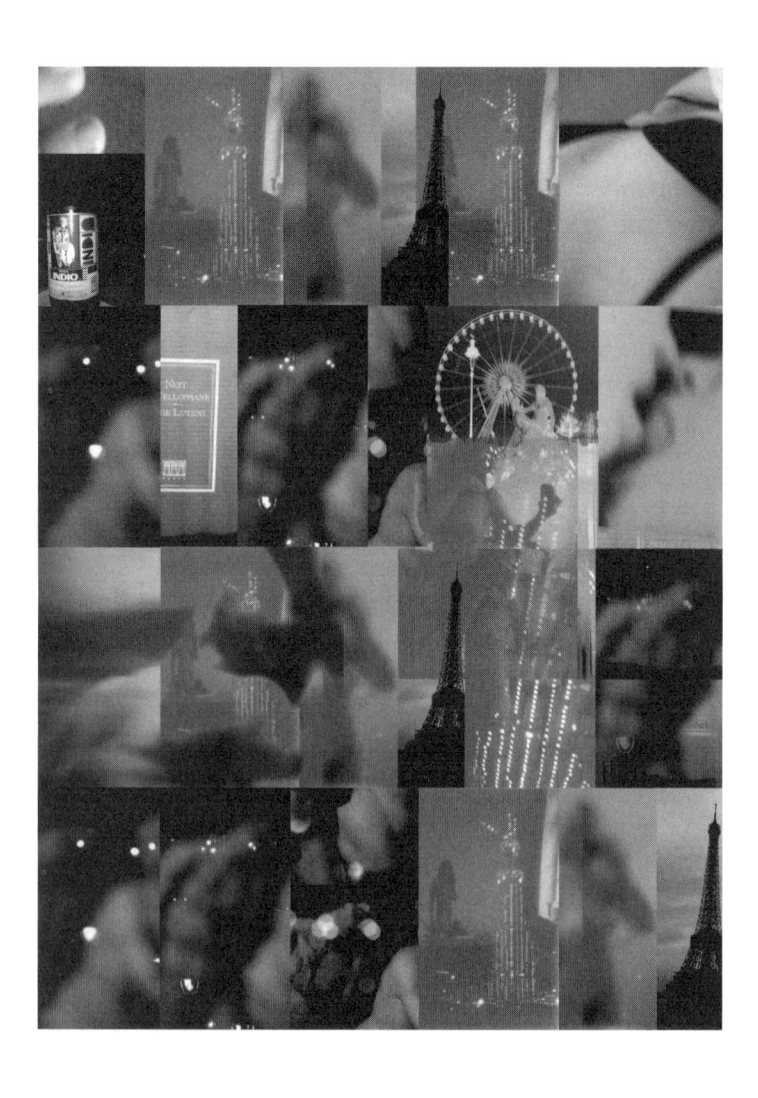

FROM **THIS YOUNG GIRL PASSING**
DONALD BRECKENRIDGE

Monday April 19, 1976

Bill had kept Sarah after the bell to find out why she was failing his class. She dutifully asked him to recommend a senior who would be willing to tutor her. He wrote a name and number down on a scrap of orange paper then offered her a ride home.

"And the photographs," Sarah glanced at Bill, "you should see them," as they continued along the narrow path, "the models are wearing casts and some of them even have black eyes," they walked by a cluster of bluebells as she concluded, "it's like pornography only worse." A chipmunk scurried across a large rock then disappeared into a pile of leaves. "Women being beaten by groups of men in suits…. How could anyone find that beautiful?" Bill stepped over a tree trunk that had fallen over the trail, "I know I don't," turned to her and held out his right hand. The cloudless sky was teeming with dozens of songbirds in flight. She placed her left hand in his, "it's like the feminist movement never happened," and stepped over the trunk. The plaster cast on Sarah's right arm extended from her elbow to her wrist. He stepped on a brittle weed and a cluster of brown thistles clung to the cuff of his pant leg. Her best friend Laura had covered the cast in tiny red hearts and flowers with fingernail polish. When a blossoming willow caught Bill's eye he stopped walking, "I think they've run out of supposedly wholesome ways," and pointed it out to her, "to sell expensive clothes to wealthy women." The willow's flowering limbs swayed as the breeze cast off a shower of yellow petals. "What does that say about the way society treats women?" A multitude of bees, undeterred by the breeze, pollinated the tree. Bill realized that he was still holding her hand, "but the models are just well paid mannequins." She frowned, "What does that mean?" "It isn't that complicated, Sarah," beads of sweat appeared on his forehead, "the people behind the camera simply script fantasy roles for women and those roles have little or nothing to do with reality." The air around them was enriched by the scent of the blooming tree. "Well," she looked at him closely, "don't you think it says a lot about the kind of people who buy them?" and noticed the faint outline of her reflection in his brown eyes. "I suppose," he nodded, "but aren't most of those designers gay?" A robin in a nearby tree began to sing. They saw each other in class, their last class of the day, five days a week, and yet she never looked the same. He was almost twice her age, "I mean, that really doesn't have anything to do with it, but it does seem strange that you would get so worked up about advertisements in fashion magazines." She smiled tentatively at her reflection while asking, "How is it not complicated?" Bill had been married for three years, "things like that are very temporal," and he was as bored by his wife's passionless lovemaking as he was repulsed by the middle-class existence that pacified her. He was as embarrassed by his wife's ideals, "next year they'll find something else," as he was resigned to them. "Like what?" "Who knows," Bill shrugged, "maybe next year they'll use vivisection to peddle their dresses." Sarah let go of his hand, "that's very funny," and began walking away.

He watched her hips sway beneath her blue jeans, "Can I ask you something?" She turned around, "you just did." He stepped toward her, "Why does that bother you so much?" She lowered her eyes, "I really thought you were different," and scratched at the rash above her cast, "So, why make jokes about something you obviously don't understand?" Her fingernails left faint whitish trails around the rash. "I was being ironic, Sarah." A bee hovered above a cluster of dandelions just inches away from the tips of her sandals. "You're being an asshole."

She had told him in the car that the cast would be removed next Monday and that she was very self-conscious about the way it smelled. When asked if her parents were concerned about her grades she looked out the open window of his Impala and laughed. When asked why that was funny she spoke enthusiastically about Truffaut's *400 Blows* that he had shown the class a month ago — then made it clear to him that the only place she didn't want to go was home.

"What is it that I don't understand, Sarah?" She placed her hands on her hips, "What is it that you wanted to show me, Mister Richardson?" He took two steps forward, "I thought that maybe we could talk and that you could tell me — " "Tell you what," she held her ground, "that I'm going to love playing in your magic tree-fort?" "You can start by telling me why you're failing my class." She shrugged before looking intently above his head. He softened his tone, "there's a beautiful lake a short walk from here," then motioned toward the trail, "are you coming or not?" She nodded sullenly and they continued along the trail. "I don't care if you call me an asshole, we can always disagree, but please don't ever call me Mister." "Why not?" "Because it makes me feel like an old man." "What about Mister Asshole," she laughed, "Can I call you that?" "That really doesn't work either," furrowing his brow, "I'd really like for you to think of me as a friend… okay?" She took his hand and asked, "How old are you?" "I'll be thirty-one this August." "Oh, that's right, you're a Leo… you are the most willful." "Not that nonsense again." "It's not nonsense Bill, you can tell a lot about a person from the sign they are born under." "For instance?" "The Zodiac is how we, as mortal beings, have passed from the spirit world into the material one." Holding Sarah's warm hand while being lectured about the Zodiac made Bill feel like he was sixteen again. "The world is divided into two opposing parts, involution and evolution. The first six signs of the Zodiac represent involution and — " "What are the first six signs?" he asked. "Aries, Taurus, Gemini, Cancer, and then you, the Leo," squeezing his hand for emphasis, "the willful lion and then Virgo, the soulful giver." "And when were you born?" With a smile, "my birthday is in February, under the sign of Aquarius." "Isn't that a water sign?" "Right, it's the eleventh sign in the Zodiac and it's a water sign, on the side of evolution. Aquarius symbolizes the disintegration of existing forms. It's a symbol of liberation." Bill's foot got caught on a root and he almost tripped. "Be careful there…" he nodded sheepishly as she continued, "the Egyptians identified Aquarius with their god Hapi who personified the Nile and when it flooded it was a tremendous source of both agricultural and spiritual importance." He was tempted to suggest that if she spent half as much time studying French as she did astrology then she wouldn't be failing his class. They passed a rusting black and white sign nailed to a tree warning trespassers that they would be prosecuted. "So," Sarah concluded, "we are from opposite sides of the Zodiac and I think that is a very good thing." The trail opened onto a small clearing. "And you consider yourself a liberated person?" They startled a pair of mourning doves foraging in the tall grass and their wings made an airy whistling sound as they flew away. "I do," with a solemn nod, "to the extent that a woman can be in a society dominated by men." He turned to her, "And how much of that has to do with the sign you are born under?" She said, "everything," with conviction. "Come on, Sarah, don't you think your environment has more to do with shaping the person you are and the one you'll turn out to be?" "No I don't," she stopped walking, "I think it's the other way around," then let go of his hand. "It's all up to your astrological sign?" "You know," noting his smirk, "arrogance is another one of the Leo's traits." He placed his hands on his waist, "it seems to me that you've got it all backwards." "How so?" A crow cawed as it flew above the meadow. He looked away from her before asking, "How did you break your arm?" "I fell off my bike," she bit her lower lip, "I told you that." He frowned, "yes, you did." She looked down at the clump of green grass between them, "So how far away is this world famous lake of yours?" He nodded in the direction they'd been walking, "it's just beyond this meadow." She tried to sound apathetic, "Are we going there or not?" He cleared his throat before stating, "the most important virtue in any relationship is honesty." She stepped toward him, "you are nothing like any of my other teachers." "I think most of your teachers are in school because of the paycheck they get every other Friday." She nodded, "it is so easy to talk to you." "If they had to sell shoes instead of teaching to pay the bills it wouldn't faze them one bit." Her curly blonde locks, "everyone in class thinks you're really cool," were rearranged by the breeze. He glanced at her chest, "it is very important to me that we are always honest with each other." Her dark brown nipples were erect and visible through the light cotton blouse. "Sure, Bill." He scratched the top of his head, "I'm really glad you feel that way, Sarah," and looked down at her sandals, "let's not keep any secrets from each other." Her toes were perfectly symmetrical and the nails were dark red. "Sure, Bill, I think that honesty — " "I think you already know that I really care about you," he looked into her eyes, "and I always want you to tell me the truth." Her smile, "sure," revealed the narrow gap between her two front teeth. "Don't you have a boyfriend?" "No, I did," shaking her head, "but he broke up with me right before Christmas." "Did he hurt you?" The trees cast shadows around the edge of the meadow. "Not really, he was a real jerk though…. I still don't know why I went out with him." "No," Bill shook his head, "I meant physically," while looking at her intently, "Did he break your arm?" "No way," her eyes widened, "I don't like guys like that… jocks or violent ones." A jet silently streaked across the blue sky, leaving a contrail behind. "What kind of guys do you like?" She began to blush, "older ones I guess, most of the guys my age are so immature… they behave like little kids." "What about married men?" She laughed out loud. "Why is that so funny?" The last thing she wanted to do was offend him, "it's not," but he had such a constipated expression on his face, "you make it sound so serious," she took hold of his left hand and examined the gold band, "Aren't you married?" he nodded before she quickly added, "I've even met your wife." Bill slowly pulled his hand away, "When?" "She's almost as tall as me and she has long brown hair and," Sarah winked, "and her name is Mary." "How do you know her name?" She felt like a lawyer on television presenting a surprise witness to a stunned jury, "Mary chaperoned a dance in my sophomore year," with a giggle, "you're not very *happily* married to Mary though."

"Sarah," he began to blush, "I asked you a question and I'd like for you to answer it." She held up her left hand, "okay," and whispered an oath, "I've never dated a married man," before placing her left hand on his shoulder and kissing him on the mouth, "but in twenty years you'll still be fourteen years older than me."

Friday March 28, 1997

Sarah contemplated his tranquil expression before saying, "I always thought that you had," in a soft voice. Bill pulled the damp condom off his flaccid erection, "that isn't true." The pounding in his chest had begun to subside. Sarah possessed a glowing intensity that radiated between them, "a lot of girls in school," her cheeks were a rosy pink, "said they slept with you," and her eyes were wide open. Sperm collected in the tip of the condom he held between the thumb and forefinger of his right hand. She pressed her thighs together and sighed. He weighed the fluid with an absentminded pride, "that certainly doesn't mean that I did." A television could be heard through the wall behind the bed. She reached behind her back with both hands and undid the tangled clasp of her bra. He leaned over and placed the condom in the ashtray. She pulled the black bra away from her breasts and cast it onto the edge of the bed. To the right of the ashtray there was a beige touch-tone phone. "How could you believe something like that was true?" To the right of the phone a red and white brochure instructed the occupants on how to exit the building in the event of a fire. A metal lamp with a beige lampshade was mounted to the wall above the nightstand; a sixty-watt bulb illuminated a portion of the room. She waited for him to adjust the thin foam pillow beneath his head before claiming, "because you never took me seriously." Long brown watermarks ran across the ceiling above the bed. He closed his eyes, "that isn't true," clasped his hands and rested them on his stomach.

Bill had saved a batch of color photographs of Sarah from the spring of '76 and would remove them from the cardboard box marked *poetry* that was buried in the bottom of the closet in his study at least twice every five years. Mary would be spending the weekend at her sister's in Bridgeport and he would be home alone and very drunk. Bill and Sarah had driven up to Sylvan Beach on a sunny weekday during the Easter break of her junior year. The image of Sarah standing on the beach with her jeans rolled up to her knees as small waves broke before her pale ankles. The image of Sarah feeding a seagull (with outstretched wings) French-fries while sitting at a dark red picnic bench. The portrait of her looking directly into the 50-millimeter lens — her blue eyes almost mirrored the cloudless sky. Sarah sitting on the back of a green bench overlooking Oneida Lake. Sarah holding a melting chocolate ice cream cone with a sardonic grin. Bill would spend hours pouring over the images until he was seeing double.

The springs in the mattress creaked, "like you were just testing the bath water with the tip of your foot," as she placed her right arm on his chest. He opened his eyes, "What does that mean?" The television on the dresser reflected their faint silhouettes on its darkened screen. She noticed the crows-feet, "that you were just interested in having sex with me," etched around the corners of his eyes, "and that you just saw me as some dumb, needy girl —" "How can you — " he tried to interject. "Who really couldn't give you anything else." "You were sixteen years old," Bill shook his head while adding, "and I couldn't believe how lucky I was to have found someone who was as… as passionately interested in me as you were then," then lowered his voice, "it was like a dream come true," as the realization that it had taken two decades to tell her that descended upon him. "You never made me feel like you were committed to our relationship." "I certainly tried," he nodded with conviction, "the sex was very important, the sex was incredible, as it should be in every relationship, although it never is… but we shared a lot of the same interests as well." Her eyes narrowed, "you never made me feel appreciated." That she would berate him about the way their relationship ended didn't come as a surprise, "I think that had a lot more to do with your upbringing and besides — " "I always felt like you were taking me for granted," she pursed her lips, "like that letter you gave me." "Twenty years ago," he shrugged his shoulders, "you can't change the past so why live in it?" Wasn't renewing their relationship a way of reliving the past? Televised laughter could be heard through the wall as she thought about his question. How could she have harbored his betrayal for twenty years?

Sarah took her arm off his chest and sat up, "you know that I kept it." Bill looked puzzled, "Kept what?" "That letter you gave me on the last day of school," Sarah rested her shoulders against the headboard. "Oh that," he contemplated their reflection in the television screen. "Oh that," she placed the tip of her index finger on her chin, "I should have brought it tonight," while watching his expression turn sullen, "Do you remember that day?" He nodded, "I don't remember what I wrote in it though." "You don't?" "No of course not… Jesus Christ… not word for word." She saw herself sprinting through the teacher's parking lot, "I guess you've done it before," and reached his car just as he was turning the key in the ignition. She was about to ask him what was wrong, "it was in the parking lot," as he rolled down the window, "on the last day of school," and shoved the envelope into her hands. He noticed the burgundy lipstick, "yes," smudged around the corners of her mouth, "I do remember that." "I'll have to show it to you sometime… maybe that will freshen your memory." Bill recalled how idiotic it felt waking up with a hangover on the daybed in his study to discover those photographs scattered across his desk. "What good would that do," he shrugged, "I'm sure that you can find a lot of faults with anyone in retrospect." "And I would get so angry with myself for wanting that life with you," she brushed his right hand off of her thigh, "you had convinced me that you didn't love her and I gave myself to you… unconditionally… and then you — " "I think you were being delusional," Bill unclenched his fists, "I was never going to leave Mary," before changing the subject, "What happened with your parents?" Sarah swallowed hard, "my mother is in a nursing home and I haven't spoken to my father in thirteen years." A door down the hall slammed. "Really?" She leveled her eyes at him, "if anyone hurt Kate the way he hurt me I would kill them." "And no jury would ever convict you," he cleared his throat before adding, "what if you got pregnant." "I wanted that life with you so badly," she hadn't taken her eyes off his chest, "and I…." "What then Sarah," he pressed his hands on hers, "what sort of life would we be living now?" "And I…" she blinked twice while looking intently at his face, "and I've never loved anyone the way I loved you. Not even my husband," she squeezed his hands, "even when things were really good between us. I've compared every man I've been involved with to you and none of them have even come close." He leaned forward, "I'm right here," and kissed her on the forehead. "I had an affair," she turned her head away, "with my boss." "The dentist?" She nodded. "At one point he wanted to leave his wife and kids for me and I told him I would quit and end our relationship if he even suggested it again." "How long did this go on for?" "The other night I realized that I was never really able to love any of them… it was more like a role that I was playing," she cleared her throat, "after we ran into each other last month I ended it with him." Bill managed to mask his skepticism, "just like that," but how many hours had she spent with her boss in a room like this, "you didn't know," he swallowed dryly, "you didn't know that we would be intimate again?" "That didn't matter," she leaned forward, "knowing that you still cared about me was enough," and kissed him on the mouth. Bill thought of taking her picture as she stood on the shore of Sylvan Beach. Sarah had removed her sneakers and socks, rolled up her jeans and stepped into the dark gray water. "It's sooo fucking cold!" He was standing five yards away when he framed her in the viewfinder and focused. She looked down at the miniature waves breaking around her ankles just before he took the picture.

"Why were you playing a role?" Bill asked. Sarah's shoulders were covered with gooseflesh, "I guess in some stupid way I felt that if I couldn't be fulfilled by one person then two might make me feel," she stopped herself from saying happy, "the thing is I could never convince myself that it was true." He shifted on the bed, "That what was true?" She frowned, "that I was unhappy," shrugging her shoulders, "or that I was just really lonely," then looked closely at his face, "or maybe I had finally convinced myself that things would never change and that I would never have another chance with you." Bill examined their entwined fingers, "When did you start sleeping with your boss?" comparing their mismatched wedding bands.

"In December." "That wasn't very long ago," he sighed, "you made it sound like — " "December of '94," she bit her lower lip, "it was three years ago... right after I started taking Prozac." "And you're still working there?" When she smiled and said, "I just got a raise," he noticed how white her teeth were. He took his hands away and stood up. "Where are you going?" He slowly crossed the room, "to the bathroom."

Dearest Sarah,
She saw him in the teacher's parking lot and ran over to his car. *We have had the very real pleasure of each other's company for more than a year now, but this relationship cannot continue any longer.* She got there just as he was turning the key in the ignition and breathlessly asked, "What's the matter with you?" *I know this will not be easy for you to understand and it wasn't easy for me to reach this decision but I need you to be strong for me and for yourself.* He rolled down the window and gave her the letter. *I have carefully thought through the plans we have made and the dreams we share for our life together and I honestly feel that I will be nothing more than a blight on your future.* When she asked what was wrong he replied, "I think it's time to move on." *The love and passion we have shared has been a real blessing and you have helped me rediscover a part of my youth that I thought I had lost forever.* "What," she pressed her hands on the car door, "what are you talking about?" *I am ashamed to admit that I could never be willing or able to leave my wife for you.* He revved the engine while asking, "How is this being discreet?" *And instead of living a lie that would have only created greater unhappiness for us in the future I think it's best that we come to our senses now and honor the secret love and friendship that we have shared.* The car pulled away as

she stood there. *I will never forget you and I will always be devoted to the memory of our time together.*

> *With much love and gratitude,*
> *Bill*

She was smoking when he returned. "Does it bother you that I'm on anti-depressants?" He stood at the end of the bed, "Isn't everyone in America on Prozac?" She exhaled, "I'm being serious," while scrutinizing his torso. "Well," shifting his feet, "is it helping?" She said, "sometimes," before placing the cigarette between her lips. "Then it doesn't bother me," the mattress sagged beneath him, "I didn't know that you smoked," as he sat next to her. "Maybe a pack every other week," she noticed a tiny bit of flesh-colored wax on his earlobe, "why were you looking at me like," picked it off with her index fingernail and flicked it onto the floor, "like you were afraid of me." Bill shrugged. "Did you hear about that cult in California?" Their clothes had slipped off the back of the wooden chair and formed a pile on the gray carpet. "Heavens Gate?" The smoke from her cigarette swirled above the lampshade. He nodded, "it was all over the news again tonight." She cleared her throat, "they thought the comet was coming to take their souls away," and placed the cigarette between her lips. "And maybe it did," he turned to her, "you know it's flying above our heads right now." She exhaled slowly, "Hale-Bop," and the smoke was pushed beneath the lampshade, "that is just so sad," where it lingered in the yellow light, "they claimed their bodies were only temporary vehicles holding in their souls and when Kate and I saw that clip on the news she said that all of those bodies, that the way they were dressed in those uniforms, made them look like envelopes." "I really loved you Sarah." Her eyes were downcast, "Then why did you end it?" Shaking his head, "I wasn't." She reached over and crushed the cigarette in the ashtray, "you used me." "That was twenty years ago." She crossed her arms beneath her breasts, "Can't you just apologize for hurting me?" "Why have you victimized yourself over this?" Clenching her jaw, "I want to know why you took me for granted." He let out a long sigh, "The risks were just impossible." She placed her hands on her knees, "Just tell me why you gave up on us." He frowned, "Answer my question." "It's not like I could have gotten pregnant anyway," she looked at him uneasily, "I was on the pill, remember that, that was your idea." He nodded, "Weren't you on the pill in college?" The off-handed way she said, "I really wanted to have your baby," stunned him. Bill shook his head in disbelief, "I wouldn't have given you that choice." "You're an idiot," she looked away and whispered, "I wanted to spend my life with you." "That's not what I thought was best for you," he examined the tufts of hair below his knuckles, "that was a mistake on my part, a selfish and — " "Is this a mistake?" He didn't hesitate, "No, no it isn't." She stretched her long legs out on the bedspread, "I'm going to see you again?" He nodded before asking, "If we had married then do you think we would still be happy?" "Why," she placed her hands on his shoulders, "wouldn't we be happy now?" and kissed him on the cheek. He cleared his throat before saying, "that's an interesting question."

FROM **URANIUM CITY**
TIM BECKETT

'm standing in front of our old house on Atom Avenue. No. 168 Atom — the numbers are visible in outline next to what remains of the front door. Up close, the house is no more ominous than any of the other houses on the street, and the sense I had yesterday of being warned away is greatly diminished, though an aura of strangeness, even menace, hangs about our old house, all the houses on the street, like a membrane you have to push through. I notice things I didn't the first time I came back a couple of days ago: the spruce tree in the front yard with four thick branches around the crown like a mutant tree, the sidewalk that runs along the side of the house before being devoured by the bushes in the back. The stillness, that contrasts so sharply with the saplings and small trees waving in the breeze like undersea plants tossed by ocean currents.

I walk up the side steps into the kitchen. It shouldn't be this easy, but it is. Someone has scrawled 'Cunt Is Good!' on the wall by the steps to the basement. A thin layer of rubble covers the plywood floor, the ceiling sags and glass from the broken windows sparkles from the rubble. Holes have been kicked and punched through the walls, the cupboards, toilet tank and dishwasher ripped from their moorings and left in the hall. Here and there, touches of normality: the black and yellow carpet which covered the kitchen and dining room floors still covers the stairs to the basement, lime-green wallpaper still lines the dining rooms, and in the living room, red and black cushions from the sunken couches by the fireplace are scattered about the floor.

Water drips steadily from the ceiling, left over from the rain storm the day before. How long will this house last before it too begins to collapse in on itself like other houses I've seen around town, support beams heaving into the ground, roof leaning down on first one side then the other. Without doors or windows, wind, snow, rain enters so easily, crossing the boundaries between inside and outside, man and nature. Abandoned areas in the city are never really empty, but this is what it is — a final emptiness of stale air, dripping water, cloying silence.

On the living room wall, the handwriting I found so disturbing the first time I came here four days ago:

"Moon, your cunt is the best I get so mad when guys talk about other girls cunts you have the tightest hairiest cunt I want to fuck you forever..."

And ad nauseum. Underneath is a drawing of a woman's torso with her legs spread, sketched in a few lines by a relatively skilled hand. These drawings, these odes to Moon, written in the same handwriting, decorate every whitewashed room in the house. Seems this guy really liked fucking Moon. The pilot who flew me in, who'd been flying in here in the years after the mine closed, told me about it: "That's what the kids did on a Saturday night hey. Got a case of beer, go to a house, get drunk, have sex and trash the house."

I didn't understand the impulse when he first told me about it, but after a couple of days here I do, sort of. At first the houses repelled me, but as I explored first one neighborhood, then another, covering the whole three miles of empty houses surrounding what was left of the occupied town, I began to be fascinated by the emptiness. I'd be mildly hungover from hanging out with the few people still left here, and as I went through house after house, looking for magazines, newspapers, any artifact of the past, my hangover mutated into a powerful if disembodied horniness. This was disturbing at first, then I gave into it, and soon what I wanted to find most was soft-core porn: *Penthouse, Oui,* the kind of magazines I stumbled across in the bush when I was a kid, yellowed and water-stained just as they had been then. It seemed right amidst the rotting carpets and collapsing walls, the spectral emptiness inside the houses.

But eighteen years is a long time, and every house I went into had been picked clean. I never found anything and soon the impulse passed.

Outside, the breeze has picked up, and trees and grasses wave in delirious motion, with a sound like the roll of a distant ocean. The front door bangs once, then is still. Inside, the silence goes on and on: even the mosquitoes won't stay inside these places. I remember my search for the magazines and wonder what it was like for the kids when they came here, kicking holes in the walls after fucking on the bare wood floor, in the midst of all this emptiness. If, for just a moment, it didn't feel like a sort of communion. Kids act on things unconsciously, on impulse; I wonder if they weren't channeling some force of nature, just like they channeled some sort of death impulse when they smashed every window of every empty building in town.

The handwriting on the wall is faded, maybe as much as a decade old. The kids don't come here anymore or if they do, they don't leave their mark.

I step back outside. Empty houses lurk amidst the poplars lining the road, doors propped half open, shattered windowframes staring out like eyes from a row of skulls. I enter our neighbor's house, then the house next to it, stepping across the fence lying flat in the grass, navigating through piles of timber and pink insulation. The rooms have been stripped bare, and sometimes entire walls have been ripped away, so one room opens onto another, or onto the outside world. The spidery handwriting, the drawings, cover the walls of every house:

"*Moon... Moon....*"

The graffiti runs along the walls of every house on the block then on into the houses on the next block down. I jump over the fences, pushing aside the grasses and saplings to clear the way, until it becomes a mania to cross the boundaries that mark the everyday, into this strange, alternate world of emptiness and decay, the world this couple, whoever they were, had reveled in as they fucked their way through the neighborhood.

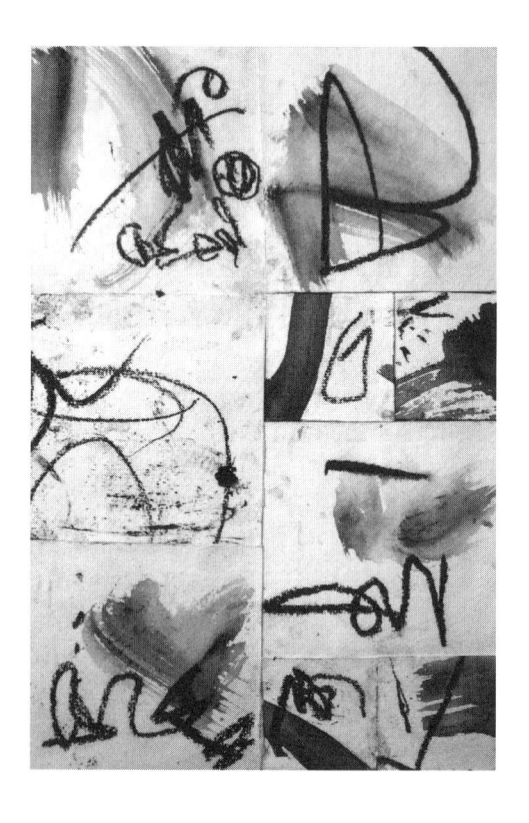

LINGERIE
MICHAEL ROTHENBERG

A naked woman in a green Edsel convertible. Scarf around her head, tangled in the steering wheel, snatch in the air. Killed while masturbating.

"I wouldn't want to be found dead while masturbating. Naked, sticky fingers stiff with rigor mortis," she says.

"You have to have a sense of humor when it comes to sex," I say.

She smiles and nods.

It's impossible not to stare at her.

"My father was a chef in Jamaica," she says. "He loved food." My father was a glutton.

Peach silk panties. Cool as my hand slips into warm flesh. Slips. Sleeps. Slippers. Sweaty feet in slippers. Snap. Strap stings against her thigh. High hips. My finger slips deeper.

I am in her apartment. Touching her things. Looking at her privately. The way I wanted to. Imagined I would. Gloating. Pleased with myself. I can't catch my breath. Can't make small talk. Naked pictures of her on the wall.

A picture of a naked woman over the toilet. I'm pissing into a pool of water beneath her round ass. Hourglass back and ass. Feet tucked invisible. Hair, long, thick, black hanging down to her ass, an upside down heart. Upside down, inside myself, looking at a photograph of a woman.

In her bedroom. Futon in black net suspended from ceiling. Macrame nest for potted lovers. Suspended from something indefinite. Something other. Net. Love chamber. Web.

Houseplants not grown especially well on narrow wrought-iron balcony. Plants. Yellow tinged edges of spider plants. Sunburned leaves of corn plant.

She stings me. Somehow. A spider.

Vining plants, green grows in rich humus. Thick, black soil, curly pubic hair. Parted. Potted. Moist.

I am the drunken man.

"You want to get a bite to eat?" she asks, suggesting Mel's.

Soft, greasy fries. Bacon slips through mayonnaise while we talk. I listen to her. She listens to me. I tell her about breaking a spiritual fast with apples and honey.

She likes to water houseplants in her nightgown in the morning, before she brushes her teeth, when she's not fully awake. Every morning, moving inside the gauze of lingerie. Rose kimono. I lift her nightgown.

"My anesthesiologist friend examines patients' genitals while they are unconscious," she says. "Say, for example, a really nice-looking woman comes in. She's on a stretcher. He looks under the sheet, checks her out," she says. "It doesn't do much for me. It's sort of creepy."

She has a window in her bedroom. Warm light filters through. By the window, on the wall, high and out of the way, there's a picture of her. Dark face, thick hair. One naked breast visible enough to fully appreciate.

I think about erotic art. Novels and sculptures of geishas, elaborate robes raised over invisible faces. Raped by Samurai. Hindu gods copulating. Mandalas of sexual gluttony. Round, chocolate breasts. Muscular breath. Sucking, dripping, overflowing. Pearls of juice. Walking through a garden. Liquid shell compressed. Easing muscle. Contracting muscle. Throat, lips…. Lumps of contracting flesh. Muscle, membrane….

"So you were a model?"

"Yes, do you want to look at my pictures?" She places her portfolio on my lap.

"Yes," I try to catch my breath. Holding my breath.

"I have a hundred negligees, but never wear them," she says. "Men are always giving me negligees. I don't know why. I'd rather sleep naked."

Nipples, face. Her face is her sex. Different positions. Walking. Standing. Looking over her shoulder. Different situations. On a beach. On a sofa.

Eating French fries at Mel's.

One picture slips from a plastic sleeve. One of her breasts slips from a negligee. She is watching me, looking at naked pictures of her. I slip the picture quickly back into the plastic sleeve, as if she could read my mind sucking her breasts. She's watching me watch her as I turn the pages of her portfolio.

Inside the liquid shell, compressed, easing muscle of groin. Oil, lips. Lumps of contracting flesh. Muscle. Dripping membranous grip, clutch, hip, hump.

I brought my dog along for protection.

I was giving her a ride home from work. I wanted to talk. She knew this.

I stopped, at my house, to pick up my dog. Take him for a ride. I wanted her to see how I lived. She'd never been in my house. I invited her in. Maybe she gloated, secretly, looking at my things, touching my things. She looked through the house, quickly, as if intruding. As if she was in a hurry. But maybe she was gloating.

When we got to her house she invited me in for coffee.

"I don't drink coffee in the afternoon," I said, "but I'll come in."

I carried the dog up terra cotta stairs.

I studied pictures of her on the wall. Her naked breast. Her house plants. When the dog sniffed around, it gave me a feeling of power. I gloated. Could the dog smell her on the white leather sofa, animal fragrance, fragrance of peach and humus, blood and chocolate?

She pets the dog. She lowers her face to his. I stop her. I warn her that's when he bites. He's nervous. I'm afraid he will bite her. He looks at her. Smells her.

Sea storm. Beach foam. Sea creatures beached and blossoming.

I tell her I enjoyed looking at her pictures. And the one picture she drew of herself. I put it back in the erotic art book she gave me to look at. Fetish within fetish. A pencil sketch of a woman's torso, signed Clara '89.

I zip up the portfolio. Absently pet the portfolio on my lap.

"I can't look anymore." I'm afraid to look in her eyes.

The book of pictures bound in black. I hand it back to her.

"Why?" she asks.

"It is too much to swallow in one breath. It will take me some time."

Strapped to an avalanche of milky come.

"Do you like Mel's?" I wipe grease from my chin, scrunch up my nose.

She doesn't answer. She wants to use me. She wants me to give myself over to fantasies of her. To imagine her entirely.

We sat there. Said nothing. We weren't going to have sex. The dog was there and she was getting hungry.

"I like to make love and I like to eat," she says, "and there's no orgasm without chocolate."

She didn't ask me to fuck her.

"Are you hungry yet?" She sets the black bound portfolio on the glass table.

"I could eat," I say.

A sandwich. Meat between two pieces of toasted white bread. I stuff my face. Mayonnaise drips down my chin, onto my shirt.

I want to unload her lingerie closet. Fill the flesh cabinet of mail order catalogues with my milky load. Unload. Ivory silk robes. Champagne sashes. Satin slips. Venetian lace. Purple, black, taupe scalloped bras. Blue floral panties. Unload. We end up at Mel's.

She reads my story so far.

"I can't believe you included Mel's," she says. "It ought to be a story about a woman in a nightgown watering her plants, standing on her balcony, a morning breeze lifts her nightgown. Her perky nipples dark against the thin white gown. And he takes her in the rich humus."

"What about the green Edsel?"

"Do you want to watch me make love to another woman?" she asks.

"Yes, I would."

Veils. Scarves. Black, blue, lace, cotton, leather corsets. Scarves. Red, black, blue, green, zebra and tiger striped panties. Black garter belts. Blush panties.

I roll the car window down slightly, so the dog won't suffocate. We go in.

Mel's, a replica of a 50's diner. Burger fat frying. French fry grease popping.

"Sit anywhere you like." The hostess points to an empty table.

We take the table near a trinity of aging Asian transvestites. The waitress scribbles our order and hurries off, ass wagging.

"Do you think we will ever have sex?" I finally ask.

She smiles. Dark brown eyes.

"No, you're married, it's not right," she says.

But I can watch her fuck another woman, watch her undress, slip out of her lingerie into the caress of another woman. Press hard tongues into an ocean foam darkness.

"Look at those three strange people in the corner booth," she says.

"Yes," I say. What is she doing to me? Trying to make me harder.

"I like to look at people," she says.

One transvestite gestures to another.

"I like to look at you," I say. "Do people take you out just to look at you?"

Neon blue scarf. Knotted fur around your wrists. Knotted, tight, behind your back, tied tighter. Knotted. Pulling myself up inside you.

My throat catches. I hold the telephone, sweating.

"What are you doing tonight?"

She is staying home to watch a horror movie. She doesn't invite me to join her. We talk on the telephone about erotic art. And this interest I have in erotica. Would she mind if I took notes while we were talking?

"No, I don't mind," she says. "Why don't you use a microphone?"

She doesn't laugh much, thinks she has a crooked smile and horse teeth. She shows me her horse teeth across the dinner table. They look alright, but I'm not a dentist.

"I can't believe you included Mel's," she says again.

Does she bring all her prospective suitors to Mel's? The waitress acts like she has seen it all before. Am I a prospect?

"You know, I'm not a gold-digger," she says.

I don't care, as long as she's got other things going. I hate single-minded people.

My mouth is dry. Her dark brown eyes say nothing. I suspect she is amused at her captive. Looking at her through a mail slot. She's looking back. My dog marks the bushes.

Why am I afraid?

Her black lace corset on the back of the door.

Is she calling me into her world? Did she win the game?

I pause against the desire to rip the corset. Then I rip the corset. Stuffing my imagination of stockings, panties, bows and lace, up her nothingness.

She shows me her closet of lingerie. Cranberry thong bikinis. Eggshell. Cocoa chemise. Spandex thong bikini. Scalloped bras, corsets. Purple, red, blue garter belts. Prizes from men who have admired her. This is her gallery of conquest. Her net. Her web.

"It's funny how men are when they get near sex." She wags a soggy fry. She measures the distance with her hand. "They get…"

"Crazy," I say.

"…crazy." She almost smiles.

She is beautiful. Jamaican/French/Swiss. High cheekbones. Lips carved from tropical hardwood. Raised in Cleveland.

"I don't like to make love without shaved legs," she says.

Why did she tell me that?

"Take these stamps and think of me when you lick them and stick them," she says.

They are stamps of seals and whales.

She says she doesn't take her makeup off before she goes to bed with someone. I want to take her makeup off and see who she really is. Blood and chocolate.

"Women are better looking than men, but boring in bed," she says.

She describes the mascara smeared on her pillow.

Her friend says she should be a telephone sex talker. I don't think so.

Teeth. Sucking flesh between teeth. She falls into the net. Heartbreak. Knotted. Web. Grunts. Sternum kinked up, she raises herself for me to enter. Massages her thighs, warming herself for entry. I slide my wrist against the moistening bristle, until I enter.

Her sex is not so much in her breath. It's in her face, serious. Her sheets a mess, smeared with mascara.

"Why don't you sit in the lobby of one of those bath clubs," she says. "You could learn a lot."

Sternum against cotton-pillowed futon. Head arched up, reaching for air.

She collects lingerie. Stiched black lips of lace, stitched with red ribbon. Bows between mesh. Sage and bow trimmed shawl on the floor. Cream panties. Star raised, she tempts me with rejection. Nothing left. Nothing.

"Have you ever been to one of those clubs?" I ask.

"Lots of times. You could watch who goes in and out of the baths. Old men and young girls…." She pauses. "I lost my virginity when I was eighteen to a forty-eight-year-old man. He knew what he was doing. It was some of the best sex I ever had."

I lift you. Raise your hips up. Bundle of lingerie tucked up under your belly. Emerald green robes. Black garter belts with red lace bows. Butter silk and satin. Spandex thongs and cotton. Sheer scarves and corsets. Apricot nighties. Panties. Magenta. Lilac panties. Bed of lingerie bunched up. I tie your ankles with a blue scarf. Your ankles are crossed. I touch the rising star with my curving erection.

Over dinner I describe to her what I remember she wore each time we met.

Day one: Black mesh blouse and beige vest. Black slippers. She took them off. I didn't warn her about broken glass.

"You want it both ways," she says.

Twenty dollars for a hot tub.

Day two: A black corset and black crotchless panties.

"I would be happy to pay," I say, "I'm learning about myself."

"If you want, I could ask my friend to come along. She's done things I've never done before. Would you like that?"

What has she never done?

Weeping flood of humus. Flood from the prison. The enormous flesh.

I'm afraid to touch her. I wouldn't like it if she said no. I came early. Her plants look better today. Creeping Charlie. Spider plant. Pictures of herself. Black gloves on the coffee table. Pictures of Paris. Calla lily on the mantel. Euphorbia by the open glass door leading to the balcony. Clock says, "6:15." Fog castrates twin peaks radio towers. Seagulls cry. Sweet smells in her apartment. Rock & Roll on TV. She's in her bedroom, just out of the bath in terry cloth leopard print bathrobe. My throat is dry. I didn't want to do this. I only wanted to….

Early. I should have come late. Made her wait. How about coming when I say I am coming. Lobelia. Petals spilled on terracotta steps. Geraniums in red bloom. Phaelanopsis in white bloom, pink lipped. Bowl of seashells, sea skeletons. Shakespeare. Plato. Einstein's tongue on the wall. White rap music. She's talking on the phone.

She sucks my cock with muscular lips. Teeth suck.

Holding the flesh slightly, licking the head, nipping the bending erection. Then she stops.

"I've been tied up before," she says. "But it didn't do anything for me."

Small, strong body. Long sleeve black lace blouse with white vest. Wide buckle around low gray jeans. Her ass not too round, friendly. Bellybutton, a warm brown oily mushroom. Buttons to unbutton.

"Discovered naked masturbating, snatch in the air."

"A green Edsel convertible."

Mel's Diner. All I could do was roll the top down. She took off her bucanneer buckle. Masturbated while I ate a sandwich and fries. I look over my glasses, my sandwich, study her. She stares back.

"I prefer sleeping naked."

She started to get into the wrong car. A green one. I drove a maroon Volvo. She wanted to surprise the dog, who would've been crouching behind the seat. She was playful. But the dog was not there. And she rarely smiles. It was a green car, but not an Edsel.

My car was maroon. She didn't remember.

"Volvo, I expected it to have a kiddie seat," she said. "All Volvos have kiddie seats and their owners have 2.5 children."

I have no children. I have a maroon Volvo. The dog is crouched behind the passenger seat. She gets in the car. I drive her home.

"Wait one second." She hurries from the car. "I have something for you."

She runs upstairs, returns with a book.

"Erotic art." She hands me the oversized book. "Tell me what you think. I'll call you Thursday."

She never called.

THE DISMANTLED BEDPOST
NICCA RAY

Flannel sheets with bulldog print the bedroom repels sex.

Her slippers Maribou the nightgown leopard the sigh between her legs
False eyelashes flutter she takes position back flat breasts to ceiling — a board.

He watches standing fingertip on zipper pulling down from opposite side of room
She smoothes her hand over belly full a Renoir nymphet
His blue jeans a pile behind him.
His chest blonde hairy the hair that wasn't there the first night they kissed twenty years ago Chanel red a smear on her chin

Their lust is a ghost tied to bedpost he grips as if it were a cane
Their gazes frozen in the knowing what is to come are the 1-2-3 motions.
He can't be sure he remembers how to let himself loose these four white walls the urn imprisons his desire

She scrapes her Maribou heel against red bulldog head of flannel sheet a rip

Lifts her head her belly rolling
His hand curls over flesh
He pushes nightie up a trickle of pubic hair
The yearning between her legs a roar

His erection
His need
The return of the blushing glow in his cheeks

She slides off mattress down on floor His grip a hand-cuff on her ankles Her lips pressing against wood tile far away from bedroom where they have spilled a thousand dreams and whispered confessions he drags her to a virgin room where secrets and struggles and friendship forever have yet to strangle his throbbing erection her breath shaky her craving to be taken she slaps his buttocks he slips inside a sudden thrust the linoleum cold on her spine pounding clutching thigh on thigh nipple to nipple cheek to cheek lashes brushing deep throat kissing the dismantled bedpost

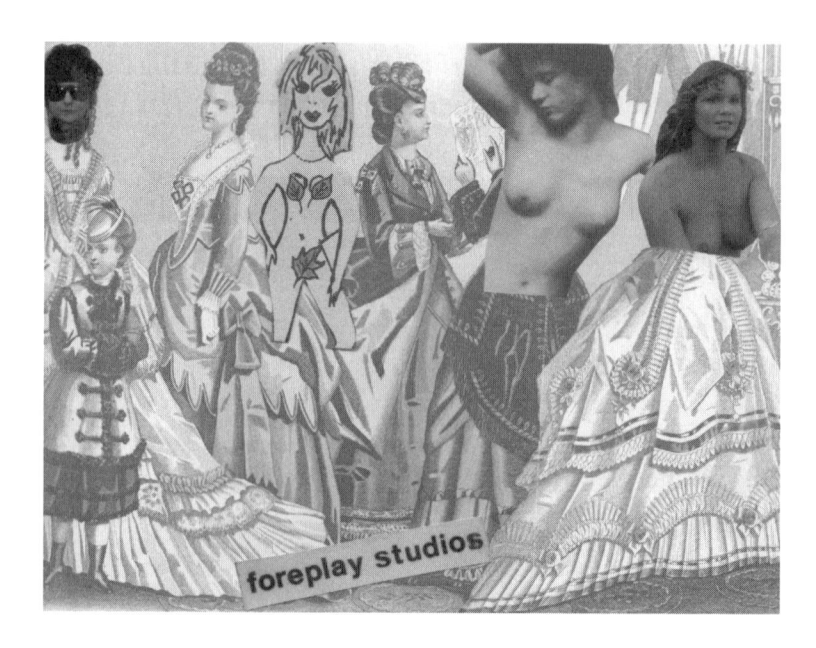

GARDEN VIEW
DIRK BLANDO

I cannot be honest about sex. So I do not write about it. I envy those great Victorians who write so eloquently about all manner of copulations, their golden words skillfully guiding wankers' hands into verdant gardens of lubricious fantasy. But I am a historian. If I cannot be honest, I do not write. Or at least, that is my habit. Now, asked to write about sex, I have been tongue-tied these many months. But I must write. For sex is now a leitmotif of my life, and, rather than pay a professional to listen to my ramblings, I can use my own skills to dispel my confusions.

Which cannot be. There is no clarity to be had. Sex is simple, animal, mechanical, the feral robot dance. Love is the gasoline, however, and this fuel, this food is extremely various. All odious, enslaving religio-statist moral propaganda aside, love and sex go together. They are sororial twins, and every human contact is a threesome in this way.

I must write now because my lover is departed. "Do you know my smell?" she asked. "No," I replied. "I don't know it because your smell is me." She did not understand. Elliptical English confuses her, and these relations are nothing if not elliptical. My lover has returned across the sea to her job, home and family in a foreign land.

We have just had one week in my city, together in a tiny over-heated room upstairs from a funeral parlor. At night we were awakened by the cries of bar patrons turned out at closing time. My baby is a light sleeper. Then, in the early morning, she might be unable to return to sleep. Then she might finger my cock very delicately, and as I move my hips in quiet response she may pull herself down my legs and wrap her lips around the tip of my member. I never learned how to take a blow job gracefully. I feel somehow at a loss unless I too can bury my face between my sweetheart's legs and tongue her parts. So I always do that, kissing her vagina and the lips. Her clit is too sensitive for direct pressure by the finger of my mouth.

In this our most recent room, doing the sacred 69 could mean singeing my hair on the oversized radiator built into a cabinet at the foot of the bed. For this sublime appetizer of the love feast, the huge bed we had in a Toledo hotel was the best; the hostel in Beacon, with its dozens of froufy pillows, was really nice too, except for the teddy bears. They seemed to be watching us in mute recrimination, and my lover dislikes toys.

Soon, when my member has enlarged, my lover climbs on top of me and places our parts into divine conjunction. She rides carefully up and down. Then, as often as not, my erection fades away, and we go back to sleep. This is because I am old, only a few years younger than that Florentine humanist who, although he had spent long years in exile, declared himself satisfied to have still fifteen teeth in his head. As an old man, I am on the young side. But driving the unmade child into my lover's womb is no longer my concern.

As we sleep we touch. She curls, I scratch her bony knees. I kiss her spine, her ribs, her shoulder blades. She is slim, with narrow hips and generous breasts, the very type of an Indian yakshi goddess. And I am a divinely contented devotee, covering her beloved body with my kisses. When we are together I must touch her constantly. We hold hands. We argue. She is asperious. I will not do as she commands, or do the things she knows are best for me. I am sullen. She insults me. In reply I can only wait a few moments, then kiss her hand, or the top of her head. "I do not care," I mean to say. "I love you."

I kiss her ears. "You know, the ears do not stimulate me," she says. Yes, but her ears, curled and differentially pink, are like delicate porcelain ornaments hung onto her lovely head. I want to eat them very slowly.

Back in our room we like to see each other in bright light. She has a wiry body and a flat stomach like a girl. She is a small size, and wears skimpy brand name briefs with erotic names. She cuts the labels out of all her clothes like some spy or hired killer. I find these on the floor: "hip hugger," and "girls' low rise briefs." I put them into my pocket and read them later.

There is no curtain on the window here, only a shade. It is either up or it is down. We want to feel the sun falling on our bodies, another dose of luxury during these bitterly cold days. The window is flush with the bed and looks out onto a graveyard. (There are no more burials; it is full.) Snow fell recently. Although it is mostly melted, some remains along the paths. A tall new hotel rises on the next street. A hundred luxury rooms face the graveyard.

"My darling, we are going to end up on the internet!"

"So? You are worried about that?"

She is not very interested in the web. I'm the one who watches porn, who finds xhamster, with the twenty-minute underwater lesbian ballet, cocksucking foursome and "double banging." This lovely anaerobic sex show is unusual. More common is the brutal anal fuck of a glossy shaved and painted woman. She is screaming in pain, the man is a retired prison guard. I am horrified. Or a laundry room surveillance video of two casual lovers. But "love" is really not involved in porn. It is strikingly rare to see a caress. And, although it is virtually certain that our morning caresses are being observed by someone in that hotel, I don't think our sex would look very exciting on film. Still I must throw the blanket over our moving hips. We are on show, whether we can see the audience or not. Although I am writing this, I guess I'm still a little shy.

We are out walking on the boulevard. It is the coldest time of the year in the city, and this is a cold year. My lover is bareheaded. I am wearing her hat. "Pull it down," she says, "or you look like a Muslim." She has insisted that I wear her hat because my regular hat is a woven Peruvian with ear flaps, and it looks too hippie. Meanwhile she is wearing her special thermal shirt, a sweater, the coat from Greenland, wool pants over that lovely underwear, and double gloves — and she is still cold.

Our last day together is a long march from café to café. In one we are again in the window, watching boulevard crowds, and her fingers feel icy. They are small, with well trimmed nails, and red from the cold. "You should wear your hat, not me. Then your hands will be more warm." I say this even though I am loath to give it up. I remember once in the airport in Europe, as we said good-bye, she was twisting her fingers in mine over and over, again and again. It was heartbreaking, and deeply erotic. Now, in the café, she is doing the same, to warm them. In the coffee shop, a new Italian place, we use the toilets. On the way out, a friend calls my name. He is newly baldheaded, and gobbling a sandwich. He informs me matter-of-factly that he is awaiting a stem cell transplant. It is his only chance to survive. He has always been cantankerous, amusing — and he is a very good artist. As we take our leave, I rub his back affectionately. He is only a few years younger than me. My lover squeezes his arm, although he has just met her and did not look at either of us as he ate his sandwich.

Again in the room, hot enough for bikram yoga, we slip gratefully into the bed. I did not pack my sex pills, so I cannot maintain an erection long enough for my love to achieve an orgasm in her best position. Still she sits on me, then lies down, rubbing her pubis against mine. I squeeze her small buttocks, feeling the bones of her hips. We are two skeletons, rubbing delightedly together. But we are not dead bones, but alive ones, enjoying scraping our bones sheathed in flesh and nerves, alive with the sensations just as living colored coral reefs squirm with life.

I like this position too. As a long celibate masturbator, I was simply too lazy to employ tools, lubricants and what have you. Often I simply imagine my absent lover riding me, and blow into the air harder than ever I can into her.

My love. I wish she would quit smoking and gain some weight.

SHE...
ALLAN GRAUBARD

She rose with the bright plumage of a word, defending herself against inquisitorial fingers that seeped, without warning, from her shadow behind her. In an hour it would be too late, in two hours too soon. Wandering naked in a thin raincoat and high heels, a wide-brimmed green felt hat and black leather gloves pulled up to her elbows, she remembered where she was, how she had gotten there and why, in the aftermath of so many conquests, refusals, allurements, teases, handshakes, toasts, her eyes all at once filled with tears and descended to the exact pin of a blindness that usurped her. That she stood there, beneath a flashing neon coffin and a revolving nickelodeon porter, palms up and outstretched, by a corner that fronted the vegetable market for the city's destitute mothers, convinced her that night was a toy for scorpions, a rag doll to be torn apart by massive circling hunters. For a moment her face resembled a puddle of rancid oil just to the left of her feet. Then she shuddered, hunching her shoulders in to mimic the base points of an isosceles triangle whose apex joined at her brow. If she could, she would spin slowly then with greater speed as certain dancers had taught her, for nothing more than to blandish the fear spreading through her nerves. She would preen herself on the presumption that centrifugal force would sustain her and that, if she desired, she could, with the twitch of an arm, hurl herself upwards or sideways in proportion to the tenacity of her exertions. She could, she knew, at the same time stipple herself into thrumming strips of truncated viscera as a warning for others not to approach. Freed from the geometry of her bones, and never again to reclaim them as they were, her neck, her arms, her legs world elongate, if still taut with the previous certainty of her image, until gravity refused her or claimed her. In either event, she would be lost into the dry ink that curdled about her. Perhaps her eyes, those delicate twin sparks of laburnum, would grace witness to her astonishing disarticulate trauma.

Her instinct, of course, was to run to the nearest bar or café where human contact was as superficial as it was enticing and where a bourbon or an espresso would reawaken her to the more humble and human avocations of her time. What she feared with such poignancy was a common enough disease: the unutterable evasion of her rage at living so meanly and always, it seemed, on the cusp of an affair, a climax, an oath to love till death. In the labyrinth of her mirages, this above all else bore the promise of special privileges of daring that she had, because of her beauty, her sudden tantrums, her immense disdain for anything less, cunningly aborted. The wound was a worm boring through her heart with an intelligence she took for her own and, albeit wondrously, gloried in by day and night. That it failed her now did not concern her in the least. Bereft of the usual accommodations she made to time, to work, to sex, her fear, no longer horrific, began to serve her. The cold sweat that broke across her smile revived her compassion for the inanity of voiceless things: a scrap of newspaper mewling in a bat-infested doorway, a trash can skewered on a stop sign by a crew of drunken police, a bald truck tire polished to the black sheen of an obsidian mirror, the scorched springs of a mattress riddled with rats mumbling click prayers to Allah as they gorged on pigeons, a pocketbook dangling from a third-flow window, an empty beer keg rising from a pothole like a periscope for nightmare subways, a child's rag doll rescued from the crematorium of indolent stares she received from men whenever she passed them in her raincoat, gloves, hat and high heels — spurious unbidden cyclones she gathered into bouquets to remind her that their desire, like hers, was of no vantage alone.

Then a taxi turned the corner and pulled up to the curb beside her. The driver unrolled his window and leaned out, asking her if she needed a lift.

"I've no money," she whispered. "No money, no heart, no clothes." And she unbuttoned her raincoat and stood there, shifting her weight from one foot to the other.

He smiled, his teeth glinting white between his lips. His eyes became two tents of green savory cactus. His hands drumheads for the garish fables he would spin when retelling this tale. Egyptian or Romanian, Polish or Chilean, his face forged maps of metallic splinter bombs, long streaks of incendiary contusions that scattered through her thought, intoxicating her.

He got out and opened the back door for her. She shook her head no and lay down in the sweet thick grime of the street.

"Rather here," she thought, "without excuse, without forbearance, in the ignorant sweat of a stranger's arms."

He knelt between her legs and unzipped his pants. She was wet and deep and took his mouth and covered him with her breath, making and remaking him into any man she wished and none she could have beyond her moans, her thrashing, her cries. As he pumped his sperm into her, he bit deeply into her shoulder, growling like a dog over a freshly cut bone thrown off by a butcher. He collapsed on top of her.

She pushed him off.

"Finish it!" she rasped.

He turned to look at her with drained dead eyes. Then he picked himself up and brushed himself off.

"Help yourself," he said.

He got in the driver's seat, slipped the key into the ignition and started the engine. He glanced back at her one more time before pulling away around the opposite corner.

A strange immaculate silence possessed her. The sky, wheeling on axes of starlight, ignited the bitter taste of his tongue. Then she gave herself to her hands, masturbating in the dark voracious cavern of the merciless careening night.

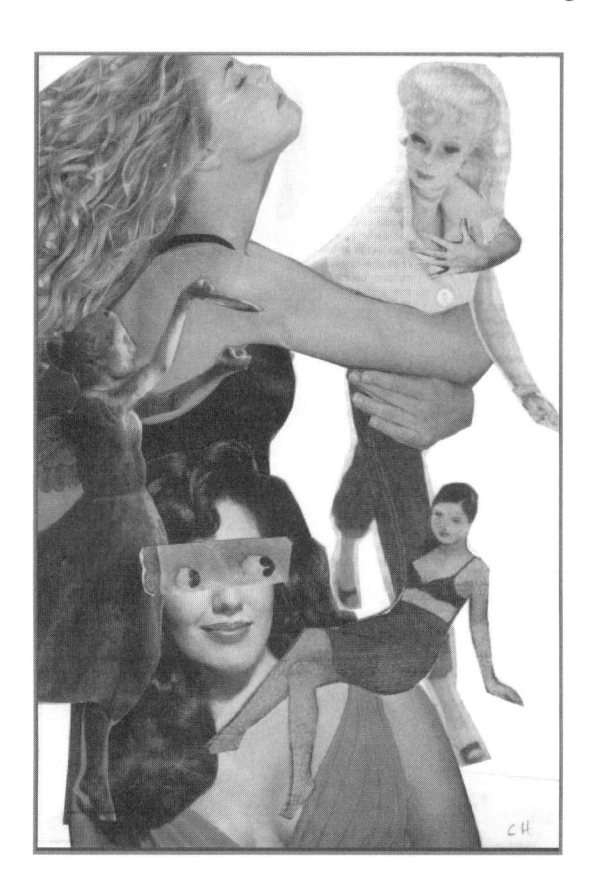

HIS FOREVER GIRL
ELLEN 'WINDY' LYTLE

When we land in Mexico City it's almost evening. I'm edgy. Probably I need food but that's not what I'm thinking, though of course Jannie Rose wants to eat. There's so much to do, and it's hot out! God, who wants food when you're in a country you've never been to, with an American Express card.

"First we'll check in and then look for the hotel dining room," she says.

I sulk. Boring. A bell cap puts our bags into the elevator and escorts us to the 18th floor.

"It's the Continental Hilton, what'd you expect," my sister says as I smile at the lavishly carpeted corridors and pots of flowers set on small polished tables. I tip the quiet man after he sets down our luggage. Knowing some five words in Spanish, I plan to try French. Jannie's nervous, I can tell, but I refuse to pay attention.

"Let's change, go outside. It's a gorgeous, warm evening. Don't worry, we'll find something — go shopping." I pull out the credit card.

"I want to eat right here in the hotel and they have nice shops downstairs and probably American food, too."

That's annoying, and even though I like the outfit I've changed into it's becoming more and more obvious this trip won't be a compromise. There's a different elevator operator this time; young (around my age), of medium height, with smooth skin and cat eyes looking at me hard as the doors slide open on our floor.

Whatever he's thinking maybe I am too, when Jannie reminds me we are actually supposed to have dinner with two men we met in Juarez. I look around the enormous, beautiful lobby for someone familiar but can't keep the elevator guy out of my thoughts and I'm too excited to think about anything else. Still, I've been trained, my sister's needs come first. We find the guys and I agree to eat with them but slip away after the appetizers pretending I forgot something in the room.

He's still working the elevator and because most guests are eating dinner, we're alone.

"Como se llama? Your name?" he smiles.

"No ra," I say lamely. His eyes are penetrating and I'm sure I'll melt before we reach the 18th floor. "Never mind. Take me back down, bajo, lobby, por favor."

"Si, si, pero. Later we go out, ok?" I nod yes, yes.

"A las diez?" he uses his hands, all ten fingers.

"Ok," I laugh, as baby bubbles start rising from somewhere near my stomach.

Jose Robles, one of my Juarez lawyers, introduces a straight looking young man to Jannie Rose and they plan a date for later — leaving me absolutely free to go anywhere with 'him,' the cool one in the elevator.

I change again quickly, into a pair of cotton pants and a stretchy top. Going up the elevator is packed, he doesn't notice me, but at ten o'clock when I breathlessly get back in, he gestures for me to wait in the lobby. Five minutes later he's standing beside me; his black hair combed straight back, his open patterned shirt tucked into a pair of perfectly ironed khakis. Handsome, really. I manage to get that we're going dancing.

The place is away from the city proper but he takes care of transportation and paying for everything seamlessly. I mostly remember the night being like confetti, all those long strips of colorful plastic that hang in every barrio doorway from Barcelona to Mexico — they hang in this nightclub, too. Only it's partially outdoors and the dance floor's below the tables as if we are sitting around the edge of a big bowl. He orders sangria — it's warm and I'm thirsty. Lovely, this sweet tasting wine with floating orange slices.

"What's your nombre?"

"Jorge." His face curls up like a little boy.

"Me gusta? Si? You like me?"

"Si, me gusta."

Suddenly his mouth is on mine and I'm inside his. We are dancing with his hair in my hair, his teeth on my teeth, his sweat mixed with mine on his arms, his neck. Again and again we dip and twirl. We dance in circles while he swallows me whole. I taste his skin, clutch every sinew and muscle, drink his saliva with his hands under my top, on my breasts and between my legs. I'm certainly wet.

"Me gusta mucho? Me gusta siempre? For ever?"

"Si, me gusta siempre."

The confetti hanging in the doorways to the kitchen, in the garden, sway gently in the night breeze and though I'm slightly scared, like when I was picked up once on a Harley, I don't want to stop anything, not now. Anyway, it's May in Mexico and I'm warm with wine and his breath in my mouth.

Around four AM we waltz outside the club, swaying. We don't end up at the Hilton but drive into what seems like a gas station. I smell the heat mixing with oil, grease and old car parts. There's red and gray paint peeling, and rust everywhere. The taxi drives inside, under the partially sagging roof, where it looks like a huge sunken stable for horses but is probably a pit where mechanics work on cars. Circling the pit about five feet high are red doors surrounded by a metal railing. Jorge says something to the driver and rushes me up the steps onto the swirling catwalk and into one of the rooms. This, I think, sobering up fast, must be a whore house. He leads me to an extremely high bed undressing me walking. I tear at him. He's on top of me, instantly my bra's half off my arm, my red pants around my ankles.

"No, no, you mustn't…. Me madre with dos babies, no, no!"

I start screaming but he is slowly and deliberately inside me making love. Part of me never wants him to stop or leave, the other prays I won't get pregnant again.

Somewhere in France, six weeks later, on my honeymoon with Jake, what's left of Jorge and me in Mexico City falls into a hotel toilet.

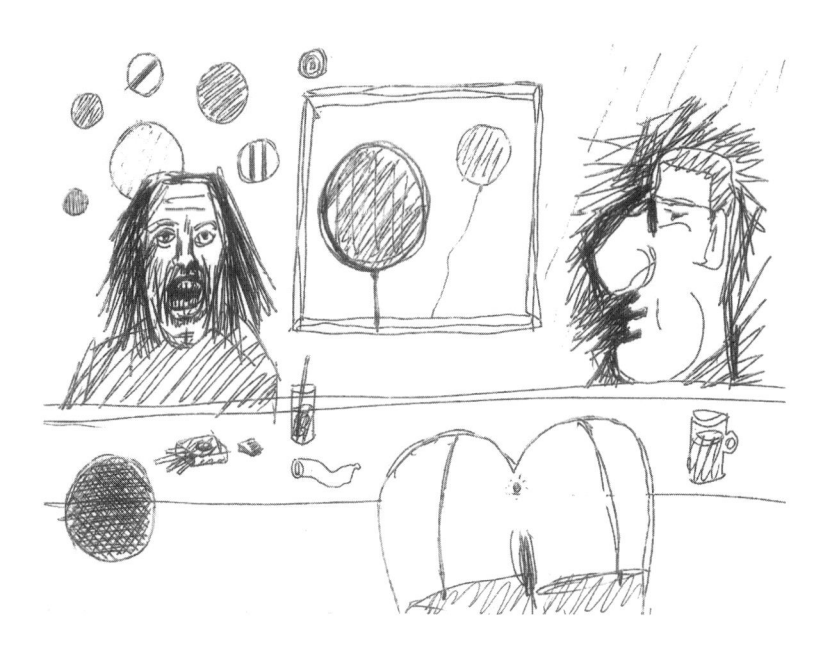

EARLY
CHRIS HEFFERNAN

Gary moved the sheets from out of the way but still remained under them as he pushed them up and took his sweatpants off and let his erection come out of the hole of his boxers and poke Sandy in the thigh. The sheets floated back down around them. He poked her again. It was warm and the sun had been up for hours but it was still early. It was one of the first times this spring they had kept the window open all night. He poked her again. Then one more time until she finally moved and made some noise and he said, "You awake?" and she made some more noise, a kind of moan as she rolled over away from him. He reached over her hips and felt around the front and went down her pants. "Gary," she said still mostly asleep, "stop."

"Come on," he said. And poked her again with his hard-on. "Giddy-up."

He laughed at this and she half laughed in her sleep. "I'm tired," she said.

"Then just lay there and don't worry," he said.

"Gary," she said.

They both lay still.

He drew his arm up and held her and let his thumb caress her. After a few moments when she didn't move he said, "Let's have sex."

She moaned again and rolled over, coming around and jostling her knees and elbows and almost kicking him as she repositioned herself. Then she put both her arms around him and left him in an awkward way with one of her arms under his neck. She kissed him then moved her head back to put it in the middle of her pillow. She didn't move anymore. He brought his hands up and began rubbing her breasts.

"Sandy says she wants me with her down in Sandy-land." He sang this to her in the melody of a song they both liked.

"Gary," she said without opening her eyes, "come on, I'm tired. And I think I'm still drunk. Aren't you sick or anything?"

"No," he said. He kissed her and continued to rub her breasts. "I took a valium last night. I'm fine."

"You had valium and you didn't tell me?" she said. She still kept her eyes closed but she was more awake now.

"Some guy gave it to me in the bathroom. He was giving it to everybody."

"Why didn't you get me some?" she said.

He moved his hands under her shirt and brought them around her back. She drew herself in and kissed him but kept her eyes closed to sleep.

"Huh?" she said. "Why didn't you get me any?"

"I couldn't just ask the guy for extra pills for people out at the bar. He was going crazy. He was mad about something and he was just throwing the pills at people. He kept shouting something like, 'Take 'em all, take 'em all.' He was fucked out of his mind."

"Next time get me some," she said.

He kissed her.

"Let's have sex," he said. "Come on."

"Shit, Gary, I'm exhausted."

"Come on," he said, "I have a big boner."

He kissed her and she kissed him back.

"I'll jerk you off," she said. "All right?" She brought her hands down. "I'm just too tired right now." She found his erection and took it with both hands and tugged at it. "If you want to wait until I'm more awake, maybe later."

"Maybe?" he said.

She slipped his boxers down over his hips and really began to tug and stroke.

"I'll jerk you off," she said. "And then you won't want anything. You won't even want a waffle."

He moved his hips to counter her movement to make the strokes quicker and more forceful.

"What the hell does that even mean?"

"I don't know," she said, "I'm tired."

"You know I love getting jerked off, but I wanna fuck, baby."

She tugged and tugged and then let go and spun herself over giving him her back while pulling the covers over her and tightening herself up into a ball. "Now you get nothing," she said.

"Christ," he said, "come on." He petted her hair and pulled it back from her face and put it behind her ear. "I'll just do you a little bit here from behind, okay?"

She didn't answer.

"Okay," he said.

He moved his hands around the sheets. He yanked and pawed at them but she had worked herself in good.

"Christ," he mumbled. "All right," he said, "because your country refuses to negotiate with my diplomats, most notably Vice Admiral Baldy, I'm gonna have to let loose the tickle machine."

"Don't even fucking think…." she started.

He released a frenzy of his fingers and hands on her sides. Immediately she bucked and knotted then bucked back the other way and contorted grunting and laughing as her body sprang up and bounced on the bed with her trying to keep her elbows locked on her hips to keep him away. "Shit," she said through her short screams and laughter. "Christ, motherfucker. All right. All right, shit, stop."

He stopped.

She lay on her back with her hand on her forehead, panting. "Shit," she said smiling and breathless.

"Can we make a sexy?" he said with a strange accent.

"Jesus," she said. She rolled over on her side and again gave him her back.

"We gonna make a sexy," he said again with the accent.

He reached in and put his thumbs on the inside of the elastic of her pajama bottoms. When she did not protest he slid them down over her hips with her panties, together and pushed them down past her knees. She brought her feet up and kicked them off. Then he made sure his underwear was all the way off and positioned himself behind her, holding her shoulder with one hand and getting his fingers tangled in her hair while he looked down into the darkness of the sheets to see where he was and find where he needed to get it to. He jostled up against her and let the tip of his hard-on find it.

"Wait," she said, "you passed it."

He kept moving slightly to find it, a little forward and back, and he was pretty sure where it was and his lap kept falling naturally down to put everything in place but he kept moving it. He moved it back up as he put himself more on top of her.

"Whoa, Buster, not that one," she said and started moving herself to get things back where they were.

"Come on," he said.

"You've go to be kidding me."

He laughed. "Come on," he said.

She pushed her hips up to get him back and down.

"Jesus, Gary, I'm too tired for this shit."

"Come on," he said. "Just to try. Just a little. I just put the tip in so you can feel what it's like."

"Gary," she said and started to say something else but he interrupted.

"Just to see what it's like. It can be for my birthday. It's right around the corner."

"It's in a month," she said.

"So I won't ask you for anything then. Not anything. Not even a CD or dinner or a drink or anything."

"Gary," she said.

"Ellen let me do it."

"Bullshit," she said.

"Ask her," he said.

"I will," she said.

"Go right ahead," he said. "She might tell you she didn't because she's embarrassed but she did. And she liked it. That's what was most embarrassing for her."

"Bullshit. Really?"

"Yeah," he said.

"She did not like it," she said.

"She did," he said.

"Well you said she was a whore," she said.

"I guess," he said, "but at least she tried it."

"Bullshit," she said.

"Come on," he said. "An early birthday gift. Just a little. Just a touch. Ellen didn't want to at first either but I gave her a touch, just the tip, and she loved it."

"How 'bout I get you a new windshield for your car?" she said.

He reached down and began playing with himself to keep his erection.

"Time's running out, honey. Come on."

"I'll get you a new windshield and I'll get you something else. We'll look online and see if any concerts are coming up. We'll spend a weekend in the city. We can stay with Bill."

"No," he said. "Now come on." He pulled the sheets back and exposed the both of them and took her waist and guided her around onto her stomach. She had her legs together and put her hands under her chin and turned her face on her cheek.

"Gary," she said.

Underneath on her belly he reached in and pulled hips up slightly and set back poking just slightly in the air at an arch. Then he played with himself a little more to make his dick harder and used his free hand to mover her legs apart.

She brought them only so far apart then stopped. He moved his fingers into her vagina from behind which made her moan and bring her backside further up and more pointed as her legs eased and he moved them wider now, with his knee. He could see everything in the light and did not have to find anything but as he held her hips with both hands used the tip of his penis to guide his way around. She moved slightly up and down. He brought himself up and closer and then used his hand to bring the head of his prick up to her asshole.

"Wait, Gary," she said.

"I'm just teasing," he said.

Then pushed the tip at it.

"Wait a minute," she said.

"It's just the tip," he said. "I'm just gonna tease you with the tip so you see what it's like."

She arched up and he leaned forward and grabbed her.

"Shit," she grunted in pain. "Shit," she grunted again.

He pushed further in.

"Fucking Christ," she said. "Gary," she said.

He felt it tight and warm like a small sun opening up underneath him.

"That's more than the, ow fuck. Gary," she said.

He began pushing into her.

"Fuck," she said. "Jesus fuck," she said. She cursed and grunted. "Gary it's fucking, ow fuck, killing me. Gary, ow fuck, stop a minute. Just stop for a second."

"You gotta loosen up. If I stop you're not gonna loosen up. That's the trick. To keep going. Most girls want you to stop," he said. "but you gotta loosen up."

"Get off," she said. "It's fuckin' killing me. Fuck. OW FUCK!"

"It's totally natural to feel like this at first."

He leaned over and grasped both of her shoulders and put his weight on her back and began pushing it quicker.

"GOD FUCK!" she screamed.

He pushed her into the bed, pushing her face into the pillow.

Her eyes watered. "It's hurting me," she said. "It's hurting me. Please," she said, "It's hurting me." She bit her fist and sobbed. "It's hurting me."

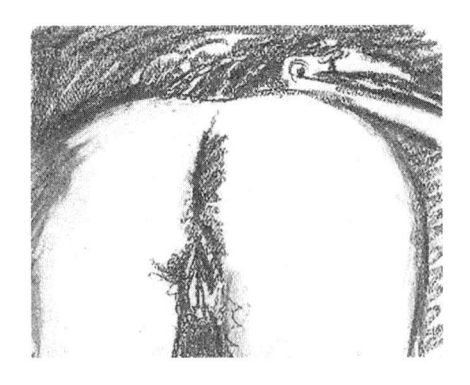

WAKING SHIVA
BONNY FINBERG

We're walking and I'm following him through the streets. No idea where I'm going. Fine with me.

"My sister had a dream that your mother was coming," he says. "She told me yesterday, *'Her mother is coming'.*"

"She's not my mother."

"No? Whatever Nanu dreams comes true. She said you will have good luck. That you will bring *me* luck. Would you like to go to Kali Temple?"

"Yeah!"

We go through an archway and enter a courtyard. A group of young guys sit outside the temple on a mosaic-tiled porch. They're smoking *ganja,* dressed like Bollywood movie stars from the 1970's. They're playing some kind of game, throwing sticks hard and fast, onto a piece of cardboard, laughing. One by one they stand, talking to Raju in Nepali. It seems like they've been waiting for him, like he's brought me here so they can check me out. They look at me with perverted smiles. I look at the darkest one, and realize it's the guy from the bus, Johnny Depp of Kathmandu, wearing a white shirt, black jeans, and black sunglasses. He sneers down at me from the temple platform. "You understand Nepali?"

"Every word."

Raju starts to move toward the archway back to the

street and I start walking after him. From behind me I hear, "You fuck?"

I finger the money, pushing it further down, hiding it from any skilled fingers that might find their way into my pocket. I'm trying to ignore the fact that I'm thinking about what I'm doing, thinking in the third person present, resolving to be less paranoid, starting now, for the rest of her life. If she doesn't watch herself from the outside so much she might be more confident, *appear* more confident anyway. But which is it? Is she watching herself from the outside, or just the opposite — stuck in the dark, overcrowded inside?

Being in a foreign country is bringing her closer to her native tongue. It follows alongside everywhere she goes like a nasty bitch chattering on like a thesaurus: *easy-target, mark, pigeon, dupe, chump, sap, sitting-duck, sucker.*

So it won't fall out, she tells herself, crossing the square with thumbs hooked in front pockets. Raju appears from about six feet away, so suddenly that she couldn't say from which direction. He greets her, *"Namaste,"* his voice dropping into that smooth lower register that reminds her of boys at school, their nervous smiles in the presence of her direct, wiry cool. "So — where are we going?" she asks. "I'm up for a long day. My dad's got company."

"Oh — your mother.... "

"She's *not*...."

"I mean...."

"Candice. Her name is Candice."

"Candice. She is here now?"

"Yeah."

"Did you ask her if...."

"*No.* I'm on my own for now. I don't know what she — and my dad — will be up to. We don't have to worry about them. They can figure out what they're doing. I'd rather...."

"Oh. I see. Well, we can go…."

"I want to go to the Shiva Temple. I think that would be perfect."

"The Shiva Temple. Yes, okay. I must get some cigarettes."

They walk toward the bus stop and he stops at a shop, buys two cigarettes and gives her one. He lights them up with a clear Bic that has a fake plant floating inside. Waiting for the bus, smoking. He's not talking and she wonders what he's thinking, trying to focus on something else, the Johnny Depp guy, how she'd blow his mind if she ever fucked him.

"Were those guys friends of yours? Those guys at the Kali Temple?"

"Oh, they are people I know — from… my village."

"*How* do you know them? I mean — did you grow up with them?"

"They are from my village. I did not know them — *do* not know them — very much. Sometimes I see them. They go to my friend's party."

"Are they bad? I mean, dishonest? They seemed different… from a lot of guys around here."

"Oh, they are not bad. Just… I don't really *know* them very much."

They get on the bus and find two seats in front. The landscape moves behind small clusters of huts, countless objects passing across the windows, people glimpsed for seconds, tiny fragments of each distinct day adding up to years, each a unique life spent between acid green fields and cramped, dark rooms where a filmy cold attaches to everything. If it isn't hot and humid, it's pouring rain. Shit in the streets. Shit on the walls. They even burn shit. Their shit is different from the shit in the tunnels. Their shit is cow shit. In the tunnels there is human shit and rat shit. Rat shit is so gross she doesn't even want to think about it. Human shit is a disgusting fact of life whose only positive is that it means you ate. She looks over at him and he stands up, indicating they'll be getting off. She notes that he never touches her casually, only the enthusiastic handshake when they meet and when they say good-bye.

They start up the hill toward the temple. She's thinking about the men chanting, hoping they'll offer a toke, when suddenly Johnny Depp appears, almost like the big bad wolf, from behind a tree. She wonders if he knew she was going to be here, wondering if there's some creepy conspiracy going on.

"Hey — wassup?" She doesn't think he'll get it but she talks the talk and if he gets it, fine, and if not, then he can deal. Still looking at her through his smoky lenses he says something to Raju, who says something back, trying to lead her up the hill. She doesn't move, transfixed by the moment, by indecision, the not-so-quiet violence behind his smile. She wants to go. She dares herself not to. Nothing yet has ever made her regret taking her own dare.

"Yo — you got something on your mind, yo?"

He moves toward her. She stands her ground even though he's touching her arm. She shrugs him off and he grips her more tightly. Raju starts in his direction. "Johnny Depp" laughs and holds her a moment, tries to read her reaction, then drops his arm. She backs up ever so slightly, without turning her back. Raju begins walking up the hill again, as though trying to pull her by an invisible rope. He's yelling something in Nepali, though no one's paying attention. But then it's too late because Johnny's got her by the arm, dragging her by the hair into the brush. Raju can't see her but hears her struggling. He starts toward the bushes and the skies open, rain emptying from the sky like a buffalo bladder, all over everything, filling the paths and pushing leaves out of its way down the hill. His hesitancy has cost time and he rushes to catch up, unsure of how he can stop the inevitable. He hears them, now deeper in the thicket; she's cursing and crying, words he's heard only in the few pirated American videos he's managed to see in the back room of a friend's teashop. He wanted to go on a pilgrimage with his family and was hoping she'd give him some money. He invited her to come and would have treated her like a sister, wasn't trying to steal her money, would have brought her to a very special place. Now he hears her scream, exultant, out of control. He stumbles upon them, only the sound of rain hitting the ground, splattering against the thick vegetation.

He should be terrified by what he sees, but he's too confused. They're wet and covered in mud and leaves, she astride her captor, hair flying in his face, his bare eyes squinting against the rain, clutching her shoulders while she pummels him with her cunt to the guitar riffs pumping in her brain, crying softly, calling him names he can only guess the meaning of by the black-tongued tone of her voice and the grimace that he glimpses before shutting his eyes against the rain. The wind above is raging while he floats, peaceful under its force.

She is howling now, her head thrown back, and the prey beneath her stiffens as some kind alchemy at the center of being transforms pain into ecstasy. All desire is for this little death, as much and as many times as possible from the first itch that needs to be scratched to the last involuntary shit. All of us, right here in this remote landscape, are filled with this.

RIDE DOWN
SUSAN MAURER

The ride down he drank anisette, scanned
His beeper, the black Caddie
Those ringlets at the back of his skull
How he looked nude, chopping wood
The mystery of the van, trashed deep in the woods
How she had been a drug dealer, coke, he said
How I said come death as he drove it home on the couch
After the condoms had run out, time after time
The rifle propped against the wall
The man next door who never left his house
His scruffy dog
The fact that he looked like a Piero della Francesca
Was not reason enough
But try telling me that then
"Hey you, stop, you are not fiction"

ALIEN FANTASY
ELAINE EQUI

I wouldn't mind being naked
in their pupil-less eyes.
Just think of them coming all that way
for nothing but a closer look
as if Earth were one big peep show
advertising LIVE FLESH, LIVE FLESH
in undulating neon telepathy.
Who could be as fascinated
by our sloppy existence?
Who could care less about what is art
as they mix semen and stardust
or goose our boredom with joyride's probe?
And busy as we are, how else to justify
leaving work except in a crazy abduction
scenario? You check your schedule
again and again. Lost forever —
those four hours — like ancient teenagers
wander in some glittering arcade.

CORSET
JANET HAMILL

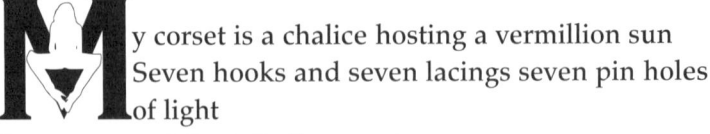

My corset is a chalice hosting a vermillion sun
Seven hooks and seven lacings seven pin holes
of light
Into my corset the tail of a comet
The dust from the first star's implosion settling
On a fire sculpted of unbreakable glass
My corset loves me a locket with paper stained in blood

Blind me and bind me one woman alone
Seven hooks and seven lacings seven pin holes of light
My corset frees me where my horses roam
Into a hermitage at the edge of the desert's darkest night
Draw me in and let me go like a temple cat
Enamored of its confinement my corset sings its memories

Of giving silk and netting and the softest raven feathers
besotted by golden arms and emerald swords

BALSA WOOD COUNTRY COURTSHIP
MARY LEARY

Midnight blue bonnet
surrounding face of the moon
is making me swoon — she and I are *so* connected.

Hips sore from sex anticipated
as the dreamer moans for me
and I hike dusty gingham, flash a little more brilliance
across his vision's field,

burying my knees in bluebonnets.

His hands have brown undersides.
There is not much pink to him.

What there is will collide with my tongue
as if there were no separation
between the soft box of me
and the warm bones of him,
the soft, fleshy envelope of him
and the wriggling, joyful notes of me.

Old stamps from faraway places
like Brussels and Mozambique
peer from our pupils. We keep
little birds in cages there,
ready to soar with the moon when she summons the fiddler
and our kisses fly thick and fast as stars

watering the sky's face
as boots stomp sawdust
and the band roars
sweet and wheezy in the grate.

I NEVER KNEW AN ORGY COULD BE SO MUCH WORK
SHARON MESMER

People hosting orgies are always surprised by how
much hard work it is.
I think the best way to have an orgy is, in fact,
to not prepare for it at all.
An orgy isn't a technological strategy as much as an attitude,
or a chance to provide your kids with a keepsake:
an AT&T orgy with Carrot Top, for example,
contains so much simple wisdom that is immediately applicable
to all areas of life.
I am so happy when an orgy does well because I put so
much work into them.
I knew I wanted a funky new conversation thing,
but I also knew I didn't want the usual drumbeats.
Too many times, people make a mad dash for the restrooms —
so much for radical sexual stylin'.
Nevertheless, the Christian symbolism we love so well is
constantly present.
In our orgy, the Mole Person took Saddam down to Moleopolis,
which is a gigantic ass vagina in the suburbs.
I got lots of noir work out of that one.
I got to orgy with a little monkey in a Mel Gibson movie.

CUNT COCK CLIT ROCK SONG
FOR SHALOM'S WALL
BOB HOLMAN

unty cocky clitty rocky
Push the button on yr throb
Pisster blister Pretty titty
Grab a pint of lube and tube it
Push and friction pull the lick and shun the bun
That shies away and eat Herr Pie
Suck it 69ishly and sexsex is easily nutritious
Cram baby, we emerge from your vagina dairy
Tonguing the crust from the SANDWICH OF DEATH
Flagellant skeletal cloud breasts
Proof behemoth of nonthought fingerbrain
Take it from me from behind with your entire body
DO IT NOW NOW NOW
DO IT MORE MORE MORE
DO IT BIG FAST DEEP
DID I MENTION BIG FAST DEEP
Of course read a poem while I eat your sweet Holy Hole
And give me a Hum Job baby, the vibrating tongue breath
Harmonious hard on forever
Do the whole of Handel's Messiah
On my cock as I use the famous dickswirl curvalicious
To your insanely tight insanely deep insane G spot
My one cock on your G Spot and my second cock on
Your clit

Asshole for my third cock and in your mouth takes two
Cocks to fit
Slam around and Now sing the Messiah whilst blow me
With overtones like a Tuvan throat singer!
Gwaa Gwaaa Gawanaaaa
It's better than The Aristocrats!
It's you and me and everyone we know
In the same bed with no clothes on
It is sex porn bushy bunny genitalia
Get off! Get off in cum spurt jism factory jizz and jizz
Some more
Why don't ya?
We got protest signs on our flesh poles, waving like the
Sea gulls
Howdy Doody is eating out Minnie Mouse and Pluto
Barks asses
Wolf pussy for dick? But of course, my Cherie Amour
Urgent urges splurge spoofy micrometer milky woowoo
Orifi orifices! Open it up with your twenty tiny tongue
Tongues
And do not stop oh no oh no oh whoops I mean yes
Much meshes sound to physicality open territory with
Dick GPS
Heat find the red liquidity lubricious licklick
Barrier shark drinks drill bit a flesh o'phobia NOT
No more eyes, you Asshole Hard-on Sucker!
Pendejo paramecium!
Get back under the covers and lemme lick labia, if you
Don't mind
Mouth slit hover drip fleur de mal
Anyhow el dia de muertos y tambien the tambourine of
Your titanic orgasmatronicalization
Phone sex chip implanted? Check on the chip.

It's fuckin chipper as a zipper
Flesh out the flesh! Flash flush and festoon your
Tiny titties and juggernaut jugs
The entire universe is after the same thing so let us do it
My rocket racket can't kick it
So don't knock it you limp dick
Excuse for a limp dick. Take a memo. Take a handjob.
Do not answer the phone let it go straight to voice mail,
Where voice means suck job
And phone means pussypuss and straight means queer
Don't answer voicemail,
Let it soak up the condom lube burger bits
Never enough guitars to cover the landscape and
End the world with crime of sex —
That you would lie there and body after body and all
Your dingdongs are ring a ding ding donging
The hard handed nipple clamped
On it and several cocka apiece in each hole
And the strap-on inserted very very
Sloooooow genteelly ah!
The odorous rectum unflinching sighs in total
Appeasement…

There is no such thing as porno poetry
And I'm jerking off to it right now
Little girl little girl, my little boy wants to play
Doctorooni now
On your muffatooni
And my lil pencil nub is exploding with cum and twat,
Cumtwat
And the howl of pleasure pop song antithesis
Turn off the wall turn off the wall turn off the wall
Turn it off motherfucker immediately and lie buried in

The femalemaleishness of it Allish —
The email impales
The e-pale pole is dark and deep and prone
Prize is never-ending roundelay eternity sex dance dick
Cunt blast boom fala
Fuckin la

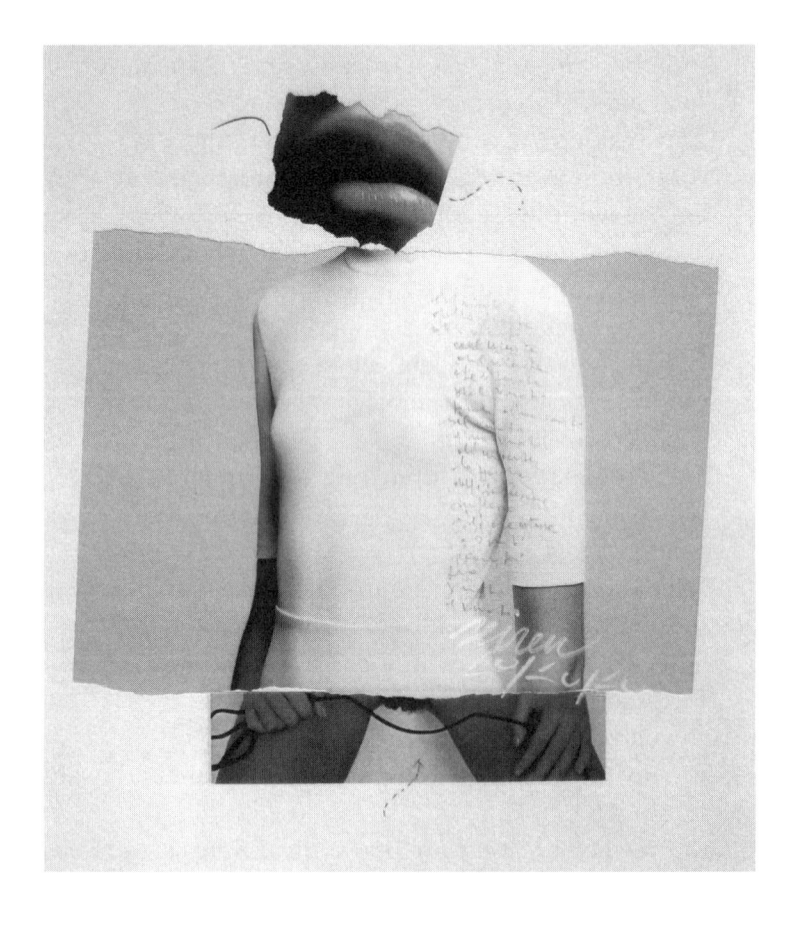

THE BODY-AND-CLOTHES METAPHOR
GERARD MALANGA

he experience has been completed — a language
event: it goes this
way: sitting front row one seat
center —
right
hair color — light blond
held in place by barrette/pony-tail/pure Connecticut
prototype.
beige cords
brown loafers fringe on top
olive-green 100% lambs wool sweater
taken off
during reading by Amiri Baraka, a/k/a LeRoi Jones
revealing red-white-blue stripe blouse
knitting intermittently/becoming more attentive
black strap watch — left wrist.
This poem is for the near future
pursuing fate: West Broadway, a Saturday
Afternoon — intense sunlight
high-contrast shadows of the woman's arms and breasts
would be outlined
thru white translucent shirt.
Stop. Ask her name. What fate wld gain
in that instance as possibility.
All language is permeated by metaphor because

words are juxtaposed, because
time has not stopped, i.e., shower cap
hung against steamed-up window. The
anatomy
of the
three diamonds

          sun-tanned
          stepping out of the surf.

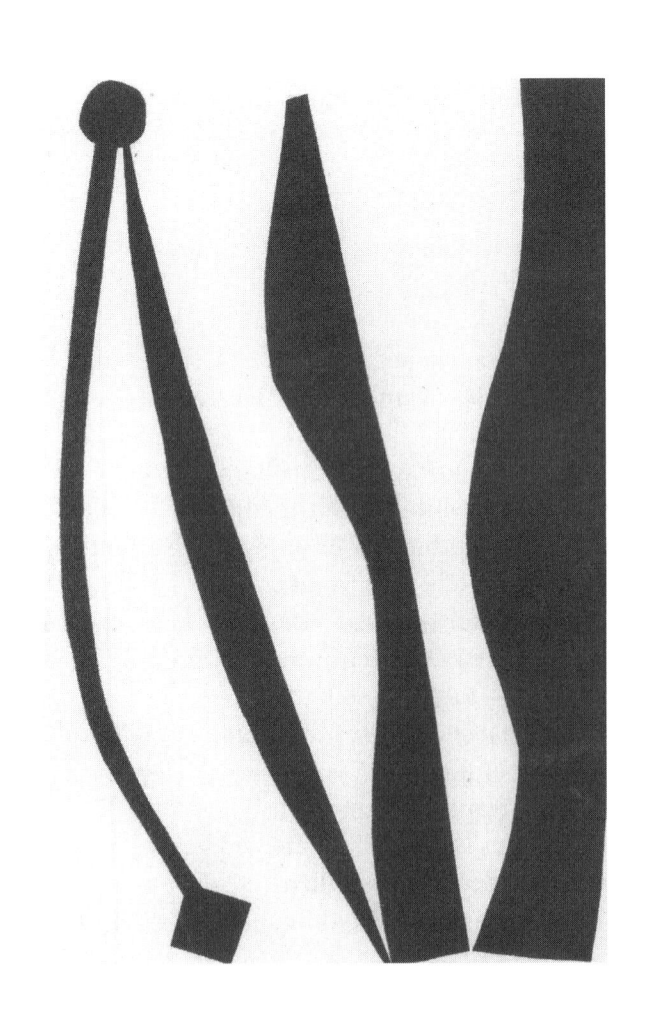

LOVELUST

ANYSSA KIM

Eight-letter-dirty-word-compounded

sheds heat
presses my knees
together
to hold it in
so I don't forget

caveman hair *yank*
lessons
on Darwin, Freud
got laid on white sheets
for all to read

be my teacher
I   want   to   play   hooky
and be real bad

it's what I like to do

I know how you like to get erect
pupils

No!   now I turn woman
wet with exclamation
point howls   in loud vowels

oh b*aaaaa*by!!!

my red crescent parts in
waves
caught by   cotton
cloud on a string
flies high   nestled in   thigh-sky
shangri-la, inside
man-made synthetic g-string   vibrations

pull it outta me
and burrow in
oh bloody hell
smack me so I don't forget
my animal side
inside   and   outside
runs wild
circles
eight-letter-dirty-words
up and down
us

KISS #479
DAN WABER

Eye p
(au,aww)sed in the sss oft
mmm(i,u)ddle of a gliss
to wishpurr inonto her
glistening slips,
"give me your tongue, pleas."
she,
by re lack sing her
sup,pull neck intoo
the ladle of my cupt
left hand,
gives me her all
I ask.
my teath (un(un(un)))guent
ly
close on her
oh!so
expoh!sed
flueshh
everso
tie
ter
I bites
her
un til she
yesses word
less
ly.

"BOOT EATING SCOOTER TRASH"*
CAROL WIERZBICKI

We're boot eating scooter trash
we're raising dust bunnies in the backyard
we leave sugar for the ants
let's fuck in my hutch

We're boot eating scooter trash
we got burlap sheets
our dogs know how to scratch
    in all the wrong places
let's rut in my rutted dirt driveway

We're boot eating scooter trash
for company we break out
    the Spam, Bud, and pork & beans
we leave our children with the Board of Ed
coast is clear — let's do it
    under the No Pest Strip in the garage

We're boot eating scooter trash
we cleaned up a little
swept the soil into neat piles
and hosed down the aluminum siding
let's skinny dip in my above-the-ground pool
    with the skin of scum on top
and sink down to the bottom
and grind 'til the silt
lodges permanently in our cracks

[*band name posted at Restaurant Florent]

SAFE SEX
TERRI CARRION

Patty let *me* ride
in the front seat of Johnny's
Volkswagen Beetle, so I could straddle
the hole in the rusted out floorboard
peer down into it, watch
the asphalt rush between my legs
as I urged Johnny, *faster, faster…*
stick shift grinding, slamming into gear
and behind me Patty scooted up
hugged the front seat
and my stomach while the Beetle
vibrated against the balls
of my feet, pulsed between
my ankles and Patty's thumbs
pressed on my ribs as a gust of heat
shot up from the hole, slipped under
my damp summer skirt, between
my thighs. Hairs rose. Patty's breath
brushed my cheek, lingered long after
Johnny came to a stop.

MORNING POEM #3
WANDA PHIPPS

odka still moves through me
wind bangs the venetians against the sill
and thoughts of you
reimagine your back through the bathroom
door high white light rounding your shoulders
now candlelight carves sweet shadows
in your face. voice/sounds like rough handling
deep strokes and sure focus
bring me back to me
and you and a separate space
ours in the ease of lingering pauses
or the rush of our seconds passing

MORNING POEM #39

if she took off her top
would that embarrass you
would you smile
and laugh nervously
would there be
room on the roof
for the orgy
if the music
was a little louder
would you remember
the color of her eyes

IN BECKETT'S BAR
BOB WITZ

Sitting at the bar
she was almost as beautiful
as a can of beer
but she said i was too short
too old
and she didnt like the clothes
i wore
rationalizing about it all later
i decided that she was about
as intelligent
as a complicated comic book
and did that matter
her body did seem
to have a kind of infinite wisdom

she kept displaying her vocabulary
as well as her prodigious memory
and i kept getting more and more excited

she was as beautiful as a bagel and coffee
sweet as a sunbeam
she had friends in philadelphia
but she didnt know who proust was

in beckett's bar
they havent swept
for 40 years
all those butts and dirt
broken bodies and bottles
twisted refuse
all those dreams
and footsteps
thousands of years lie there

in the dimestore when
beckett goes to buy razor
blades he sees the young
lightheaded girls who sing
as they move
like those old attic vases
and they talk and smile
moving like mysteries
and music through the stillness
of his mind

theres my double
a boring man asking
a waitress boring questions

late at night
beckett sleeps in his bed
his bed floats above the roof
held up there by dreams

becketts eye moves slowly
thru the smokey barroom light
to a door open to the rain
that keeps falling

she was blond
a kind of honey
color down below
with a taste of sweat and wheat
erect nipples
firm white ass
didnt say much
and she was efficient

color that cigarette
the smoke light grey
the lips red
the red of lipstick wine fire
the mouth dark
like time

beckett gets plenty of sleep now
and when he sleeps he travels
thru snow
and the branches are black
against the frozen blue and
they move like hills and mountains

EROTIC POEM (UN POCO LOCO)
STEVE DALACHINSKY

She tells me that my new erotic poem is too clean
that i'm too clean
i tell her that i don't know how to write erotic poems
the sax player bends over & grabs her horn
i pat her ass & tell her that i just don't know
how to write erotic poems
that i really don't even want to write
erotic poems
but that my new poem's a good poem none-the-less
she smiles & nods her head
arching her back ever so slightly
in time with the music
she heaves her chest forward &
says she understands
the sax player plays a heavy tune
i say that i can't just write about certain things
i see & block others out
she says she's strong the sax player
& that i should write
just what i write but that this poem is
too polite
too clean
i kiss her on the mouth
caress her breast
& say i understand

when in truth & fact i actually do not

i just can't write erotic poems

she smiles gently rises walks away
the tune is over
the sax player puts away her
horn.

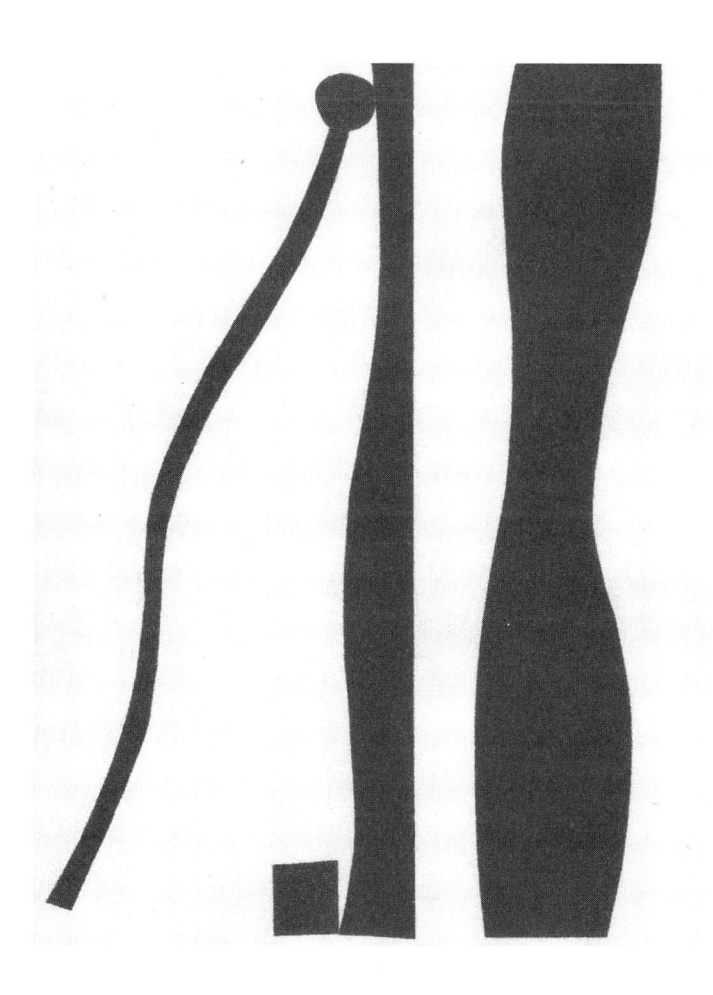

CONDIMENT
MICHAEL LA BOMBARDA

I want you
In the conventional way
With your clothes off
And submissive —
A sole rubber band
On the night table
To intensify the pleasure
Of our congress.

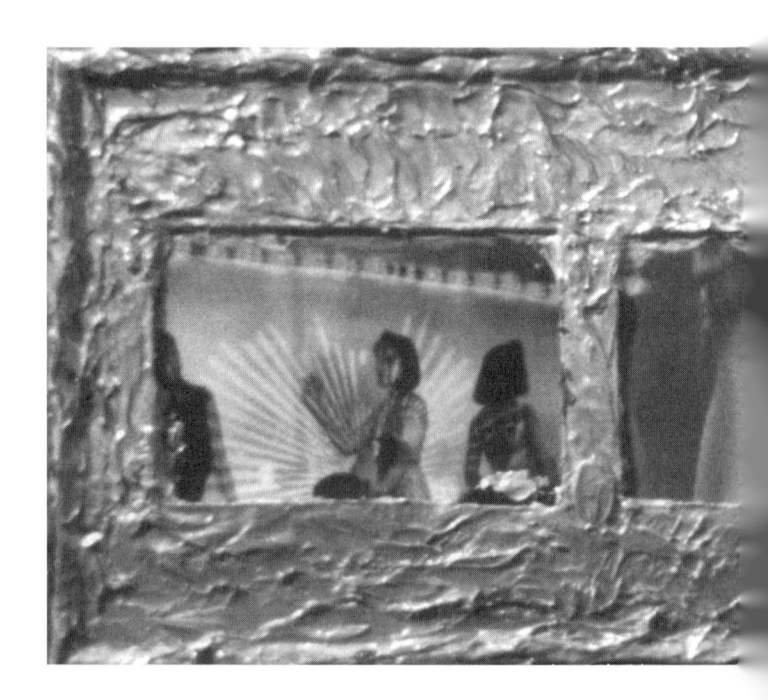

A COMMON PROBLEM
TIM HALL

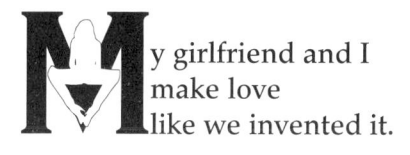**y** girlfriend and I
make love
like we invented it.

You should see us
lying there
fighting over who gets
the royalties.

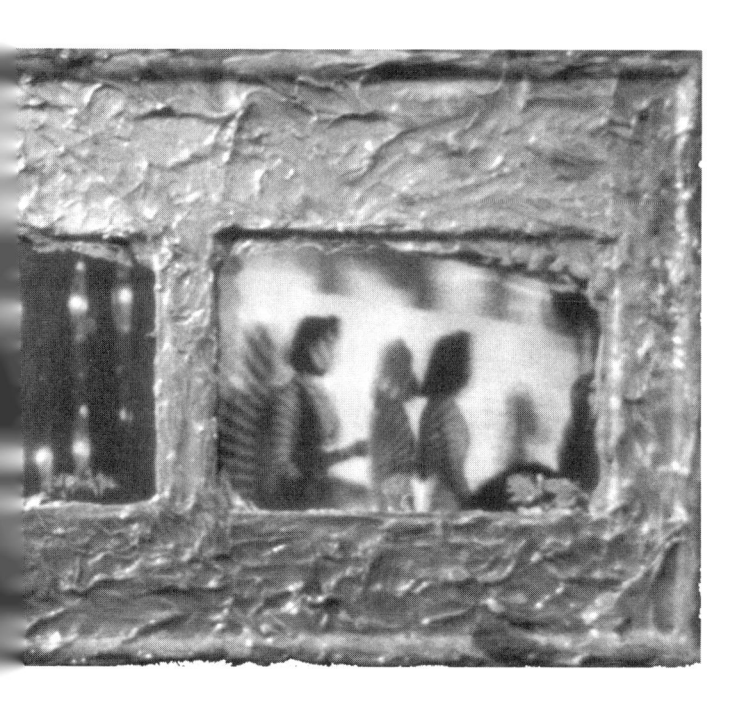

EVERY CITY IS ITS FOOD
KAT GEORGES

Chicago: hot dogs
Los Angeles: tacos
Cincinnati: chili
New York: pizza

American cities:
you eat standing up
easy, quick meals
couple bucks and
You're gone

American people:
you fuck standing up
easy quick deals
couple sucks and
You're gone

In Paris, every meal
Has slow multiple courses.

Gotta love Paris.

THE LINGERING TASTE OF PORK
HAL SIROWITZ

I'm a vegan, she said.
I watch very carefully
what I put inside my mouth.
They say you can tell
by the taste of a man's
sperm everything he
has been eating, And
I hate to be accusing
you of infidelity, but
last night after you
had an orgasm in my mouth
I suddenly tasted Chinese ribs.
It must have been take-out,
because it still retained the grease.
Whatever you put in your
body, I sample, You can't
imagine how horrible
it was for a vegan — one step
higher than a vegetarian —
to come across the animal
kingdom in such an intimate
manner, A relationship has
to be built on trust. You
trust me not to sleep
with other men. I trust

you to stay away from pork.
But if you lie about
the small things, like
what you have eaten
for dinner, how could
I trust you when you
tell me a big thing,
like you'd love me forever.

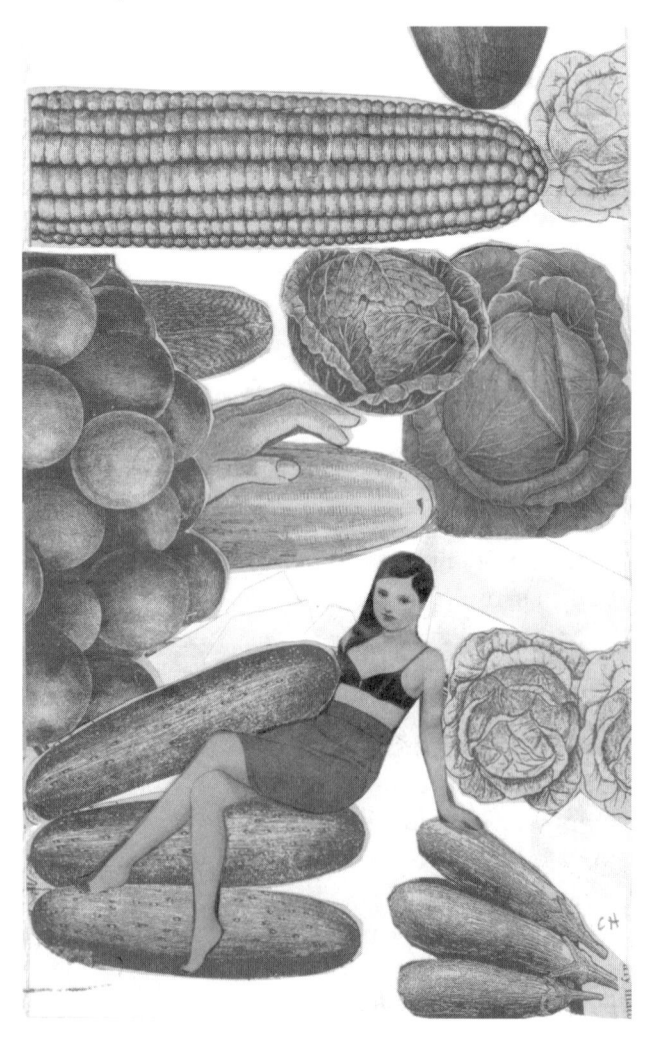

MY BEAUTIFUL PUNK
MERRY FORTUNE

Broken Morning, good morning
I leave you a poem of something
You might recognize, like the color of old coffee
The feel of fire, or even my eyes
or the coffee of itself

Or a picture of a blow job
In the eye of a blow job
In the heart of a blow job
Or the blow job itself

Or two blow jobs, and one bathtub
A birdsong, Messiaen. A bath day
And a birthday, or a bird day
and the bird itself

Sudden morning, good morning
And stay whether perfect or old
Or young or tall, or lost or needing
A subway card, or the fare itself
Or my hand to take your arm
Or life itself

Suddenly on my knee
A perfect form

An entire garden there on your lower lip
And I can see it!
Clear as a bee or something
Slow and stitched

Maybe untouched by sadness
But with great potential
For sadness itself, and then

Running and not laughing
But cracking up over something
A society or something
brevity or cake

Very irreverently
Very irreverent
Like mucous itself

Her highness the queen
Her highness the queen mucous
And spit! Hilarious spit!
Gobs of gobs and lots more spit!

I love you like spit itself
I love you like morning itself
I love you like a good hard spit into the morning itself

LOVE AND CONCRETE
ELIZABETH MORSE

Next to piles of paper
On the too-solid desk
You stand in shirtsleeves.
July's fevers disarrange
Your black hair like sleep.
You insist my heart is a mirror,
That we will fold into each other
Just behind the glass.
You are letting me take in light.
I think of steam and palm fronds.
Late afternoon's rich blue
Peeks in. I cannot tell you
About my sequined past,
The ecstasy of not feeling.
I have traded all that in for calla lilies
And lace curtains.
I am steeped in your gaze.
Your lightning runs
Through to my feet.
It's just too hot for floating.
Icy water laps at our toes.
I want to say:
Look, we are aging like the stones,
Like moist pieces of ground.
In other cities, other rooms,
In breathless evening breezes,
I will find you.

SEX ON DOPE
HORTENSIA

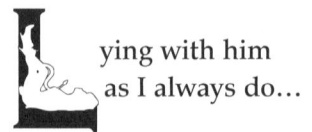 ying with him
as I always do…

sticky black tar
is on my white hands
and sheets and as I
heave into the bucket
behind the bed he
holds my long hair

kissing
my mouth
his tongue
wrenching
my guts

oh god not again
he is inside me —
an erection that stops
at nothing and goes
nowhere and I so
blissfully out of it

whatever it is,
that is.

ANOTHER NIGHT IN GOTHAM

i want to sleep with you he says,
we did i say
and we've been sleeping for hours —
i mean really sleep with you he says,
look i say
we just lost consciousness in the same bed
christ one of us could have easily
killed the other and didn't —
if that isn't closeness, i would be hard
pressed to say what is.
but he's already hard
and pressing into the small of my back.

after i come and
before he does, i get bored.

from the window, i can see the top
of the Empire State building and i can't
fathom why they picked those colors.

NO ONE IS AT THE FRONT DOOR
MARGARITA SHALINA

No one takes it up the ass
no one reeks of perfume
i thought, i heard
no one at the door
no one makes me nervous
no one knows i await
no one comes through the
night of this first death and
the night of no other
singing a night porter's lament

no one is a carnival stripper
with a year's accumulation of clients
barring their teeth, falling into unconsciousness
again, absent again, forgetting again,
depressed again, drunk again, vomiting again, high again
and again, to go on
a portable plywood stage again, communicating
with the nothing that is not there
the leers and fear

i come from no where, reside in
these hours, these days of
no one's abandonment, horizon, or hope
yell into the air at no one and
no one will respond
i'm no one
and who the fuck are you?

CAVEAT
LEE WILLIAMS

I'm not just fucking you
—You know —

I'm fucking
— Or is it we? —
That muskrat
stealing across your lake
his nose a
bullet
aiming for the vacant interior

I'm fucking Eve
— Not that I want to —
But I'm terribly worried about her
in her hospital bed, the tumor the size of a watermelon
crashed and exploded on an linoleum floor.

You're fucking Michael I presume
Michael with the plate in his head
and Dacron on his heart
and vent down his throat.

I'm not just fucking you
—You know —
if you even care
Who are you fucking anyway
while you're fucking me?

Are we fucking this beautiful day?
shapeless blue
so new
as if there never was a sky until today

So come on
Let's enter the abyss
Just put our tippy toe on the edge
and tumble over
Raggedy Andys
Cartwheeling
in the bright blue air
over and over
cos you know what?
We're never going to reach the bottom

We just keep whirling down

LAST TIME
LYNN ALEXANDER

The last time we parted we were getting into our cars
and I remarked how it was such sweet sorrow,
and we laughed, already thinking about next time.
But that would be our last time
and now it's strange to think that your eyes
flashing blue in the dark as you moved inside me
will never look into mine again.
I always want one more look
knowing it's going to be my last,
I want to consciously walk through a doorway
knowing I'll never be back
and hear the click of a lock once I'm past.
It was our last day, but neither of us knew that.
You start your car, adjust the rearview mirror
and watch me wave as you drive away.

THE NOOSE
JEROME SALA

Dreamt last night
I was getting hung.
I said: not again!
Though I wasn't afraid
cause, since I'd been through it
so many times
knew the pain
was no worse
than getting knocked in the head
with a baseball bat
or smashing your skull
through a car window
with the difference being
that with a hanging
you know what hits you,
but you forget anyway
— and pretty fast.
I woke up wondering
about the sex of hanging.
Don't some people strangle themselves
in order to beat off?
Don't you die
with a hard on?
What causes this response?
Must the top half of you

always feel bad
for the bottom to feel good?
Does the flow of blood
to the brain have to stop
for you to attain ecstasy?
And is that what's implied
when people say someone
is well-hung?

CONSTANT COMMENT

The porno star said he was getting "tea bagged"
by which he meant someone was licking his nuts —
an experience he felt was illuminating
only the word he used was "warm."

And the viewer could not help but think of his own teabags
sitting peacefully in their warm box
waiting for a cup of hot water, followed by
a dipping, a
      stirring
sensation — like a musical that slowly works you up

until the end, where the two stars are dancing in fishnets
      and straw hats and canes
in front of a curtain with a spotlight on it
that looks like a golden moon
so that the audience can hardly catch its breath.

THE OTHER WOMAN'S CUNT
LARISSA SHMAILO

I'm not jealous; I'm merely concerned.
That other woman
Who says she's thirty-three
Who never noticed you before you started seeing me;
The one who glares at me and smiles at you
Like an old cat gone in heat:
It's her vagina, dear, you know, that dried up old thing
She uses for storage space? She's got stuff down there,
    I mean.

Toilet paper, styptic pencils, chewing gum, receipts,
Kitty litter, her brother's dentures, a bowl of
    Cream of Wheat,
A scratch and sniff ad for some very old spice,
Subways seats (for the disabled),
A flamethrower, her poetry notebooks, a set
    of formica tables
(Baby, that woman's got
a diner
in her vagina)

She's got:
Twelve truckers trucking
Eleven doctors docking
Ten grocers grossing

Nine hookers hooking
Eight fleas a leaping
Seven lice a laying
Six scabies scabbing
Five transsexuals
Four lesbians
Three cop cars
Two falling drunks
And a biker with clap and herpes

Her vagina is an attic in the summer, a New York
    studio for rent
Her cunt is so old....
(HOW OLD IS IT?)
Sedimentation records of her twat show that ancient,
    I mean ANCIENT cultures live there.

I'm not fussy
But her pussy is messy.

A cluttered vagina
Can't come to no good.
A littered-up clitty
Can't do what it should.
So don't eat out, baby — come home.

PARTICIPLE PRESENT
PETER CARLAFTES

i am a man
i watch the women
on the street
from my
window
and i see
this one
run
her fingers
through her hair
and that one
rub her
right breast
in a
circular
fashion
and the next one
rub her
own rear end
and
these moments
in reflection
make me wonder
if the future
holds
any more
than they
do
and
i wonder
will we know

BEAUTIFUL UGLY GIRL
SEAN FLAHERTY

I am watching, spying,
catching
an ugly girl
who knows
she looks beautiful:
her curves, the dress,
the heels
she knows
the woman is the thing

VOODOO
PATRICIA CARRAGON

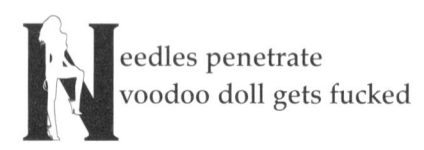eedles penetrate
voodoo doll gets fucked

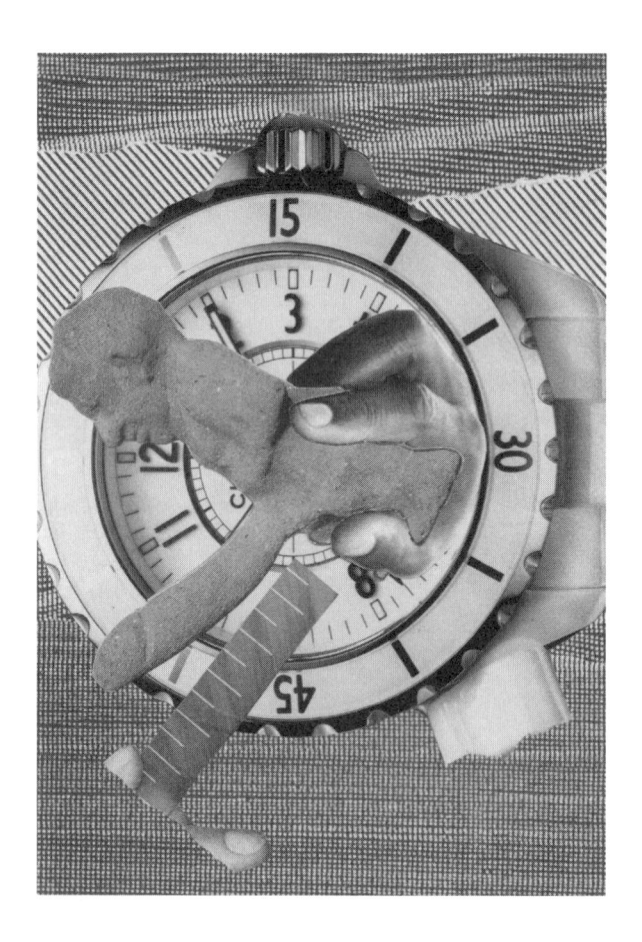

FLOWER MESOSTIC
GOOSEBERRY = ANTICIPATION
HOLLY ANDERSON

Mornings you made me jo**G** the
timber r**O**ad with
y**O**u.
cha**S**ing your
young bon**E**s was
a form of **B**liss.
ravishing th**E**m, too, as
da**R**kening clouds blew
ac**R**oss the lake and sun
to**Y**ed again with our bare skin.

THE DIVINE INTENTION
SPARROW

God intended us to have sex in groups of six. (Notice that even the words "sex" and "six" are similar.) That's why He gave us the social impulse: the urge to gather in groups at taverns, churches, football games, etc. Six people should congregate in a public area, begin hugging and caressing, then have sex — in full view of everyone. This discourages sexual misconduct.

God told this to Moses, who was shocked, and rewrote His instructions in the "Ten Commandments," thus altering human history.

AFTER READING FREUD

After reading Freud for seven years, I suddenly noticed that the cross (emblem of Christianity) is obviously a phallic symbol. Conversely, the Jewish star clearly depicts a vagina. This explains why, for 2000 years, Jews have been "fucked" by Christians.

READY

I was ready.
You were ready.
She was ready.
But were we equally ready?

HAVEN O' LUST (NEO-VICTORIANA)
ROBERT C. MORGAN A.K.A. LEPSO VAN HEUSEN

I.

Telepathic bugger of reason, O virtual saint of the
neurotic lovelorn.
Ah yes, to think of the old days, the wild and wind-
less into airborne strife, the night-tide dusk offering a
quaint reconciliation of amorous memory.
Celestial foot-softeners, penchant moods of echolalia —
returnest thou!

II.
Rip softly thy nocturnal glee, for methinks thou
art at play twixt the seasons of spit and twat,
O grow for the glory, mate, thy cheeks do fondle
more the more they swell to the point of burst
If not for the crush of saints, given to eves of rapture
thy member sanctified, straddled on a throne of praise

III.
Ah *oui, mon ami*, the tickles and chortles amid the throngs
do nothing to dissuade me from thy plough-by-night anthem
Those who prey against that red roguish countenance.
Neigh!
Not a singe of it, quite the contrary when it comes, though
dare I say, who turns thy brotheling faucet into a polite scorn?

policies undone by Donne, the poesy prince of Latamour,
Aye!

IV.

The night is spent, dove's drool, o'er the clover, soiled
sinister toes and fingers, degraded as to raise thy truss —
Afore the Requiem, thy kingdom comes, saccharine, alas,
in bed at dawn, downy comforted, up thy sassy main
a Tudor's ransom, fickle arse, neigh the coarse, by belly.

V.

Leeched in frog-site, eventually soldered to the fin
Break-up the coil, stoking the gorge in truest form
Where's the knack? your gift tonight— O fool o' mine
Look! tis a peak in the buffet, loins amid lambs in frolic,
hence, the gates go unlocked on the way to Herculaneum

VI.

Ah, so many times I lay on my feather bed with yet another
one spent wound around the bedpost, lost in swirling
untold passions, who utters a faint cry, the sentiment so
humbly bestowed on me, my sweet — and thus, I gaze
upwards to the crystal chandelier, a Gaulois twixt my
fingers, a demonic moist member cleverly coiled amid
those satin sheets, breath abated for an hour of oysters,
savored twixt a sea of intrepid cunnilingus

VII.

twirl a whistler 'round a feigned twaddle
till glory reaps thy forlorn conscience
then to hear Meister Eckhart enunciate
the soul's dung: "And Behold! All is One"

FROM **A FANCIFUL GLAMOUR**
JEANNE DICKEY

March 1, 1999
Franco Fumigalli
c/o The Windhover Poetry Festival
Portland, Vermont

Dear Franco Fumagalli,

Picture this, even though you were there. A downtown street. A lowdown street. One that's becoming hip, because it contains one club, that Club, not known by so many, just those in the know. The Poets stand on a balcony, looking down, while comely waitresses slink up the stairs with trays of glittering cocktails. In the center of the pit, loveliness. The soul of a writer, in a deep turquoise dress with a plunging neckline, a delicate purse, dazzling earrings. This plump but lovely groundling casts her eyes upward, toward her favorite poet, who glides down the stairs to meet with her. She weaves through the crowd, into the corner, with her pomegranate margarita.

This was our song, after all. The beautiful meeting we would look back on, forever, and reminisce about when our love threatened to grow stale. Trust me, as a woman I know that romance must evolve slowly, like a treasured piece of music. And so I breezed into a corner.

Tiny, false flowers sprang up in my absence. The Hyacinths. The Parsleys. I thought about their cricket faces and pimpled shoulders, the sharp, crusty elbows that fought for a space within your circle. No wonder your eyes looked vacant, searching for me, a natural beauty and a standout in any crowd. I sipped my drink and risked a few delicious glances at you.

You may already have a sense of what happened later that night. Seeing no crack in the wall of Hyacinths and other sycophants, I decided to wait for you by your car. I had a hunch about where you would park, so I headed for the nearest garage, and on the way, I hatched a plan.

I know many of the garage employees, as I often park here when I make deliveries. I give generous Christmas gifts and have many friends. You must understand by now that I am a woman of enormous power in this city. This garage happened to be managed at night by one Dennis McCaffrey, who had a thing for me. In fact, I did give him somewhat of a special Christmas gift one year after a particularly risque party. I approached him at his stand, and he looked up from his book, which a quick glance revealed was a true crime account of a boy born with fins instead of hands and feet, who grew up to murder his family.

"Hey, you look foxy today, Ms. Rank. Where you at tonight, a party?" I might add that Denny McCaffrey is one of those slight, red-headed Irishmen who likes to act like he's black.

"I'm sort of at a party," I said. "You know, a business thing."

"Gotta take care of biz-ness," he said, saluting me. "I don't see your little flower van here tonight."

"I took the subway," I said, and then I asked him for a favor. "Do you know Franco Fumagalli, the boxer? The one who also wrote a poetry book? Is he parked here tonight?"

"Right over there, white Volvo," he said. "Tough guy."

"So he is," I said. "I'm supposed to leave with him. I'm not feeling well, and he has some obligations, so he told me that I could sit in his car and wait."

Denny laughed as he dangled the keys before my eyes. "Cause it's you, OK Fa?"

Franco Fumagalli, how much do I love anything you've touched? My palms caressed your white leather seats, feeling their heat. Your heat. I pressed my nose to the back of the driver's seat, where your neck would be. I took off my shoes and ran my toes through your rugs. I regretted that I hadn't perfumed my feet, as the mingling of our scents could have brought us deeper intimacy. A few times, I thought I heard you coming, and I ducked, my belly churning with a sensation I've never known before. My fingertips electrified, I was breathless by the time I noticed Denny watching me.

I hope you forgive me for what happened after, with Denny. I was thinking of you the whole time. Afterward, I opened your glove compartment, and finding only your registration and a worn copy of *Leaves of Grass*, I left a gift. The poems I left concern very intimate details of our relationship, but I hope you can see the humor in them, and the love.

Franco Fumagalli, do you remember the movie, *Cocoon*? I'm thinking of the part where two people peel off their human skins and radiate pure light. As light, they make love. I know the forces ripping us asunder are stronger on your side. Your fame. Your reputation. They're weighing you down. Franco Fumagalli, we need to meet, alone, somewhere you can shed your renown, I can shrug off society's judgment of my size, and our pure souls can unite. Perhaps we can meet at Grand Central Station, at the bottom of the escalator, and then ascend to the stationery store in the Met Life Building to browse the new journals that have published your poems. I'll set the date two weeks from now.

Done. On March 15, you and I will linger in the company of suburban commuters, those whose lights are elsewhere, outside the City. Among the thousands of footsteps, ours. We'll drink vodka tonics and, perhaps, while we're both reaching into a bowl of tiny salted goldfish crackers, our hands will touch.

I've made my bed, Franco Fumagalli, and it's ready for you.

> Yours in sin and sainthood,
> Farolyn

A SUPPLEMENT TO MY FORTHCOMING BOOK: *HARRY SMITH'S ANTHOLOGY OF AMERICAN FOLK MUSIC: THE SECRET SEXUAL TAROT OF MID-CENTURY AMERICA*
ALFRED VITALE

I'll start with an apology. The book you have in your hands, *The Unbearables Big Book of Sex,* will come out before my own, and so you will have to wait to see the whole text of the book mentioned in the title above. But as an act of contrition, I present a sort of "director's commentary" on the project and some important extras that will help you when my book eventually appears. Consider this the bonus you get for buying an Unbearable book. And I will enter an instrumental anecdote up front: I was told years ago by Rollo Whitehead that I need to put footnotes, for his benefit, in everything I write. At first I laughed and resisted,[1] but Rollo made a strong argument using Balinese shadow puppets and Nyquil, and eventually convinced me to aggravate the bottom of my pages with footnotes.[2] Now onwards with my story already, so you can begin the arduous process of ignoring it.

It was a long time ago, in hyperbolic terms. I had been working on my master's thesis, "Jarry's Pataphysics and the Aporia of Boswellian Humor: A Bataillean Appreciation," a tome which did not sit well in the gray cinderblock walls of the Department of Rational Economics at a major university where I had been a graduate student for three years. (I know…you're already thinking this is a metafiction… that I am blurring the already blurred boundaries between parody and truth…that you've uncovered my conceit. And yes, if you've read any of the other Unbearables' books, you'd see my trademarked style and think, "oh here we go again." But you'd be wrong. This is no short story, this is an excavation of a historical narrative, and one which you are damned lucky to be made privy to.) And during that time I was courting three presumably supple young women who were undergraduate seniors all majoring in contemporary literary studies, and all very much interested in pataphysics (do you see the utility of my thesis yet?). Now, at that point I had already achieved much in the realm of the sexual, and thus was courting these three women simultaneously… as in going for the elusive four-way that for lesser mortals would have been the stuff of porn or payment, but I had reasoned thusly: anyone can have a three-way (and lord knows I had many) but it takes a true master craftsman to obtain the pleasure of three women at once. "Could he handle that?" you're thinking. Of course he could. Or at least he presumed he would… or die trying (and what a fine death, no?). A pioneering spermo-gnostic would have it no other way. But, alas, I was younger then.

It is at this point in our jumbled missive where I want to remind you of what I said earlier. If you've ever heard me spout out my mythos, within which I am constantly caught up, you'd know that I was once a flamboyant heterosexual who was driven by his libidinous life force… his visceral élan vital (and my last name is no coincidence). And so you'd come to expect something like that from a man who was once King Dick for a day. But I remind you that this is a narrative of historical significance, and I have to work hard to be free of your expectations. After all, as historian Frank

Kermode has said, "The only powerful constraint habitually felt by writers of history (if we leave out of account the refined strictures of philosophers of history) is the reader's set of expectations."[3] So constrain me if you will, but I will be risen, and then I will come again.

Reader, if you have come this far, then please return with me to my thesis. As I began to lure the three sweet voluptuous nymphets closer… letting them read my dog-eared copy of *Wiggling Wishbone,*[4] huddling with them in sepia-toned cafes as we conjured up comparisons between Pere Ubu and Peter Griffin, their latte breaths each flavored by a different syrup, all combining and exhaling in unison like a carmel chai wind across my cheeks… the lyrics of our conversations forming a chaos pattern leading to the strange attractor that I carried down below, with innuendoes and suggestions winding like a caduceus… an almost tangled web that I believed we were about to weave. Until a flippant remark wafted by, from no discernible source, saying "the key to Harry Smith's anthology is not *Kaballah,* it's the *Kama Sutra.*" Now, most of the words in that ghostly sentence of no origin were not only familiar to me, but were indelible to that which formed my inner monologues. On one arm, I have a tattoo of a naked Radha embracing an equally naked Krishna as drawn by a 17th-century Sri Vidya tantrika for a related text called the *Koka Shastra,*[5] and on the other arm, a diagram from the anthology of American folk music[6] liner notes. I was intrigued, and unwound myself in a whisper, walking slowly backwards from our little round table to see who might have been discussing such matters for which I was enamored, to say the least. I saw only the empty gaze of mathematicians and policy makers discussing regression analyses and getting up repeatedly to ask for more hot water. Finding nobody to blame for this accusation, I set back to the mission at hand. But it only takes a horrible instant for the air of hypnosis to pop like a bubble, and my delicious desserts began to speak of other things and I only hovered by like Kaa patiently awaiting another moment that did not come. So while alone, later... kept awake by the copious caffeine of hours earlier... I took out the Anthology and considered, for a moment, the sexual possibilities engendered within. With the opening notes of the first song, and the opening of the first pages of the liner notes... with all of Smith's oblique song summaries and references to older ballads... something seemed right. There were 84 songs in all, spread out in three sections: Ballads, Social Music, and Songs. Smith had been an occultist and kabbalist, eccentric, animation pioneer, painter, ethnographer, poet, shaman, collector of string figure stories and paper airplanes and Russian eggs and vinyl saved from the ravages of war time scrap.[7] The 84 songs were said to be arranged in some way to form a cohesive whole, but nobody had cracked the code. Was it numerological (as I had assumed) or was it encrypted? Was there something geographical about the artists, or something in the instrumentation? It remained a mystery. But that shady and isolated sentence from a few hours earlier might have been onto something. And so that night I listened to the anthology's songs... and tried to seduce the sensual and perverse from their grooves. Letting the music talk dirty to me, and then looking at the liner notes to stimulate my imagination, I started to feel something stir. The titles began to awaken slumbering associations that I had accumulated over a lifetime of sexual adventure.

It took almost eight years of intense exploration... hundreds of hours in musty east village bookstores, tracking down leads on those who knew Smith... spending evenings in the burnt out remains of former Yippie strongholds where the crumbling stone steps to the building had stains colored by 30 years of CBGB vomit… losing massive amounts of blood from papercuts received while clambering through collections at libraries… trudging regularly to Queens to dig through Ron Kolm's last available archive-cum-bathroom… finding every scrap of anecdotal information I could to formulate a substantive hypothesis about the Anthology that I now know was in fact held secret by the keepers of its wisdom.[8] And here it is: Every single song that is included in the Anthology refers to arcane sexual practices that had been lost to folk wisdom. In essence, this is not the story of folk music so much as it is the story of how those folks fucked. Like tarot cards, each song was the signifier to something greater signified and symbolic… and totally sexual. And that, my friends, is what you'll read in my book… the elaborate, surprising, and titillating exposition of lust and depravity that our forbearers enjoyed as told through washboards and guitars and dulcimers and accordions and fiddles.

Now it would be wrong of me to bring this up without actually sharing at least some excerpts. But that's not why I'm going to present them. I do so because I want you to buy my book when it finally sees the light of day. In the interest of space, as I've just rambled on far too long, here are just a few of the songs and their secrets. These don't have any of the illustrations, of course, but you can use your imagination for that. I'll start with the very first song, sung by a man with the auspicious name Dick Justice: 'Henry Lee': Named after a 19th century economist, a Henry Lee was the soliciting of vice presidential candidates for lewd acts requiring draft horses. Although the Henry Lee was thought to be the stuff of legend, it seemed to enjoy a brief renaissance between 2000 and 2008.

For me, the first 27 songs comprising the "Ballads" section gives us the basic repertoire for appropriate fin-de-siècle debauchery, like the Major Arcana of the Tarot. Song number three: 'The House Carpenter': also called "getting nailed," the house carpenter called for trepanation to be performed while reading *Collier's* magazine.

Song number five has a long history in Appalachia: 'Old Lady and the Devil': an intricate wife swap role play involving three participants, enacting the role of the lady, the devil, and her husband. There was no actual sex involved, technically, but after the husband gives his wife to the devil, he enjoys a fortnight of sitting at the dining room table and scratching his balls with impunity.

Some of the songs are called "blues" and we all know the reason they are called "blues," right? Sadness, pain, depression and angst, right? Well... actually that's a smokescreen for one of two possibilities: according to the late delta singer Blind Gums Powell... either blue balls, or the throbbing blue vein astride the top of the penile shaft. The variation is likely regional. Thus from John Hurt's "Spike Driver Blues" (song # 80) I learned that in Mississippi, a Spike Driver was hobo slang for a man who found pleasure by vigorously humping mud until climaxing.

Whereas in Tennessee, the blues was testicular. Song number 66 is the Memphis Jug Band's "Bob Lee Junior Blues" and it was Joe Maynard[9] who told me that when he was a boy, it was customary to name your testicles after your maternal grandfather.[10] I assumed this to be the case for a few songs in the Anthology, but I was proven wrong when I visited a sorghum farm outside of Dyersberg where a photograph of a Bob Lee Junior had been found in a box hidden in a barn. Song number 66: 'Bob Lee Junior Blues': Despite the Tennessee custom of naming one's testicles, the Bob Lee

Junior Blues did not refer to this practice. Bob Lee is instead said to refer to General Robert E. Lee, and the junior to his notoriously small penis. A Bob Lee Junior Blues is when a very tiny, yet uncircumcised penis retreats into the scrotal sac until it looks like a clitoris nestled in bloated labia. Its owner can only then have sex by surrendering to General Grant at Appomattox.

This is not to be confused with song number 40, which represented a rust-belt version of the blues as demonstrated by the Cincinnati Jug Band: 'Newport Blues': A Newport Blues is essentially a "Cincinnati Bowtie," with a twist… the twist being performed on the scrotum itself. Most of the time, a Newport Blues was administered vengefully and well-timed, so as to prevent a two-timing man from a climax. This song has an additional layer of meaning, because a Cincinnati Jug Band is a Cincinnati Bowtie that is given to an exceptionally fat man.

Harry Smith recognized the importance of veiling these secrets, given the cold war McCarthyism of the 1950s, and it was his dedication to keeping these secrets present for erotic semioticians to discover as absent that gave us the compellingly lyrical, sexual heterotopias we can purchase today online or at music shops that don't suck.

I'd like to end here with a rationale for all of the above. Kermode, again, clarifies….

A passion for fragments tempts one into psycho-analysis. Objects, part-objects; the envious spoiling of the object, its fragmentation in infantile fantasy, and consequent reparation; absolute fragments as paranoid-schizoid, implicate fragments as depressive. But it also invites blague, the developed relation between art and jokes or put-ons. And while one could argue that an excessive addiction to blague is regressive, it is of more immediate interest that it commonly depends for its effect on the ambiguity of the fragment.[11]

Postscript

Ron Kolm is invading my brain and telling me to stop writing now. But everyone else in this anthology is swinging their own genitalia proudly or with deliberate pathos, so I think it's only fair that I do the same... succinctly so as to not be that guy who writes the really long piece that Ron is too nice to circumcise. So I will sew up the story from where I started....

The three ladies were eventually transformed from the stuff of my foursome fantasy to the stuff of being too big for my bed or my couch and so had to become the stuff of my living room floor on top of the fake Oriental rug I got on CRAIGSLIST. Am I a lucky man? Probably. But I confess that there is a downside: the human body is really stretched to its limits with three partners. Logistics become the divine order, and someone winds up just giving up and laying there awaiting some type of treatment out of necessity. Ultimately, you spend most of your time jockeying for position and being faced with more cognitive and aesthetic choices than you bargained for. Fun is replaced by function, taste and touch are replaced by issues of confidentiality and the potential loss of bone density. You want to brag, but no matter how you describe it you will more often receive pity for your gluttony rather than an elevated high-five of appreciation for the opus.

And it's no better with four partners either, even if it is more symmetrical.

Notes

1 No I didn't.

2 And yet I resisted further. Don't furrow your brow. This doesn't prove anything.

3 F. Kermode, *History and Value* (1987), 111.

4 b. plantenga, *Wiggling Wishbone: Stories of Pata-Sexual Speculation* (1994).

5 A set of medieval Indian writings based on the *Kama Sutra*... sort of like the articles in *Playboy* that you tell everyone you read.

6 If you have not heard of this collection, stop reading. Then take your Emo CDs and hold them up to the mirror so you can see how feeble they make you look. Aren't you embarrassed. What happened to you? You used to be so cool... such a rebel. Now you're just some person who hasn't heard of a pivotal piece of American musical history.

7 Seriously. I refuse to describe it further because it's just terrible to me that you don't know what this is! It helped him get a fucking Grammy award right before he died living at Naropa as the Shaman-in-residence, you scrawny philistine.

8 The forthcoming book will elaborate on this. Mike Golden, of course, knows what I'm talking about. His book, *Conspiracy Jones,* has helped me once again.

9 Unbearable editor of the legendary sex rag *Pink Pages* who, like the aforementioned Mike Golden, hails from the home of Davey Crockett.

10 Using that logic, my balls would be named Nunzio Arcuillo.

11 Copiously copied from Kermode, 1987, 142.

FROM CATEGORIES (AMAZON KINDLE, 2010)
RICHARD KOSTELANETZ

The epithet INNOVATIVE EROTICA would characterize such alternatives as a short seduction narrative with paragraphs no more than one word long (that became both an audio and a video with kinetic abstract shapes representing the two characters); a book-length narrative with paragraphs no more than two words long, printed with either one or several entries per page respectively on both spine-bound book paper and newsprint; an erotic narrative printed on fifty feet of continuous acetate; a perfect-bound book of hand-written visual-verbal representations of women known; several hundred single-sentence stories about "Lovings" for print and/or performance; real names and only names handwritten on gold-surfaced cards in a limited edition 8 1/2" x 11"; sixteen narratives in sixteen different typefaces interwoven one sentence at a stretch (that were not only realized on audio-tape with sixteen different amplifications of my own voice but can also be performed live by spectators selected from an audience); over two hundred sheets of single-page "More Portraits for Memory"; a chapbook in which the words "come here" are erotically (re)designed through pages to constitute a narrative; and a strictly audio fiction portraying female orgasm. Perhaps I've realized yet other ways of representing heterosexual experience differently. (Recurring subjects are sex, art/writing, and New York City.)

LIKE A VIRGIN, UNTOUCHED FOR THE VERY FIRST TIME
ANITTA SANTIAGO

When Madonna sang "Like a Virgin" in 1984, the operative word, of course, was "like." And in her career-retrospective *Rolling Stone* interview last year, looking back on the hit song, she poses the question, "how can you be *like* a virgin?"[1] *Like* is a question of representation, and if the music video's answer was "wear a white dress," the controversy after the MTV Video Music awards performance suggests that the white dress wouldn't cut it. But Madonna was not the first woman to tell about recapturing virginity while donning a white dress, nor the first to endure controversy for it. This experience was, in many ways, the story of the life of Margery Kempe, Medieval mystic, wife and mother of fourteen.

After the scourge of God had ruined her beer business to chastise her pride and greed, Margery Kempe experienced a conversion that came with a literal distaste for sex. In *The Book of Margery Kempe*[2] her sacerdotal scribe writes:

> After this time she never had any desire to have sexual intercourse with her husband, for paying the debt of matrimony was so abominable to her that she would rather, she thought, have eaten and drunk the ooze and muck in the gutter than consent to intercourse, except out of obedience. (46)

Out of obedience, she would have sex with her husband only with sorrow and tears over the fact that she could not live *like* a virgin. She tries to convince her husband to live a celibate matrimony, "that they had often displeased God (she well knew) by their inordinate love, and the great delight that each of them had in using the other's body, and now it would be a good thing if by mutual consent they punished and chastised themselves by abstaining from the lust of their bodies" (46). But husband John seemed to think that while that was all well and good, he might use her body a little longer, though she made sure to clothe it in a carefully concealed hair-shirt. After two years of suffering sex with her husband, Kempe experiences three years of temptation to sleep with other men, and offers herself to a man who propositions her on St. Margaret's Eve, only it turns out he wasn't serious and rejects her. It would seem that Kempe was struggling with living like a virgin on many fronts.

It may have been the hair-shirt, but for eight weeks Kempe's husband has not touched her, and as they travel from York, John asks:

> "Margery, if there came a man with a sword who would strike off my head unless I made love with you as I used to do before, tell me on your conscience — for you say you will not lie — whether you would allow my head to be cut off, or else allow me to make love with you again, as I did at one time?"
>
> "Alas, sir," she said, "why are you raising this matter, when we have been chaste for these past eight weeks?"
>
> "Because I want to know the truth of your heart."
>
> And then she said with great sorrow, "Truly, I

would rather see you being killed than that we should turn back to our uncleanness."

And he replied, "You are no good wife" (58).

John's question involves rape and castration. He must either have sex with Margery against her will or have his head cut off. What is interesting is how he re-scripts the rape so that it is not John who is forcing sex but a strange, sword-wielding voyeur, and the matter rests on Margery's choice. She can either will to have sex against her will or "allow" her husband's castration. In this hypothetical situation it is John who is the victim. Margery's answer is about as blunt as they come, and when John tells her she is "no good wife" because she will not defend her husband's life (or penis) and refuses to ever again under any circumstances pay the "debt of matrimony," he is perhaps unwittingly paying Margery a compliment. Consider that what Margery rejects is ever turning back to "our uncleanness." As a married couple, there is nothing sinful in their having sex. At the end of the scene, in fact, Margery asks John if they can make a vow of chastity at the hands of the bishop, which he refuses on the grounds that now sex with her is no mortal sin, but after a vow of chastity it would be (which most of all indicates that John refuses to give up on the chance of bedding Margery again). The "uncleanness," therefore, has to be understood as a relative condition, returning to the uncleanness of sexual contact after a newly reacquired virginity. That Margery is, according to John, no good wife is no real insult as it is her status as a wife that Margery has been struggling with and against.

That John poses his question, *are we ever having sex again?*, under the conditions of violence is telling, and in the scene directly following we have a good picture of why

Margery struggles with being a wife. On the road to Bridlington, John tries to strike a deal with Margery, that he will agree to the chastity if she will have dinner with him on Fridays and pay his debts before going to Jerusalem. In other words, she would cover a monetary debt to be forgiven of the *debt of matrimony*, and share food instead of sex. Margery at first refuses so as not to give up her Friday fast, for which John threatens, "Then I am going to have sex with you again" (59).[3] Shayne Legassie in *Differently Centered Worlds: The Traveler's Body in Late European Narrative (1350–1450)* notes that in setting this scene on the road, the writer of *The Book of Margery Kempe* casts what would be a normal scene of domestic relations (i.e. the husband demands sex of his wife) into a familiar generic scene of the woman traveler on the road and the threat of rape. The strange voyeur of the hypothetical question is not necessary. John himself poses the threat of rape and it is Margery whom we now see in the victimhood of matrimony as she staves off her husband: "She begged him to allow her to say her prayers, and he kindly allowed it" (59). Legassie also points out that it is not just her chastity at stake here but her ability to make the desired pilgrimage to Jerusalem, which she could not make without her husband's consent. Where John imagined himself victim to rape/castration and Margery's consent, in reality, it is Margery who is the actual victim of rape and her husband's consent, to travel, to pray, and to not have sex she does not desire. John is not a bad man, but he is no good husband. The status of husband in Medieval English society, like Margery's status as wife, is itself the problem.

When Margery prays, God tells her that she can give up the Friday fast and make the deal. Virginity takes the form of a kind of emancipation for Margery. She can get away from her husband, even to great distances. But in the course of

Margery's travels *like* becomes a problem. After receiving permission from the Bishop (with the necessary consent of her husband) to wear the virginal white clothes in acknowledgement of her vow of chastity, Margery is constantly ridiculed and slandered. She is a non-virgin in white who wails loudly during the Eucharist or at anything that reminds her of Christ, including newborn babies and handsome men, and she makes many priests uncomfortable with her calling out against vocational hypocrisy. But it is precisely the fact that Margery can only be *like* a virgin that allows her to be an authority on sincerity of heart, because it is only in her heart that she can reclaim virginal status. In her conversations with God, she laments her lost virginity and God consoles her, assuring her of his love and re-scripting her wifehood, claiming her as his wife. She receives Christ in her heart *like* in her body as both husband and child, so that her experience as wife and mother gets reshaped in the spiritual as the image of her chastity. In these spiritualized effects of likeness, however, there remains the problem of the physical. Everywhere she goes Margery encounters accusations that her whole spiritual demeanor, the chastity and the weeping, are just an act. Priests continue to worry over her gender and sexuality, and at times she is requested to take off the white clothes, which she does out of obedience. Though she often has consent to travel without her husband, she cannot travel alone (a woman traveling alone has long suggested the streetwalker), and the search for a traveling companion is often an ordeal.

Even her confessor, who has throughout trusted in her holiness, and has even spurned the conversation of those nobles who refused to talk with him if he continued to deal with her, continues to worry after her fifteen years of chastity about her sexuality. She sees Christ in the lepers and feels a tremendous desire to kiss them as an expression of love for Christ. This moment marks the real transformation of her conversion:

> Now she began to love what she had most hated before, for there was nothing more loathsome or abominable to her while she was in her years of worldly prosperity than to see a leper, whom now, through our Lord's mercy, she desired to embrace and kiss for the love of Jesus, when she had time and a convenient place. (216)

Conversion allows Kempe a spiritual immunity whereby she no longer fears disease, though this immunity comes through a valuation of disease. Kempe loves the diseased person because she views him as Christ. Conversion has not only re-scripted disease, but also Kempe's sexuality. Throughout the narrative, we have read the danger of Kempe's sexuality, whether she is seducing another man, seeing clergymen naked, or suffering others' accusations of promiscuity. We do not read Kempe's desire to kiss the lepers (or are not meant to) as sexual desire, but spiritual desire. But the spiritual does not take us into the abstract, into metaphor, because she needs the physical contact with the lepers in order to have contact with Christ. Kempe still desires physical contact, only her physical contact is spiritual, where the one term does not negate the other.

Though Kempe's sexuality is thus re-scripted, it is also prescribed (restricted) by the male authorities (in this case, her confessor) who are constantly regulating Kempe's spiritual health, travel, and sexuality.

Then she told her confessor how great a desire she had to kiss lepers, and he warned her that she should kiss no men, but, if she would kiss anyhow, she should kiss women. Then she was glad, because she had permission to kiss the sick women, and went to a place where sick women lived who were full of the disease, and fell down on her knees before them, begging them that she might kiss their mouths for the love of Jesus. And so she there kissed two sick women, with many a holy thought and many a devout tear, and when she had kissed them, she spoke very many good words to them, and stirred them to meekness and patience, that they should not resent their illness, but thank God highly for it, and that they should have bliss in heaven through the mercy of our Lord Jesus Christ. (217)

It is important to recognize that in this prescription against kissing male lepers, the confessor limits his recognition of her desire as a spiritual desire, in so much as he fears worldly sexual desire. His prescription is centered on Kempe's sexual identity. Kempe's desire has a spiritual precedent in St. Francis, but the prescription comes in to limit her contact with the diseased based on the fact that she is a woman. It seems that her confessor does not mind the physical danger the leper is to Kempe, but he is very cautious of the physical danger Kempe as a woman is to the male leper. This prescription, however, based on the worldly fear of sexual desire, has ironic sexual and spiritual repercussions as it not only has the priest endorsing non-normative sexual contact (if his problem is that he fears Kempe's kiss may be sexual, his redirecting it to women seems to open it to the possibility of being homosexual), but also has women standing in for Christ in the spiritual physical contact. In this light, we can read more into Kempe's exhortation to the women not to resent their illness. Kempe recognized her loss of virginity as uncleanness, and leprosy, too, is biblically defined as uncleanness. Disease and sexuality share liminal dimensions, concerns of bodies in contact. If Kempe initially saw in the lepers Christ, through contact with the female lepers she can perhaps see in them herself. Kempe knew what it was to resent her "uncleanness" but now comes to find *like-ness*, which was once a curse, a blessing. If her living *like* a virgin has called for constant assertion of boundaries and regulation, it has also allowed for the exploration of ways to compromise and re-regulate them.

At the end of the leper chapter, Kempe consoles a virgin who is undergoing sexual temptation. She prays to God to give the virgin strength to resist temptation, and, so says the writer, "it is to be believed that he did so." If Kempe no longer resents her "uncleanness" she maintains a commitment to virginity, and seems to have succeeded at acquiring the virgin touch. She can empathize with the virgin, perhaps strangely in a way that another virgin could not. Her commitment to virginity makes her virgin likeness perhaps different from Madonna's 1984 virgin likeness, but I think she can still offer at least one possible answer to Madonna's question. How can you be *like* a virgin? What does it mean to be *like* a virgin? For Kempe it seems to mean living within the sexual politics of her era and constantly trying to recreate them through virginal conversion. It is an embodied spiritual resistance.

Notes

1 Austin Scaggs. "Madonna Looks Back: The *Rolling Stone* Interview." *Rolling Stone* 29 October 2009: 51.

2 *The Book of Margery Kempe.* Trans. B.A. Windeatt. New York: Penguin, 2004. All references and quotations are to this edition.

3 Shayne Legassie, *Differently Centered Worlds: The Traveler's Body in Late Medieval European Narrative (1350–1450).* Diss. Columbia University, 2007. In his chapter, "The Body of Margery Kempe: Gender, Genre, and Historiography in Pre-Modern Travel Studies" (pp. 188–249), Legassie argues that the reason *The Book of Margery Kempe* is not considered a representative of Medieval travel writing is because of limited notions of genre that read travel narratives along the model of Mandeville's travel, coordinated on a distinct sense of *home* and *away*. Kempe's narrative gets critiqued for not being chronological, and not starting from a single space of home into one travel adventure, but, so Legassie argues, this is because Kempe conflates home and away. Her narrative, he proposes, can be read as a response to gender inequality and "the patriarchal nature of home itself" (193).

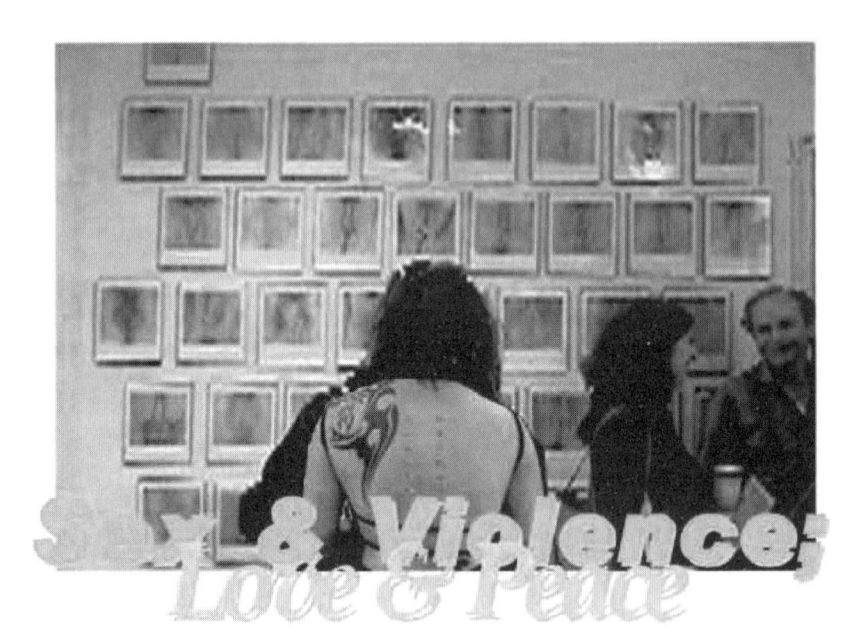

Sex & Violence;
Love & Peace

On October 16, 2004, a wall of vaginas, entitled by photographer Alexandra Jacoby as *"Vagina Verité"* participated in the women's group show called "The Exhibitionists" at the Tribes Gallery in the Lower East Side. It caused a sensation at the art opening where I videoed the event. I went home and showed the tape to my live-in boyfriend who became very agitated. We had not had sex since the demise of the World Trade Center. It had been three years. However, when he saw the wall of vaginas, it became a powerful conduit for us to have sex.

During the "unofficial" Iraqi War, I experienced domestic violence with my live-in boyfriend. He is an alcoholic and we had been together for 8 years. His drinking and chain smoking got worse to a point that his judgment became totally impaired, especially his jealousy streak. When I talked on the cell phone to a guy, he became angry. He grabbed the cell phone and broke it in half. I got angry and screamed "Get out!" I started to call the police on another phone where they arrived. The cops told him to leave the apartment. He left and eventually I have my peace without the LOVE.

by Susan L. Yung

BISHOP BERKELEY AT THE PEEP SHOW
KIRBY OLSON

Flying south from Seattle towards San Francisco, looking thru an airplane porthole: I peep out and see clouds floating like smudgy typos above a typography of mountains, lakes, a network of barely visible lumber roads. In the distance, a jagged mountain with snow clinging to its sides. In a few arable valleys, we see the rectangles and squares of farm fields, with a barn neatly set to one side. We cannot touch these items. Before the invention of the airplane, we could not see things in this way: we could only imagine the earth's surface from our usual standing height: between one and eight feet. From 20,000 feet in the air, the small things: ants, cows, rocks, plants, all disappear, and all that is left are general outlines, general forms: here scabrous mountains, there irrigated wheat fields, and on past Ashland, dry rolling hills which look like buffalo prairie.

My nerves tremble, as I am going to speak at an academic conference at Stanford University. I order a whisky. Unused to alcohol, I nod out. Everything disappears — a mere black hole takes its place — nothingness, a refreshing rest from something-ness. When I awake again and look out the porthole: things themselves are refreshed, their outlines clearer, their colors sharper, now the fields below are plowed in circles, to prevent erosion perhaps. An angel says hello through the porthole, waving wings. (A curious thing about angels, ever since I started reading Milton, I always look to see what sex they are, but never see anything specific.) Then, a stubble of trees to the north of California, looking like the unshaved face of Paul Rubens (a.k.a. Pee Wee Herman) in the mug shot after his arrest for whacking off in a Florida porno theatre.

At a peep show, I gaze through the opening. On the other side, six or seven women playfully gyrate, mimicking fornication, fellatio, sodomy, cunnilingus. Completely nude, or with only a scarf or a g-string, the normal clues to identity have been carefully removed from the peep show dancers. I don't think of these women as having families, or church affiliations, or career aspirations. They are women as they appear in dreams, as divine archetypes, as signs without any other signification that the goddesses of ancient Greece had when they appeared before a pool of water in the hills around Athens. The strobe lights and pounding disco music further disorient me, putting me into a trance state. I could close my eyes and imagine a barn, or a mountain, and this image would replace the image of the women dancing the who-knows-what in front of me. For these images, I do not need to pay a quarter. To see the women, I do. 25¢ for about twenty seconds. I am also supposed to jerk off while I watch this spectacle, though the police make weekly raids, and if I am caught, I will end up as another kind of spectacle. I really shouldn't be here at all, which is of course why I am. And because I am researching a paper on Bishop Berkeley's philosophy of perception, and have decided to do a little field work. Berkeley's philosophy posits a single subject and single object. For example, one individual (subject) looks out over a distance of miles at a castle on a far hill (object). But Berkeley says that there is no such thing as distance. He says that the object is only known through our perception of it. Without the eye, the castle might as well not exist. The castle, according to Berkeley, sits on the pupil. We do not see the castle, in fact, at all, but rather the *image* of the castle, brought to us at the speed of light. Light is faster than any known substance on earth — if it is a substance at all — it is presumably even faster than thought. Light speeds past thought and tricks us into thinking we are seeing the castle. Berkeley wants to slow light down, so that we can see that this is no more the castle that meets our eye than the rustling of a pile of leaves *are* leaves. What we hear is the *rustling*, and not the leaves. What we see is the *image* of the castle, and not the castle properly speaking.

Similarly, Berkeley, at the peep show, would not see the women. He would only see the images of the women, dancing on his pupils. The client is a kind of reader. He watches the women and between them they form a mutually comprehensible language, the same as the reader of this essay must step inside the language and reinterpret it for him or herself, making the language his or her own. Berkeley says the world is a divine language, through which God is trying to tell us something. We must read very carefully, as learning the language of nature is at least as difficult as learning ancient Greek. What are the women at a peep show trying to tell us? When we've seen their simple grammar of images, their set of tropes, it all seems as wind-up toy as a chicken who carries a ping-pong ball across a short distance to pop the ball in a tiny basket to get some feed. But it is certainly no less complicated than Mick Jagger strutting across the stage like a rooster; nor is it less complicated than any other genre based on the simple neural firing which simulates desire. If it's degrading, it is because it turns us into animals, which is fowl I suppose, but isn't that what makes popular culture divine — its reminder of our origins? Some readers, and some clients, might decide to close the text. Many men, and more women, are convinced that the sex show workers work under duress, and we should feel sorry for them. But there is some evidence that this needn't be the case. At Seattle's *Lusty Lady*, for example, there is profit-sharing, and the business is women owned. Many other places are sickening in that the women do not seem to be moving on their own, but rather as if they were attached to strings manipulated by unimaginative idiots. In Houston, I saw a show which made me think the sign above the door, "Live Girls on Stage," should have read "Dead Girls on Stage." It was just not worth the quarter. Was the difference simply a matter of aesthetics? What distinguishes a good experience from a bad in the peep shows is probably the same thing that distinguishes good art from bad, in general: did the artist enjoy making it? Is there inner compulsion? Is the artist *paying attention*? At the *Lusty Lady*, I've seen some of the same modern dancers I've seen elsewhere on Seattle's artistic stages. Sometimes they ask me through the glass what I'm reading lately, while still gyrating. This ruins the effect for me, frankly, splitting my attention, and then the interaction often turns into comedy — making funny faces at each other, or devolving into discussions of Busby Berkeley, when I'm intent on carrying out investigations of Bishop Berkeley. Some of the women in the peep shows are lawyers who do it for fun — as an alternative to aerobics. I refer the disbelieving to *Caught Looking*, published by the Feminist Anti-Censorship Task Force (Real Comet Press, 1988). One argument they offer against censorship of the sex shows or pornography is that just now women are finally educated and able to join in the sexual dialogue, and it is just now that laws are being passed against the whole topic.

At the peep shows I've been to, the women look back. A leer at a certain part of a woman's body will focus the woman's attention there. When eyes meet silently through the distance of the glass, the gaze is mutually engaging — if one is bored by a woman, she immediately knows, and the relationship goes kaput.

Can we call what occurs between strangers through glass a relationship? Since St. Paul, who said it is better to marry than burn, and that we could only have one relationship for life, the idea behind marriage has been a kind of domesticated desire, like having sex on tap in the house in the same way we have hot water and electricity. Although gas and electricity can be domesticated to the extent that we can control a switch, desire is less easy to domesticate. By definition, desire may *have* to be undomesticated. Dionysos, the Greek god of ecstasy, always appears as a *stranger* (see Marcel Detienne's *Dionysos*). He wears a mask. At the same time, Dionysos flips out if he is not recognized. That is the essential structure of the myth, and it is the essential problem in love today. Women and men insist on not being treated like objects, but rather on being known as individual humans — but to make love there has to be an element of strangeness, of the unknown, of the wild and undomesticated. It is a circle which we keep trying to square, and which runs the market economy — if only we buy this perfume, if only we take this trip to Cancun, if only we get a new and better apartment, or this mink fur, *then* the cultural myth of domesticated Dionysian love will take place. In marriage, one is supposed to have both a close, trusting relationship, and to fantasize enough about the other to have Dionysian sex. I can manage one or the other, but not both, because "desire is suffocated in incestuous claustrophobia" (see Slavoj Zizek's *Sublime Object*, 120) in "true love:" and in wild sex, all I think about is that I'm going to die from AIDS.

The peep show is a partial safety valve for this Mexican stand-off. It is a sexual contract, safe, and not binding. It is a professional service, rendered with a high degree of charm and skill. What do women get out of it? A Jungian answer is provided by Nancy Qualls-Corbett in *The Sacred Prostitute* (Inner City, 1988), where she tries to resurrect the destroyed pagan era, stomped out by St. Paul, of the period of a woman's life spent in worship of the goddess Astarte. She inscribes her being to the goddess in a carnal act of mutual pornography, a living love lyric to the deity. Then, this profession was not a choice, but rather a religious duty. Today, one chooses this profession. It is not for everyone, but then neither is the sanitation field, medicine, or evangelical Christianity. It is a choice, and it is women's choice, just as it is the choice (for now) of an author to say or write or dance what he or she pleases. Sexual orientation may not be a choice, how we feel about a specific person sexually may not be a choice, but what we choose to read is. The reader at the peep show, if (s)he decides to spend not only the quarter, but the mental energy which is truly required, identifies with the women or with one specific woman to the point that (s)he becomes her. The subject (Berkeley) can become so entranced by the object (peep-show dancer) that he can become a new subject (Berkeley as peep-show dancer). It is through this sort of identification, this sort of intersubjectivity, that I would try (with some success, I believe) at the Stanford conference — to show a positive side to the "male gaze" — and try to explain how in fact men were becoming women as they looked upon women at peep shows. Is this transmutation, and not the sexual exploitation of women, what had Florida's reactionaries mad at Pee Wee Herman? Pee Wee was breaking the Platonic-Biblical taboo against mixing, too, in which each person must be one thing. For a man to pretend to be a child is about all most lawful authorities can bear. For him now to become a woman is *not* cute — it makes the walls of the big city shake — and not with laughter. It is these sudden transmutations which are thought so disturbing to order, and which are therefore outlawed.

The walls of the cities are rattled enough from the sixties, many say. But I say let the walls of the city shake, rattle and roll or else we will lose beauty altogether in the search for a tyrannical security.

"Beauty," as surrealist André Breton said, "will be *convulsive,* or not at all."

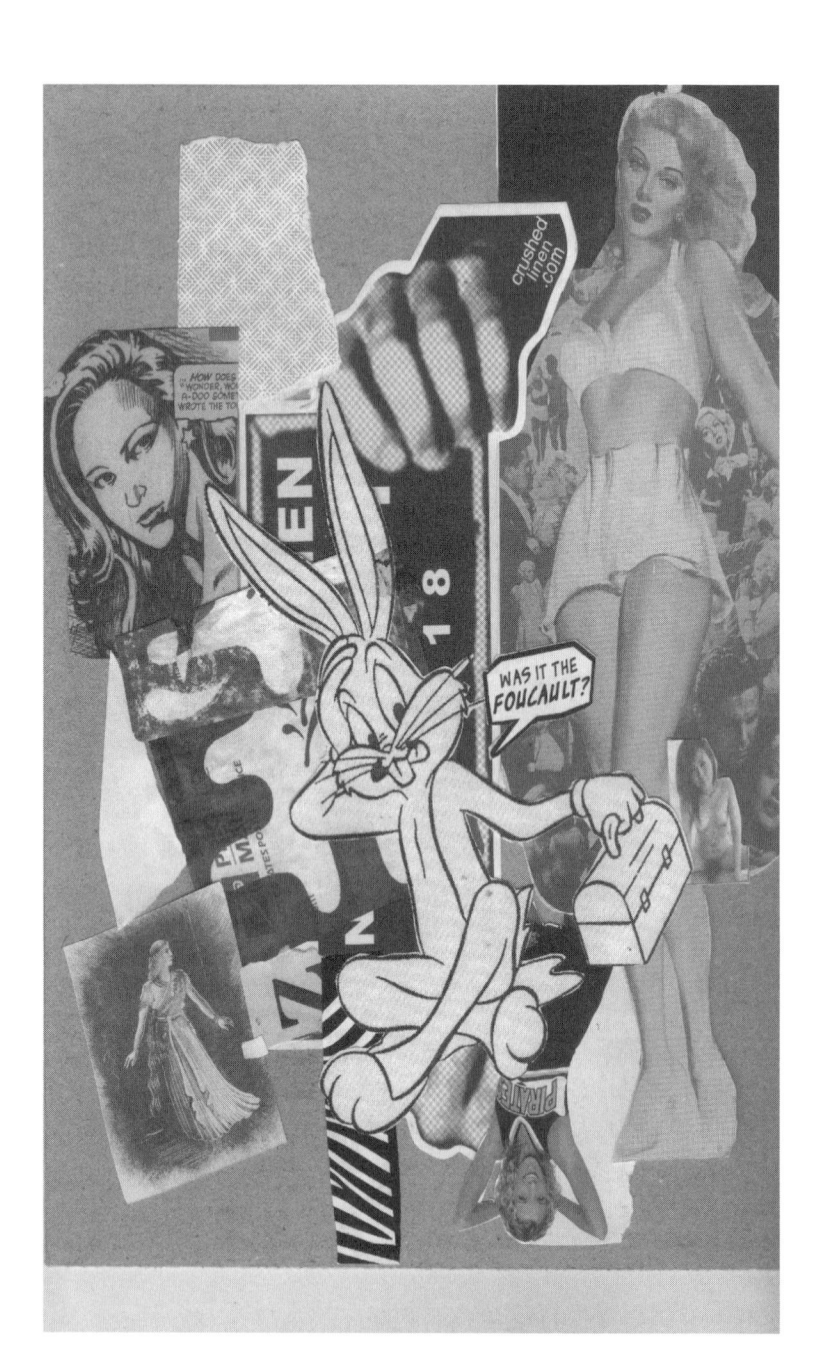

WILHELM REICH: THE EMOTIONAL PLAGUE & THE AUTHORITARIAN FAMILY
PETER WERBE

The juxtaposing of anti-sexual statements by the Vatican and certain leftist leaders and groups [not included here] isn't meant as an exercise in cynicism, but rather to illustrate in graphic terms the role sexual repression plays within all authoritarian systems.

The Church, for example, is easily identifiable as a repressive institution. Its power to regulate moral conduct grew as did the centrality of its wealth and authority within the feudal system of the Middle Ages.

The Catholic Church was the international agent of feudalism, on the one hand, sanctifying its rigid social relationships as God-ordained and being the largest single landowner, on the other, holding a full one third of the soil of Christendom.

Its religious ideology tied people to the structure of feudalism's political economy not just through investing it with divine characteristics, but also by developing a hold rooted in people's basic psyche. This would tie them to hierarchical systems of domination and submission even when that particular form of economy, based on land ownership, had long been replaced by the rule of capitalism.

In all regions where religion flourishes, it functions as an important part of the control system and is heavily supported by the reigning political structure. Although the neurotic mystics who founded religions did not necessarily intend that their creeds be used to entrench systems of domination, when the crippling power of religion became apparent, all rulers were quick to adopt and support it.

Denial of the flesh appears as a constant in the world's major religions and the importance of this mechanism of sexual repression can be seen as the key to the reason why people have been willing to passively accept the dehumanization of their lives since the rise of class society thousands of years ago.

Some explanation is needed as to why soldiers go enthusiastically into battle for purposes not their own, why workers slavishly labor to make others rich and powerful, and why all of us accept the whole of what civilization is today: the denial of human community and the affirmation of the State, hierarchy, and the general blunting of life's potential. Always the readiness to submerge one's desires to the grand schemes of the Leader, the State or religion.

THE THEORIES OF WILHELM REICH

Social psychologist Wilhelm Reich suggested that the root of this "emotional plague" lay in the suppression of infant and adolescent sexuality — from harsh toilet training to punishing masturbation to teaching that sexual intercourse is "bad and dirty."

The child adapts to the punishments, threats, and scolding by repressing his/her sexuality. Further attempts by the child to affirm its sexual desires become revolts against parental authority and are met by further condemnation and punishment. The punishment assures that forbidden activities are infused with guilt feelings and ultimately produce an adult in which sexual drives and *all thoughts of rebellion against authority* produce anxiety, feelings of guilt, unworthiness and inadequacy.

In describing this process in *The Mass Psychology of Fascism*, Reich poses the central question: "For what sociological reasons is sexuality suppressed by the society and repressed by the individual?" His answer is:

"The interlacing of the socio-economic structure with the sexual structure of society and the structural reproduction of society takes place in the [child's] first four or five years and in the authoritarian family. The church only continues this function later. Thus, the authoritarian state gains an enormous interest in the authoritarian family: It becomes the factory in which the state's structure and ideology are molded."

What is produced is known to us all: passive, docile, fearful, dependent, obedient, malleable, respectful masses — in short, *the civilized human being*. Without the passive multitudes, the idea of the State, with its 8,000 year history of tyranny, ruling always in the interests of a few to the detriment of almost all, could not have lasted a single month.

The validation of Reich's analysis of the role of the family can be clearly recognized in crude advocates of the state such as Adolph Hitler who said that the family "is the smallest but most valuable unit in the complete structure of the state" (*Mein Programm*, 1932).

Also, the family is not *just* the training ground for the authoritarianism that benefits the State, but its essentially undemocratic internal structure is a model of the State apparatus itself. At the head of the family stands its ultimate ruler in the form of the father; this is mirrored in the political realm by the chieftain, emperor, king, president or commissar.

The ruled or "governed," both in the family and the State, usually have nothing to say about the administration of things or, at best, are given some formal say (elections or family discussions), but ultimately all important decisions are made by the father or leader. The enormous fear, respect, and deference granted rulers through the ages mirrors that forced upon us within the authoritarian family.

Swords have not been at the neck or guns at the breast of us as we reproduced society after society that has dashed the Living in us. "There is a gendarme inside every Frenchman" goes an old saying: In other words, the most powerful cops are inside of us.

Human families left to their own designs might have evolved to any possible form, including that of a non-authoritarian, non-patriarchal, democratic structure such as developed in isolated geographic regions such as Polynesia or the Philippines. Since such a family-type would not serve the needs of the reigning society, religion's function is to imbue its compulsive sex morality with the quality of being above human affairs, pronounced from Heaven, existing before mortal humans and after.

Religion not only continues the process begun in the family and maintained through education wherein the individual is taught to submit to authority, but also wraps the family in the mantle of sacredness, which insures its perpetuation as a social institution of control from one generation to the next.

A Craving for Leaders

Our reduction to child-like states of anxiety and dependence creates a craving for leaders, not a situation where they are foisted upon us. There have been many social upheavals, rebellions, and revolutions against leaders and social systems (too numerous to count, in fact), but each time, after the blood and carnage were washed away, the basic relationship of rulers and ruled has re-asserted itself.

What was at issue was that the old society and its leaders had become *too* denying, *too* brutal, *too* incapable of providing for daily survival; the society or leader had ceased to be a good father/provider and the masses began searching for a substitute.

Was there anything in 300 years of daily life under Czardom in Russia that did not call every day for a revolution — autocratic rule, staggering poverty, serfdom, religious domination of social life? Yet the great masses of Russian people loved the Czars and worshipped them almost like deities.

It may be appropriate at this time to insert the important notion that there have been rebels and rebellions that have questioned all authority, from the family to the State, and for short periods of time conditions of genuine liberation have held sway over large numbers of people.

In the 20th century, activities of revolutionaries in the Ukraine (1917–1921) and in Spain (1936) come quickest to mind. Their suppression in those cases was accomplished militarily at the hands of leftist governments in the process of consolidating their political power and control of the State.

The elimination of these revolutionary social movements was considered to be of exceptional importance since it was recognized by the new reigning political powers that people in the act of rebellion have slipped (if even momentarily) from the shackles of authority

New rulers who have just gained social power through a social rebellion have as a priority, almost on a par with suppressing elements of the recently toppled regime, the repression of these very elements of the revolt that brought them to power.

It's a tricky situation for the new rulers since to stop it too short would mean a containment of the revolutionary energies they are banking on to thrust them into power, but to allow the rebellion to go too far would bring into question the legitimacy of the authority of the new rulers.

George Washington and V.I. Lenin needed the revolutionary activity of the American and Russian masses, but neither of them wanted to go as far as the Tom Paines, the Daniel Shays, or the Russian factory committees or anarchists wanted to push the situation.

THE LEFT AND SEXUAL REPRESSION

The role of religion within authority's Holy Trinity (the compulsive family, religion, and the State) with its blatant anti-sexual ideology and its historic record of service to totalitarianism is easily understood as an institution of repression and most revolutionaries quickly reject overt religious mysticism of all varieties. What is at first surprising is that identical or even *more reactionary* pronouncements about sex leap from the mouths of those same leftists who claim to speak for liberation and revolution.

However, an analysis which looks beyond the rhetoric designed for public consumption by both the Church and Left quickly understands the hidden purpose of the repressive sexual views: the reproduction of patriarchal, authoritarian society.

Throughout the so-called socialist world, the sexual ideology of the leader and the state plays the same role that Christianity plays in the West: sexuality is discouraged in youth, homosexuals are persecuted, and authoritarian families are exalted. Even the structure is the same: in place of saints, leaders are venerated through the omnipresent statues of Lenin, Mao or Kim. In place of the Bible and prayer books, schools in socialist countries provide for compulsory reading of the teachings of the Leader and "good communists" are thought to be those who have the maximum amount of the Leader's thoughts inscribed in their minds.

Reich described the process of inhibited sexual excitation being replaced by religious exaltation exemplified by such occurrences as priests ejaculating during mass or women reaching near orgasmic states during frenzied religious revivals. Extending that analysis to the political realm, it is hard to miss the religious mystical tenor of mass political rallies dominated by the revered leader and structured to produce child-like emotions of dependency in the person attending.

At Hitler's stage-managed Nuremberg rallies[1] or the anthill, choreographed, mass demonstrations in Peking or Pyongyang, participants are reduced to insignificance by the giantism of the setting while their actualizations as people come through the celebration of the Leader or the State.

Also, the very content of the pronouncements by the Vatican and the left on sex share a similarity beyond the fact that both are repressive, anti-sexual statements. Both carry with them a fall from grace by the offending individual ("You are not a good Catholic" or "You are not a good communist"), bringing the entire weight of the dominant social institution down on the head of the sinner/counter-revolutionary ("condemned in the New Testament" or "against the Revolution").

Individuals find it generally hard to buck the weight of such condemnation. To do so means to become a pariah, a rebel, and suffer all of the consequences such a decision implies. In normal times, when a society is functioning relatively smoothly, few opt to take such a road; it is just too perilous, both physically and psychologically.

And it is precisely this fear, this timidity, which has allowed every society its ability to continue functioning even though the vast majority of its members have no real, sensuous, human reason to reproduce it.

THE EMOTIONAL PLAGUE & ITS SOLUTION

Reich characterized this dismal view of human behavior with its willingness to submit to authority as "the emotional plague," yet he did not despair of altering the situation. In *The Murder of Christ*, he states, "It is possible to get out of a trap. However, in order to break out of a prison, one first must confess to *being in a prison*. The trap is man's emotional structure." [And one must assume he included woman in this formulation.]

It is, he argued, only persons structurally capable of liberation who could then begin a successful struggle to abolish authoritarian social structures.

"The feeling was of a vast room, with the beams serving as might pillars of infinitely high outer walls. Now and then a cloud moved through this wreath of lights, bringing an element of surrealistic surprise to the mirage. 'The effect, which was both solemn and beautiful, was like being in a cathedral of ice,' British Ambassador Henderson wrote."

The impact on the individual in such a setting has always been taken for granted in liberal and leftist literature when describing the Right, but the same criteria is never applied to left-wing government rallies *where the form is identical.*

Note

[1]Hitler's architect, Albert Speer, described the setting for the Nuremberg Nazi Party rallies in his book *Inside the Third Reich*, thusly: "The hundred and thirty sharply defined [searchlight] beams, placed around the field at intervals of forty feet, were visible to a height of twenty or twenty-five thousand feet, after which they merged into a general glow.

AVATAR EROTICS
JACK BRATICH

Overheard at the Affect Diagnostic Clinic:
Q: How long have you been sexually active?
A: I don't know, doc, but I've been sexually reactive
since the age of eleven.

It's all too easy these days to take up one of two positions on eros in the digital age. One, out of the mouth of
overgrown babes, proclaims a freer sexuality and an
increased libertinism with social media. These noncreative
anachronism role-players are battling against Puritans
while on a stage made of silicone in a theater owned by
Maxim. The other finds a "lost youth" whose online explorations are filled with stranger danger and sexual predators
(meanwhile the real exploiters — marketers, corporate platform owners, and other privacy violators — receive
Hollywood blockbuster treatment). But what would it mean
to take insights from each of these without the moralism of
regulators or the self-deluded notions of libertines? What
new dances are possible?

At the turn of the second decade of the new millenium,
scandalous news stories conveyed the challenges of Eros in a
Networked Era. Sexting, of course, has drawn the approba-
tion and the titillated gazes of moral authorities. This rather
pedestrian peer-to-peer porn stirred dormant moral panics
over youth and mediated desire (whose lineage stretches

from Victorian indignation over love letters to the fear of young sexuality in early cinema houses to the outrage over the primal possession undergone by the 1950s teen set).

More crystallized anecdotes come from the rich world of Japanese pop culture. Dating simulation games abound, some of which feature the very real possibility of being rejected by the digital object of affection. In one case, a Japanese man named Sal 9000 had a public and online wedding in which he married his digital beloved, a character from the videogame "Love Plus." Which one is more of an avatar anyway? This case appears tame, as it at least involved an interactive figure. Compare it with the phenomenon of *dakimakura* — men who exclusively date body pillows containing anime and manga characters. One interpretation of these minority reports of desire is that they represent pathological excess, limited to a few individuals. But we might see these figures as prophetic, embodying virtual futures as if they were vehicles for a hidden animus. J-pop, the recession-ridden nation's major export of the last 20 years, sends us signals from the depths of the libidinal techno-unconscious. Let's bathe ourselves in this digital basin to see what kind of ablution is possible.

> *Status update: Elka Mikelov "is fed up with fucking avatars! Especially the ones in my bed"*

Our networked eros revives an old chestnut, the problem of the image. The image isn't what it used to be. Long devalued as paltry representation, now the image returns with newfound powers, namely to stimulate, resuscitate, and circulate affects rapidly. More importantly, these sensations spread among *familiars* rather than strangers. Images do not capture desire, stealing it away from a truer version among the enfleshed. This made sense with the old erotic image, namely the porn film (be it in the theater, on the TV screen, or on the computer monitor). The standard porn scene recreated mundane situations (pizza delivery, shared cab rides, chance street encounters) as fantasies. But they still remained, as images, separated from everyday life. Now, in an age of convergence culture, porn chic has gone mainstream, and reinvested those mundane scenes with the *actualization* of fantasies. Filmed VIP rooms, celebrity home-made sex tapes, spring break wild youth videos, amateur living room productions, sexting, porn tube: these all embed the images themselves into everyday behavior. They comprise a porn ecology.

Even this development doesn't reveal the key element of digital eros: *participation* or the merging of social communication with voyeurism.[1]

Spectatorship belongs to a different era. Voyeurism is no longer a pleasure derived from a distant spectator position, but from a temporal merge of the face-to-face with the Facebook-to-Facebook. Of course, digital life boosters will justify this trend by trotting out examples of people meeting and loving across larger geographical divides. What they forget is the converse — digital eros requires creating chasms between the most proximate.

The most telling example of this intimate isolation is the reported drift of male gazes away from traditional porn to their friends' Facebook profiles. Why spend attention-energy on a stranger when very available and proximate women have provided so much material? This should be a lesson to all those who still adhere to the belief that dressing up as Lady Gaga is purely an act of free expression. This faith in intentions allows everyone to sleep easier at night — for the self-objectified posers, a rest-inducing forgetfulness; for the masturbating subjects, a peaceful post-lurk-and-jerk slumber.

As psychoanalysists have insisted, the phantasmatic has less energy than the Real. Feeding it energy depletes us. What happens when this phantasm meets interactive technology? No longer cinematic image, but digital avatar.

With a participatory spectacle, we are interactors with avatars. People encounter each other as enfleshed online profiles, as corporeal information. Is this a more effective prisonhouse of desire? Is our humanity diminished? Perhaps, and it's a good thing too! Remember that avatars originally referred not to representations or projections, but to *incarnations*. The process did not begin with the human and go towards representation, but from the Divine down to the earthly. What is certain is that they embody the *inhuman*, even that which might be hostile to the human. Can loving the avatar augment rather than diminish us? For this we need to remember and extract the inhuman from the erotic.

> *textsfromlastyuga*
> *Q: What's your favorite part of me?*
> *A: The missing one.*

Social theorist Slavoj Zizek finds the clearest expression of contemporary desire today in the annual event called Masturbathon. Participants engage themselves simultaneously, a collective set of solo performances. But even this image is antiquated, as it depends on physical, geographical proximity. Today's scene would be more accurately captured in a network map of all the individuals currently masturbating at their computers.

But wait! We have something close. Chatroullette, a program that allows videochatters to connect randomly with others, quickly transformed into this oneiric communication. A Chatroulletter of this type is an epochal figure: an agent of self-pleasure who hopes someone sticks around to witness and assist. The chatroullette masturbator with even more agency keeps one finger on the nexting button, flipping through the parade of witnesses in order to find new stimulation.

> *Status update:*
> *Lance Penellette "is looking to get his lack-on"*

Another mutation, less crass but for that reason more mischievous, could be called the Chat-coquette. Classic coquettery involved an expertise in appearance and withdrawal, a set of skills devoted to becoming a subtle object of attention. These artists enacted what psychoanalysts only later formulated: desire is not for another, but for another's desire. Now, we send avatars out there to become strange attractors, with more "liveliness" and interactivity, but less mystery and flair. No need to be tied to a body or even to the rarity of public communication. Instead, the coquettish avatar makes vortices of disappearance within a self-produced glut of images and information. Dropped signals rather than dropped hints.

What is lost in Chat-coquette is a sense of play. Even the crafty codes have been replaced by The Rules formulated by clumsy eros bureaucrats. The time of this amorous subject is segmented, mini-bursts of info-packets and then their sudden halt. Rapid noncommunication and unacknowledged severance leaves little sense of intricate ambivalence.

The online coquette has less to do with seduction (getting the attention of other), and more with pre-empting *self-attention*. The ability to forget, a Nietzschean noble value in many contexts, is here a self-programmed repression. Pervasive nexting sees a return of the ego with its self-delusion of choice and control. "I" choose when to move on, rather than being compelled to forget because of vulnerability. This is forgetting not as indifference, but a hyperdifference, a dagger difference.

Status update:
Les C. Kressi "needs to increase his rate of profligate"

Much has been written about a contemporary "attention economy." Attention, a vector of will, energy, and cognition, is the elusive source of value in a hypermediated ecology. Attention is now scattered while seduced, augmented, and directed — devoted to giving and receiving stimuli rapidly to a wider, variegated public. This is a wholesale diffusion, a command to become profligate as a prerequisite for sociality.

Now the attention economy meets the libidinal economy. What is networked eros but a dispersion of *asymmetries* of attention, ones that require constant modulation of attitude and time: "I can keep this one on hold, I am still waiting for this One, this one is in zone of curiosity, this one's potential has yet to be tested, this one is exhausted, etc."

As Paolo Virno points out, the contemporary multitude is becoming accustomed to not having customs. Disruption, shocks, surprises — these wild vacillations make up the rhythms of everyday life, from reality TV programs ("Expect the Unexpected" says Big Brother) to the sudden privacy changes by Facebook owners. These external programs get internalized by amorous subjects, resulting in the explosive relationships that get valorized as chemistry and drama. How easy it is to get attached to being out of control while clinging to an ego that seeks to stop the chaos. Endless matrix bubbles, made of tears, along with endless bubble-bursting, make up this collective passion.

> *Status update:*
> *Sam Saraphul "smells like libertine spirit"*

From the anhedonic margins, we are reminded to challenge a reigning delusion: that enslavement to the passions constitutes liberty rather than its opposite. *Jouissance* is a cultural imperative, now expressed as an individual's demand: I am owed pleasure! I have a natural right to feel good! Any loud neurosis will apparently do.

The demand for passion is its own type of mania, one that forgets its etymological roots in suffering. Passion is better thought of as *pashu-n*, a self-fastening to one's snares.

The pleasure trap begins to answer Spinoza's guiding question: Why is it that people will fight for their subordination as fiercely as for their freedom? Well, it tastes sweet for starters. But like the aspartame that turns into formaldehyde when metabolized, enjoyment can carry its own future toxins. A slavish devotion to gratification underpins many desperate claims of sexual freedom. Many libertine assertions are akin to someone announcing they do freestyle dance, but only if there's a stripper pole on the stage. And this is no analogy.

What is released in these paroxysms is not itself pleasure but a whole host of conflicted and vexed drives. Repetitive behaviors, trauma re-enactments, compulsive regression: all these can be unleashed. Parasites that fed on the psyche's internal darkness now run free to play and fight with their familiars.

Status update:
Thomas Kulakali "is watching LSI: Libidinal Minds"

Networked desire is a full-time job, an affective online labor organized around accelerated stimulation and release, overexcitement and depletion. Like all contemporary immaterial labor, it involves the incessant learning of protocols. But these are emergent codes with no manuals, only piecemeal training through constant disruptions that tax the nervous system. Lessons require a continuous reactive questioning and modification: should I make myself visible on the chat? What did her wall post mean? Who's this new friend posting cloying comments on the beloved's wall?

Unsurprisingly, youth have become very aware of all this. Their self-reflection has hypertrophied, especially in an erotic world defined by pathological calculation (for the feminine, The Rules; for the masculine, The Game). Entangled in one's own tingling strategies, all while feeling in control via knowledge. Networked eros demands becoming a slave to knowledge. Love as forensics, at times a prefigurative cold case. These are Love Scene Investigators, but the body is missing.

Status update:
Morrissey Kressi "is a feminist at heart.
His other body parts however…"

Casual observers of youth culture have noted that many teens find it easier to give a blowjob than to hold hands. We are witnessing a reversal of the 1970s "erogenous zone" thesis. Previously, any part of the body could become sexually charged if enough energetic attention was paid to it. Now, the disenchantment and dis-eroticization can take place in any body part, including genitalia, which now become nerve endings to be stimulated as tension-relief, ego-indulgence, trauma-re-enactment, and *intimacy dissuasion.*

Even in flesh sex, radical dissociation is all-too-frequent. One only need take note of how a partner seems to disappear internally. Genital interaction entails becoming noncommunicative and not because anyone's speaking the Tantric "secret language." This is mutual introversion, an unspoken agreement to not disturb the other's "safe space."

When something *is* shared, it's as strapped-in spectators on the scene. The erotic connection is equivalent to sitting side-by-side in a tilt-a-whirl. Yes, you're experiencing affective jolts simultaneously, but only via a mechanism external to both participants. The only things shared are the reactions.

> *Status update:*
> *Ann O'Dyne "is tired of opening her box*
> *only to discover it belongs to Pandora"*

Eros has traditionally involved the dissolution of ego boundaries, but we must ask "into what" and "what returns?" Eros no longer opposes power (in some Reichian fashion) but gives content to the techniques of control. The deterritorialization of the self is now necessary to keep a mobile, flexible population at work and play. We find it in reality-TV programming, which operates by breaking down individual egos (open up, confess, tell us who you are). We also see it when privacy dissolves in the drive towards celebrity-status and self-promotion. What we are left with are continuous vacillations between defensive egos and nervous breakdowns. You want excessive control? How about an eating disorder. You want excessive submission? More of the same.

But what about the return, the search for ground, the reterritorialization? Some can't handle constant stimuli so they turn to stabilizing pharmaceutical solutions. Others desperately seek grounding, and so ferociously cling to ego boundaries (thus drama ensues). The result is a sadism culture, from humiliation entertainment like prank shows to the verbal war of all against all known as snarkasm.

Still others seek a preservative, a chastity protection that rivals any homeland security checkpoint. Most of these are routed through patriarchal lineages. The "Love Waits" movement preserves virginal youth but as a command from the Phallic triumvirate: Big Daddy (God), Little Daddy (familial father), and Baby Daddy (future husband). In a ray of hope, mini-goddesses like Lady Gaga call for a celibacy based on feminine independence and a refusal of phallic attachment for completion.

We have so far immersed ourselves in the "worst" composition of bodies, the basest elements of contemporary eros. But it would be an injustice to remain in this pit, satisfied at having traced the contours of our samsaric traps. As we know, simulations can be escapist worlds or experimental models. The *Tibetan Book of the Dead,* for instance, is a manual for the living. Life is preparation for dealing with the bardos, the suffering scenarios of attachment that postpone our spirit's return to new form. Reading the book allows us to recognize illusion for what it is. We do so while living, making it easier when going through them after death. Can we think of love in the same way? The avatar as preparation, as exercise. Not as simulation-as-replacement, but as model for the possible.

Most events are ambivalent, a continuous stream of fluctuating signs and effects that both enhance and deplete. Can constant stimulation produce a new subject capable of absorbing these barrages? Is attention a nonrenewable resource or is there something about this directed affect that allows us to rethink the Source itself? This is the crux of the networked eros. If we begin with the mingling of bodies, with suffering as crucible, we can begin a transmutation of and within eromania. By dwelling in this crucible for a while, we just might locate the golden pathway.

Status update:
Tara Phi Ying "is through with being a trophy wife"

We have already noted that contemporary image-powers are unlike the traditional Spectacle, insofar as the latter presumes a split in the erotic between fleshly reality and image-fantasy. Our erotic mutants are hybrids of fantasy and reality. The Image is no longer projection, distraction and escape. The virtual has turned the image into an introjection and *inscapism.*

Let's take another look at something as debased as reality TV, but now as crucible for fairy tales. Most analysts focus on how reality-TV is escapist, a fairy tale as flight from the mundane. However, contemporary reality programming is more like the archaic faery tales — a spell of transformation within the hearer. Reality-TV is an immanentization of the fantasy, a restoration of the fairy tale to its function as life guide. But what has happened to it during its journey? The spells can return as binding mechanisms or their opposite. Reality is now both the democratization of escape (a fantasy in every pot!) and the immanentization of power-image.

Status update:
Mork Shamichaels "is a monk with a harem,
looking for an ascetic coquette"

From projection-spectacle to introjection-vessel: we can catch a glimpse here of the subject needed to endure this transformation. The erotic traps of a thousand little threads are not to be negated or repressed. Rather, the power needed is one that can absorb and overcome. To learn the art of reception (even of a text message), to take something well, to be capable of *not* reacting — this is a desire for passion without becoming *pashanate*.

Not apathy, which defends the ego by becoming-numb to affects. A detachment from being possessed, but one in which external causes are absorbed as internal (but not as our individual interiority). What is needed is observation with ardor, a fiery discernment *with* attention. Knowing, for instance, how to distinguish the Will to Surrender from the tumultuous and centrifugal desire for a Master. Along these lines, a willful discrimination allows us to devalue those sources that depend on our sadness and depletion for their power. Only then does the transmutation of the worst poison (networked eros) into the sweetest nectar become virtual and a virtue. The Sun, I am part of that.

Status update:
Lee Berkayas "has found 50 ways to love your leaver"

Social media's organization of eros depends on a collection of isolated individuals who interact via intimate disconnection. What about an erotic connectivity that enhances powers? Eros, as philosopher Teresa Brennan notes, is as much a synthesizing force as an individual pursuit of ego-loss. Eros is tied to the life drive, a living attention whose goal is "to establish ever greater unities, and to preserve them thus — in short, to bind together." Eros is no longer defined around an excessive pursuit of sexual freedom but better yokes, where the bonds are like the chemical composition of attachments and detachments. A bond as *fasciare*, whose connotations include "to bandage," "to dress," "to cocoon." This living attention, combining into a common notion, is what thwarts fascism, the other *fasciare*. Sure, the molecular prevention of fascism requires the liberation of desire from repression, but it's only an inaugural ceremony. How it circulates, its new shapes and circuits, is the test of any true freedom. These metamorphosis-machines might even involve restraints, a set of restrictive powers which themselves eventually undergo transmutation. We ask, "do we contribute to the disordering of the Other's affects? Or give back to them the connective energy of the Commons?" A vector is haunting Second Life, the vector of commonist love.

> *Status update:*
> *Otto Nomisone "doesn't feel any chemistry*
> *between us, only alchemy"*

Eros belongs only partially to the base pleasures reserved for what typically gets called sex. It is there, in the base, that poisons are bound and transformed through living attention. Not negation, but pushing through; a transmutation of the worst, of the chains through the chains. There is a liberating power of fear, sex, desire, as long as the objective is Divine. How does the avatar allow this homeopathy?

Social Media assist in this process by publicizing, accelerating, and proliferating avatars-as-players. Networked eros taps into the shadows, revealing the heretofore occulted personal dramas and sensations. The digital age is an apocalyptic working-out of the private *pashuns* in public. We are no longer even dealing with the personal, but the pre-, trans-, and superpersonal: pulsations, fantasies, images, information, energy patterns, life-forms, elementals. The avatars play in basins only to absorb and extract the inhuman (no longer animal but anima).

It's always *something* healthy that seeks suffering, as Nietzsche reminds us. Only one who has undergone/gone under can transcend. The metamorphosis requires a vital body that can withstand the subtle divine. A cocoon is capable of handling dissolution. It turns its many-threaded ensnarement into nourishment. Abandon with Abundance. This divine dance composes a love that contains and releases multitudes.

Note

1. Of course, porn has its own interactive elements, from dolls to Second Life islands. One can even imagine an island in Second Life devoted to re-enacting celebrity sex tapes.

WHEN WOMEN WROTE SEX
ROBERT SIEGLE

I t's not something I knew much about at the time I came across Lynne Tillman's *Weird Fucks* and the first Kathy Acker pieces stacked up at St. Mark's Bookshop. Not sex, I mean — I thought I knew some things about it — but women writing sex. I knew some of Gertrude Stein's pieces (*Tender Buttons*, anyone?) were out there, I knew that Anaïs Nin had written some things, it was between the lines in Jane Bowles, and there was also some French writing. But I was an academic; my reading had for years been first the graduate reading lists about which we were expected to have encyclopedic knowledge, then the lower-level course lists for the required courses new faculty typically teach. Somehow, Nin & Stein never made those lists; they show up now more often.

Looking around me now, reading the work that twenty-year-old students write, can write now, I am amazed at the difference this thirty years makes. There are lots of obvious reasons you could list — sex is now everywhere and more open in a square-inches of skin kind of way, the internet enables 24/7 dial yr kink, and the religious right froths a bit of salaciousness back into pornography, back as baristas of the Jeremiad Café. But I think there's a more interesting point to be made, and it's how sex was written about when women cracked the monopoly of male writers' all too often wet dream school (all wet, often) of sexual writing. You could make similar arguments about gay writing — work by David Wojnarowicz and Dennis Cooper comes quickly to mind — but, to be honest about my process of reading my way into downtown writing, I found that material on the second trip in from my neck of the boonies.

I am, that is to say, a test case of an interested reader of fiction working within the constraints of the distribution system in existence in 1980–85. Coming to New York to hunt for it, I found presses I'd never heard of, magazines whose editorial eye greatly exceeded their powers of distribution, writers whose work failed to show up on the so-called New Fiction Radar machines of those outside a few key cultural centers. In fact, my book was, in its grant-getting research and writing stage, called *Unread Renaissance* because it mostly was just that; outside the magnetic poles of the literary landscape. Not only did "we" in the academic periphery not know about Acker & Tillman, we didn't even know how to read them. We had been machined in a very patriarchal, old school kind of normalizing.

So take this writing of Acker and Tillman as a case study with the proviso that there were others, and other others. But from writing's others came work that included the politics of its emergence, and of women's sexuality's emergence, as the frisson that laced (bad word choice?) their narratives. This was not (mainly) the narrative of arousal, and certainly not the giddy euphoria of Jong's zipless fuck mercilessly lampooned for its infantilism by Acker's "hello i'm erica jong" routine. Theirs was a narrative realization of the slogan, "the personal is the political." Or, if you like, of Deleuze & Guattari's theory-bomb bumper sticker: there is only the social.

In other words, we see in this work emerging 1975-85 the destruction of two flows that fed the prevailing master code: the persistence of the individual self as a sufficient frame of reference, not to mention its serving as the central apparatus of capture in the West, and the phallomorphic form in which that persistence commonly took place. Or takes, since these flows continue to prevail in much of the land, though increasingly as ice sculptures in the late northern spring (i.e., gone or vestigial in the hotter climes, menacing and cold in their brittle aggressive clarity).

Luce Irigaray's *This Sex Which Is Not One* takes the piss out of these flows, parodying the implicit form by which the male anatomy and pleasure graph mimes the metaphysics and poetics of the West (the one in logic, being, theology, meaning, you name it; the congruence of, say, the graphs of male climax and Freytag's pyramid of dramatic action). By taking "seriously" the otherness, diffusion, and multiplicity assigned "the feminine" in disdain by the canonical misogynists, Irigaray slyly triggers the epiphany that postmodern ideas of art, self, *und so weiter* snap to the grid of the feminine. Sometimes humorless readers miss the joke and think her a feminazi (a favorite word of my banker ex-father-in-law) or an essentialist. But these reactions are part of the politics of embeddedness, that sinister infection by which we soothe the inner child by bedding down with The Man. Therein entwined, this is how Irigaray, Acker, and Tillman's generation of writers would seem.

But (mostly) not so to the audience that embraced them rather than turning stonelike in the face of them. To read Tillman again in this light is a reminder of just what that historical moment felt like. At a fourth of July party in *Weird Fucks*, the narrator remembers that "Firecrackers kept popping off and everything feels slightly evil. For the urban dweller whose adventures are limited to sexual ones the Fourth of July has nothing to do with America's independ-

ence. One's own independence being severely circumscribed anyway, we play out the hunt we can in limited
ways." Things feel evil because "adventures" were cut from
the script generations ago; the hunt is what the phallomorphic predatory self does in patriarchal capitalism. There's a
whiff of zipless fuck in the air as women try out the subject
position once monopolized by boyfriends who, in this age,
are likely to be a recurrent figure in Tillman's fiction, the
impotent boyfriend.

But what happens? Too often, more of the same: we're
not talking about some free utopia here, but an evil zone in
which "independence [is] severely circumscribed." By what?
In *Haunted Houses*, we read Emily hunting for the right
metaphor: "Love is … like an occupation, being occupied by.
He swept over me, she wrote, his body larger than mine,
and I am helpless against him. I let myself be taken. Her
own words unsettled her, marching in as they did from
what, if she spoke it, might seem enemy territory. She could-
n't tell anymore, she didn't speak it." In the no-man's-land
of postmodern sexuality, pun intended, you can't tell anymore where pleasure, power, identity, any of it, come from,
but they bring with them the entire history and politics that
make sexuality less than liberation and more like an occupation. "Language fails me… I fail language," another of
Tillman's characters realizes at one point. Viral language carries viral form, (pre)shaping everything, and these becom-
ing-aware characters in Tillman's work know that as the old
form and shape begins to fall away, it's less Jong's flying
than little satoris of the vertigo of code-switching going.

Sexuality carries these characters into a bodily awareness of how "male" pleasure is and how "circumscribed"
the self is. Starting to let go of gendered egos and sexuality
makes characters "giddy with possibilities," but also

sobered: "Make up her mind, her face. Dress it up, rearrange the pieces, move the furniture, change the décor. The design…. It was as difficult to know what to fill her days with as her body, or mind. It wasn't like learning the alphabet; it was more like unlearning it, not taking it in and not spitting it out." Everything is "up for grabs" when the alphabet is known as such rather than, say, as "human nature" or as "femininity." Ideology freeze-frames, sexuality through the sheer intensity of desire can let loose the flood for the apocalypse of Man.

Kathy Acker's fiction is committed to the same mission with all the stitchery at the surface, as when characters realize we have to "stop believing in human beings," or when she stitches in Deleuze and Guattari's remark that "there is no position of desire not capable of destroying whole sections of the social machine." At a pivotal moment of *Blood and Guts in High School*, Acker writes as if summarizing this historical moment's realization about recognizing the alphabet of cultural programming for what it is and laboring for some line of flight that could leave behind its crippling syntax (yes, sin tax): "at this point in the *Scarlet Letter* and in my life politics don't disappear but take place inside my body." Indeed, they take place nowhere with more decisive power than in the bodies they occupy.

When women (re)write sex in 1980, it isn't pure and free and idyllic. It is a raw, painful, and deeply-layered palimpsest of forms and shapes for sexuality and ego, univocal and phallomorphic until the subtexts and the crowds in their margins begin to be seen and heard in the fiction. It doesn't seem to me that sexuality liberates anyone; but, in writing sexuality, these layers and voices are freed from obscurity and marginalization to reflect Irigaray's fundamental question: "is this the way culture is seeking to characterize itself now? Is this the way texts write themselves/ are written now? Without quite knowing what censorship they are evading?" It does seem to me that all three of these writers know with fair precision what censorship they're evading, given the archness of Irigaray's irony and the cultural inventory we find in the fiction of Tillman and Acker. Writing matters, and perhaps some day the cultural historians will swarm downtown fiction at the dawn of the Reagan Era when, ironically, its underpinnings come to be thought and written.

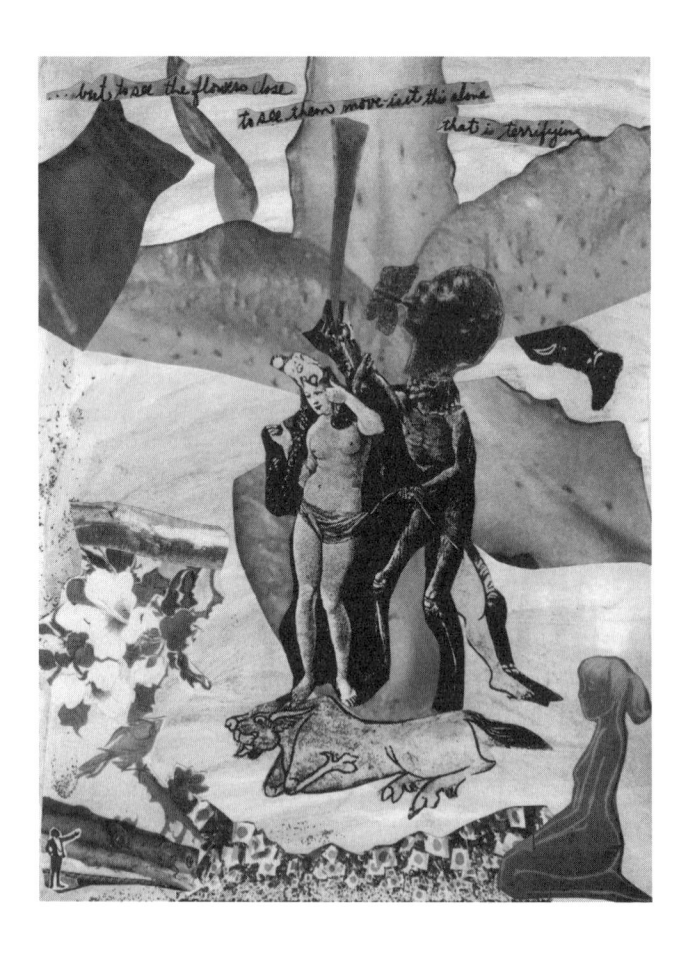

FEMME FATALE
MICHAEL LINDGREN

For the record, when my advance copy of *The Sexual Life of Catherine M.*[1] arrived, I did not slink out of the store with it concealed in a pile of innocent-looking books and papers. No, I strode casually out with the cover, naked female breasts and all, in full view of employee, supervisor, and customer alike, ho hum. Then I got it home and pounced on it.

To back up a bit: the book in question, a memoir by a French art critic named Catherine Millet, has sold over a half-million copies in Europe, mainly by force of a tumultuous reception by the French media. The translation arrived on these shores last month, courtesy of elite literary publisher Grove Press, with the reputation as the most sexually explicit book ever written by a woman (although one reviewer voiced his suspicion that the book was really the work of a transsexual).

So, in view of all *Sexual Life's* advance hubbub, the question: how shocking is it? The answer: fairly, but not terminally shocking. By her own account, Millet was relentlessly, inexhaustibly promiscuous, and her encounters, which include seemingly every kind of act physiologically possible, are described at length and in explicit detail. On the other hand, she seems to have experienced little genuine physical danger; her partners all fall within a fairly narrow middle-class milieu, and she never even mentions, for example, the threat of rape, unwanted pregnancy, or AIDS.

Is *The Sexual Life of Catherine M.* pornography, as some of its critics charge? The answer here is a definite no. As graphic as the book's sexual content is, it is clearly not intended to titillate or arouse (although that may well be a secondary effect), but rather to convey one woman's experience of an unusual life. What is radical about Millet's book is not the extent or variety of her promiscuity but rather the utter completeness of the schism she effects between sex and emotion. "Feeling desire and having sexual relations were two separate activities," she writes at one point, and in fact the only emotional pain she suffers comes exclusively at the hands of men with whom she is not intimate.

The book's style was described by the *French Vogue* as "gracefully pristine," which is either a serious misjudgment (not out of the question) or an indication that Millet's prose has not survived Adriana Hunter's translation. In the end, though, what matters is Millet's cool, detached tone and her refusal to attach any moral judgment to her action; in reading this messy, provocative, occasionally frustrating book, you may end up learning more about yourself than about the narrator.

Note

[1] *The Sexual Life of Catherine M.,* by Catherine Millet (New York: Grove/Atlantic, 2000).

LOVE AMONG THE RUINS: HELLENISM, PEDERASTY, AND HOMOSOCIALITY IN H. RIDER HAGGARD'S *SHE*

MARVIN J. TAYLOR

I n 1892 Charles Gilbert Chaddock dramatically limited the way in which male-male desire could be described when he coined the word "homosexuality" in his English translation of Richard von Krafft-Ebing's *Psychopathia Sexualis*. Growing out of nineteenth-century German studies of sexuality, which used scientific principles to classify social behaviors into easily identifiable gender and sexual types, the term "homosexuality" represents the introduction of this sociological methodology to England, which in turn created modern English gender and sexual categories. Throughout the nineteenth century, however, Hellenism and references to ancient Greece had served as a language by which male-male desire — as opposed to the modern configuration of male homosexuality — found expression. But the rise of modern social sciences, the near hegemony of sociological typology, and the recent configuration of what Eve Sedgwick calls homosociality have clouded our ability to unravel late-Victorian explanations of sex, gender, and culture that are indebted to this Hellenistic tradition. This inability is readily apparent in H. Rider Haggard's novel *She*, when Haggard, like many other Victorians, invokes ancient Greece as a model for England, for the empire, and for male-male desire. By examining how

Haggard uses references to Hellenism, and to Greek pederasty — the pedagogical structure for training young men
to become warriors — I will question our ability to apply
the concept of homosociality transhistorically.

She belongs to a nearly forgotten nineteenth-century
"masculinist" tradition, which invoked Hellenism and Greek
pederasty as a model for male-male interaction. Andrew
Hewitt argues that there were other possible meanings for
male desire that cannot be understood if viewed exclusively
through the lens of an always already gendered culture.
Hewitt explores texts that "perceive male-male Eros as a dis-
tillation of a fundamentally masculine social instinct, and
that therefore resists any attempt to explain homosexuality
as a form of effeminization" (Hewitt, 80-81). Profoundly dis-
trustful of medical, sociological, or psychological interpreta-
tions of male-male intimacy, "masculinist" writers returned
to the paradigm of Greek pederasty in an attempt to
reground nineteenth-century culture.

She is a text obsessed with preserving and promoting
male culture as the means for bolstering the narrative of
the British Empire. Haggard invokes the male culture of
ancient Greece when the elder Vincey first speaks to Holly
about his son, Leo. He gives a genealogy of his family, saying that Leo

> will be the only representative of one of the most
> ancient families in the world, that is, so far as families
> can be traced. You will laugh at me when I say it, but
> one day it will be proved to you beyond a doubt, that
> my sixty-fifth or sixty-sixth lineal ancestor was an
> Egyptian priest of Isis, though he was himself of
> Grecian extraction, and was called Kallikrates (*She*, 11).

Vincey directly links Victorian England and ancient Greece with the tradition of male-dominated empire building. Vincey goes on to chart the gradual decline of his family from their royal status until they became "merchants" and his father "dissipated most of the money" (*She,* 11–12). The Vincey family becomes a metaphor for England itself, with Vincey's fears about the degeneration of his race extending to the degeneration of England and its ability to summon the strength of the ancient Greeks in order to rule the burgeoning empire. With the industrial revolution, the rise of the working class, the seemingly endless extension of suffrage, the erosion of the status of landed gentry, Victoria's extended reign, and the imminent education and enfranchisement of women, the "degeneration" of England seems to mirror the Vinceys' at every turn.

Faced with these threats to the landed gentleman's right to rule, Haggard seeks to recreate ancient Greek pederasty in Victorian England in order to reinscribe male culture and save the empire. Chief among the references to ancient Greece is a long quotation from Herodotus's *History,* which Ludwig Horace Holly, the narrator of the novel, provides in a footnote. When the dying, elder Vincey refers to his ancestor, Kallikrates, as the grandson of a famous Spartan warrior, Holly provides this gloss, which is notable for its length:

> The Kallikrates here referred to by my friend was a Spartan, spoken of by Herodotus (Herodotus, ix. 72) as being remarkable for his beauty. He fell at the glorious battle of Platæa (September 22, b.c. 479), when the Lacedæmonians and Athenians under Pausanias routed the Persians, putting nearly 300,000 of them to the sword. The following is a translation of the passage, 'For Kallikrates died out of the battle, he came to the army the most beautiful

man of the Greeks of the day — not only of the Lacedæmonians themselves, but of the other Greeks also. He, when Pausanias was sacrificing, was wounded in the side by an arrow; and then they fought, but on being carried off he regretted his death, and said to Arimnestus, a Platæan, that he did not grieve at dying for Greece, but at not having struck a blow, or, although he desired so to do, performed any deed worthy of himself.' This Kallikrates, who appears to have been as brave as he was beautiful, is subsequently mentioned by Herodotus as having been buried among the *ireues* (young commanders), apart from the other Spartans and the Helots. — L.H.H. (*She,* 10)

Ostensibly supporting Vincey's patrilineal heritage and establishing the male, political, and ethical status of his ancestor, this citation points to the central anxiety of Haggard's text: the young Kallikrates is "the most beautiful man of the Greeks of the day — not only of the Lacedæmonians themselves, but of the other Greeks also." The uneasiness clusters around the word *ireues,* which Holly translates as "young commanders." While not technically incorrect, this translation is misleading. The word *ireues* is a Spartan term that meant both "young commanders" and the younger men in the Spartan pederastic structure.

For the ancient Spartans, the Eirens were not only "young commanders" but also, as Plutarch notes, youths "who have proceeded two years beyond the boy's class"; that is, who are older than twenty and specifically defined as "boys… courted by lovers from among the respectable young men" (Plutarch, 28). In *Greek Homosexuality,* K. J. Dover notes that the use of *eran,* the verb from which Eirens derives, was associated with

Eros in the classical period and carried with it the connotation of sexual love (Dover, 43). What becomes clear is that young Kallikrates, whom Herodotus describes as "the most beautiful among the Greeks," was not only a brave young commander, but also and importantly, an object of male desire. Haggard's translation attempts to eliminate the erotic potential of Kallikrates's body while emphasizing the military and social use of male-male desire.

Haggard's reference to Kallikrates is complicated further by the phrase "not only of the Lacedæmonians themselves, but of the other Greeks also." This statement establishes a hierarchy among the Greeks in terms of their beauty in which the Lacedæmonians — that is, the Spartans — are ranked higher than the others. Certainly the Spartans, if not known always for their beauty, were regarded as the bravest and fiercest warriors — in fact, we are told that Kallikrates means "strong and beautiful" (Dover, 10); Spartan culture was organized to produce just such warriors, as both Xenophon and Plutarch note.

It comes as no surprise that Haggard should invoke this passage from Herodotus in 1886, when many English men were searching for a narrative that would bolster the always tenuous stability of the empire. By invoking ancient Greece, Haggard participates in this wider Victorian discourse: stressing the martial aspects of the Eirens, he heightens the militaristic aspects of the pederastic model and swerves away from the possibility of male-male sex. Like the other Victorians, however, Haggard's evocation of ancient Greece fractures around the issue of sex in the pederastic structure.

A conservative who distrusted democracy and the university system in general, Haggard invokes ancient Greece in a manner that departs from the by-then standard Oxbridge notions of people like Benjamin Jowett at Oxford who introduced the study of ancient Greece, especially of Athens, into the curriculum, hoping that a variant of the Greek democratic model of government would be adopted in England to bolster middle-class male political power (Turner, 103). Between 1828 and 1833, the British government saw three major changes in the structure of politics that had supported aristocratic rule: the repeal of the Test and Corporations Acts in 1828, the passage of the Catholic Reform Act in 1829, and the Reform Act of 1832. These Parliamentary acts eroded the monopoly landed gentlemen had enjoyed over power in England, paving the way for dissenters, Catholics, Jews, and well-to-do tradesmen to vote and hold office. Greek democracy provided a model for polity in which a broad spectrum of men could interact, and seemed perfectly suited to the political climate with its extensions of suffrage. But invocations of Hellenism did not stop at political and educational circles. Greek studies and ideas were also appropriated with little concern for historical or archaeological accuracy, appearing in popular culture and abounding throughout the century in literature and the visual arts, and subtly influencing nearly all aspects of Victorian culture. Unlike Jowett's democratic Hellenism, which promoted Athenian democracy and the study of Plato, Haggard — always more militaristic and imperial — echoes the work of Walter Pater and John Addington Symonds and invokes Sparta as a model.

She represents a complicated response to both Pater's elevation of Spartan culture and its opponents' fears of male-male sex. Unlike Pater, Haggard forcefully invokes Spartan pederasty, but he also rejects the public school and university models of education in terms that suggest he believes them to be effeminizing. He invokes the model of Spartan pederasty in two major ways: when the elder Vincey details how Leo should be raised, and when he depicts Leo and Holly as Spartan warriors.

From his early childhood, Leo is raised solely within male culture, and his training follows closely the elements of Spartan pederasty. What we know of Spartan pederastic education derives mainly from Plutarch's *Life of Lycurgus* and Xenophon's *Constitution of the Lacedæmonians*. In brief, Spartan boys were removed from their homes at a young age and went to live in barracks with other boys and citizen/soldiers. Here they were trained as warriors, increasingly given responsibility as they passed through a series of stages until they reached adulthood, and then becoming the teachers of the next generation of boys. Men, often referred to as either "inspirers" or "lovers," selected a boy, referred to as a "hearer" or "beloved," with whom they found a bond and whom they wanted to educate. Spartan soldier-citizens lived in this arrangement until the age of thirty, at which time they were considered adults. As a boy progressed through the various levels of his training, he, too, had boys for whom he served as an "inspirer."

This trajectory matches the plot of *She*. The elder Vincey selects Holly as Leo's "lover," to use the Spartan term, and gives very specific instructions about how Leo is to be trained. Vincey himself acknowledges that this education is "a somewhat peculiar one. At any rate, I could not intrust it to a stranger" (*She*, 12). Holly, a self-styled "misogynist," was carefully chosen by Vincey as Leo's inspirer; he is very careful not to allow the boy to be under the influence of women. It is unclear what the Spartan attitude was toward the society of women and the raising of young warriors, because Spartan culture was primarily stratified along class and status definitions as well as gender; Spartan women had more autonomy than male slaves, for instance. Haggard, by contrast, definitely sees women's influence as detrimental to the development of young Englishmen.

On his twenty-fifth birthday, the time comes for Leo to open a chest his father left for him. Inside are several texts in Greek, Latin, and English, handed down from father to son in the Vincey family for 2,000 years. The fragments and translations tell the history of a Greek Kallikrates, grandson of the Kallikrates mentioned in Herodotus, who became a high priest of Isis before being banished from Egypt. He and a band of followers traveled south into Africa, where he met his death at the hand of Ayesha, a woman who loved him, because he had fallen in love with another woman, Amenartas. Following his death, the pregnant Amenartas escaped from Ayesha and made her way to Greece where she delivered a boy, naming him Tisisthenes, "the Avenger," from which the name Vincey eventually derived (*She,* 30–31). The story is passed down through the Vincey family from father to son and several attempts are made to seek out Ayesha and avenge Kallikrates's death. A letter to Leo from his dead father explains this history and sets out the quest that Leo should undertake to find Ayesha. Hearing this implausable tale, Holly is torn between his disbelief in the story and his abiding relationship with Leo. Holly thinks it foolish to go in search of Ayesha, but notes:

> as a matter of fact, I had no intention of allowing Leo to go anywhere by himself, for my own sake, if not for his. I was far too much attached to him for that.... Leo was all the world to me — brother, child, and friend — and until he wearied of me, where he went there I should go too. (*She,* 46)

Holly's conflation of "brother, child, and friend" perfectly describes a Spartan pederastic relationship.

In the passages from Herodotus immediately preceding the description of Kallikrates, we learn that Kallikrates was a partner in a pederastic relationship. Holly, it turns out, is patterned after Aristodemus, the most powerful of the Spartans who fought under Leonidas at Thermopylæ, and Kallikrates's lover. Herodotus describes Aristodemus as by "far the best of the Lacedæmonians," meaning the strongest, who fought at Platæa. He was also the only Spartan "of the Three Hundred [who] survived Thermopylæ" (Herodotus, xi. 71). Haggard describes Holly as unnaturally strong, hyper-masculine, but also ugly. The equation of Holly's ugliness with hyper-masculinity and strength becomes vexed when Leo is equated with both beauty *and* strength. The text presents the possibility of adopting a Greek model of male beauty and strength rather than relying on the more traditional equation of brawny maleness with a heroic ideal. Haggard's explicit citation of Herodotus to describe Kallikrates indicates that Haggard must have known he was patterning Holly on Aristodemus. His deflection of the possible sexual relationship between the two Greeks is symptomatic of his evocation of a desexualized pederasty for purely pedagogic purposes.

Leo is the perfect example of the imperial hero, and his body, which is like a Greek warrior's, announces his superiority. The narrator first notices him because of his beauty:

> One of these gentlemen was I think, without exception, the handsomest young fellow I have ever seen. He was very broad, and had a look of power and a grace of bearing that seemed as native to him as it is to a wild stag. In addition, his face was almost without flaw — a good face as well as a beautiful one. (*She,* 1)

Leo is constantly referred to as "a statue of Apollo come to life" (*She*, 1) or a "Greek god" (*She*, 2). But Leo is not merely the god returned to earth. He is the reformulation of Greek warrior culture in England, as Holly tells us when he sees Leo and Ayesha together:

> It was a pretty sight to see her veiled form gliding towards the sturdy young Englishman, dressed in his gray-flannel suit; for though he is half a Greek in blood, Leo is, with the exception of his hair, one of the most English- looking men I ever saw. (*She*, 211–212)

Leo's depiction as Apollo reborn in nineteenth-century England echoes Pater's invocation of the Spartans as the "peculiar people of Apollo" or, as Dowling says, "the virile, sane, beautiful, pæderastic, all but English Dorians." (Dowling, 5).

The most remarkable description of the male body, however, comes when Ayesha takes Holly and Leo to view the embalmed body of Kallikrates:

> There, stretched upon the stone bier before us, robed in white and perfectly preserved, was what appeared to be the body of Leo Vincey. I stared from Leo, standing there alive, to Leo lying there dead, and could see no difference; except, perhaps, that the body on the bier looked older. Feature for feature they were the same, even down to the crop of little golden curls, which was Leo's most uncommon beauty. It even seemed to me, as I looked, that the expression on the dead man's face resembled that which I had sometimes seen upon Leo's when he was plunged into profound sleep. (*She*, 238)

In this highly charged scene, Holly's gaze turns to Leo's body, and the effect is a homoerotic description of Leo's "crop of little golden curls" and of an expression on "the dead man's face" that Holly had seen before. This description implies that Holly has stared at Leo's beauty before, even when Leo was sleeping. There is a more serious problem in this scene: when Leo is shown the body of Kallikrates, the viewing is intended to prove to him that Leo is really the reincarnated Greek. By extension, it also proves that Greek ideals can be reborn in England. When he sees the body, Leo exclaims: "It is all so horrible; and that — that body! What can I make of it?" (*She*, 241). Leo's horror arises from the male gaze being turned onto the male body, which, when viewed, objectifies men and creates the possibility of homoerotic desire. And yet, despite the anxieties, such scenes suggest that the text constantly holds up Leo's body as the prototype of the imperial hero, subjecting it to the male gaze as the model body that Englishmen should emulate.

The most important and highly sexualized pederastic moment occurs just before Leo and Holly leap across a chasm. Holly agrees to jump first:

> I acquiesced with a nod, and then I did a thing I had never done since Leo was a little boy. I turned and put my arm round him, and kissed him on the forehead. It sounds rather French, but as a fact I was taking my last farewell of a man whom I could not have loved more if he had been my own son twice over.
>
> "Good-bye, my boy," I said, "I hope that we shall meet again, wherever it is that we go to."
>
> The fact was I did not expect to live another two minutes. (*She*, 304)

This kiss, given on the edge of the vaginal chasm, represents Holly's benediction to Leo as his pederastic charge. Leo, now a man, as his newly whitened hair attests, has foregone the influences of women and has become an inspirer himself. The scene goes further, however, for Holly leaps across the chasm but almost misses the other side; he is left hanging, holding onto the giant phallic "spur" of rock, and Leo must save him. In an erotically charged scene, Holly muses about Leo's "powerful arms," wondering if they will be "equal to lifting me up till I could get a hold on the top of the spur" (*She*, 306). When Leo lifts Holly, Holly feels "as though [he] were a little child." After Leo succeeds in saving Holly, the two lie there "panting side by side, trembling like leaves, and with the cold perspirations of terror pouring from [their] skins" (*She*, 306). Holly now has become like "a little child" and is no longer the "inspirer." As though this scene weren't suggestive enough of male-male sex, they lie there "for some half-hour… without speaking a word" (*She*, 306). The price exacted of Leo for his love of Ayesha is the loss of his boyhood.

This highly charged scene atop the phallic "spur" and at the climax of the novel uses the possibility of male-male sex to promote camaraderie, the virility of Englishmen, and their victory both over the colonies and over the effeminizing potential of women. It is a classic use of male-male desire to promote empire.

Just how anxious Haggard was about male-male sex is not as clear as it might seem, for while Holly rejects Oxbridge Hellenism as suspect, he worries that attachments to women symbolize the decline of culture. At the very least, attachments to women are signs of weakness and detrimental to the male camaraderie necessary for governance and military rule. This notion is clearly expressed when Holly berates himself for neglecting the sick Leo in favor of Ayesha's company:

> How I cursed my selfishness and the folly that had kept me lingering by Ayesha's side while my dear boy lay dying! Alas and alas! how easily the best of us are lighted down to evil by the gleam of a woman's eyes! What a wicked wretch was I! Actually, for the last half-hour I had scarcely thought of Leo, and this, be it remembered, of the man who for twenty years had been my dearest companion, and the chief interest of my existence. (*She*, 194)

"The gleam of women's eyes" for Holly represents a break in the order of the world that potentially leads to the death of his "dearest companion and the chief interest of [his] existence" — another man. Holly's infatuation with Ayesha threatens to break his bond to Leo, a bond that has more than once saved both their lives in the trials of their quest. This startling passage sounds homoerotic as well as misogynistic to modern readers. Haggard juxtaposes the love of men for women with the love of men for one another, which he suggests is more important. The text specifically places the Spartan male, pederastic relationship of Holly and Leo in direct conflict with the modern homosocial triangle of Holly-Ayesha-Leo. Rather than having a Sedgwickian displacement of the erotic charge between Holly and Leo displaced onto Ayesha, however, she is seen as a detriment to their intimacy. Haggard, far from being overcome by fear of being labeled homosexual, attempts to recuperate male-male desire via Spartan pederasty to revivify male culture. His project fails, though, because, as the title posits, She, meaning metaphorically all women, is always present in the modern world in a way that women were not in ancient Greece.

It is tempting to apply Sedgwick's homosocial continuum to the Victorian evocation of pederasty. Despite acknowledging that the homosocial model may not be transhistorically applicable (*Between Men*, 26–27), Sedgwick supports her argument by citing ancient Athenian pederasty as an example of a culture where "the continuum between 'men-loving-men' and 'men-promoting-the-interests-of-men' appears to have been quite seamless"(*Between Men*, 4). In a move worthy of Haggard or the other Victorian Hellenists, Sedgwick attempts to ground her conception of homosociality by linking it to ancient Greek pederasty. Following the work of K. J. Dover, she over-emphasizes sex between the partners in the pederastic model, equating the man-boy relationship with the modern conception of homosexuality among equals — "between men" of the same status who are, therefore, like modern gay clones or examples of what Sedgwick calls "homo-style" (*Epistemology*, 159). Elsewhere, in *The Epistemology of the Closet*, Sedgwick again grapples with the relationship of pederasty to homosociality. This time she proposes that the pederastic structure of male-male desire is equal to gender difference, noting that age difference between the man and boy substitutes for gender difference (*Epistemology*, 160). In both attempts to explain the relationship of men and boys in pederasty, Sedgwick employs modern conceptions of gender to describe male-male desire. In the first instance, she assumes that the man and boy are the same, invoking the narcissistic model of male homosexuality; in the second instance, she attempts to see the pederastic relationship as differentiated, as though the boy were gendered feminine. This invokes a heteronormative understanding of homosexuality that suggests misplaced object choice.

Sedgwick's shifting and ambivalent description of how pederasty relates to homosociality points to a problem within the concept of homosociality. When she positions pederasty as the apex of homosocial desire, Sedgwick conflates Greek pederastic relations between men and boys with a modern construction of male homosexuality.

Not surprisingly, it is the addition of Ayesha into the pederastic relationship that causes anxiety. Haggard, naïvely, attempts to invoke Greek pederasty as a militaristic, class-based, pedagogical, and political structure that joins Holly and Leo (or England — the holly tree — and ancient Greece, as their names connote). Only when Ayesha is posited between them does the Greek model become suspect. The text *She,* as the title implies, constantly places women into the male-male culture in a more essential position than women held in ancient Greek. The result strongly genders culture, creating the possibility of a gendered erotic charge, and making possible a sexuality based on gendered object choice; that is, homosexuality. But Holly's fears in the passage are not about homosexuality, but rather about Hellenism and male-male desire. Only by seeing beyond the modern concepts of homosociality, homoeroticism, and homosexuality can we understand the subtlety of Haggard's use of male-male desire.

Sources

Dover, K. J. *Greek Homosexuality: Updated and with a New Postscript.* Cambridge, MA: Harvard University Press, 1989.

Dowling, Linda. "Ruskin's Pied Beauty and the Constitution of a 'Homosexual' Code," *The Victorian Studies Newsletter,* Spring 1989: 1–8.

Haggard, Henry Rider. *She.* Ed. Daniel Karlin. Oxford: Oxford

University Press, 1990. All citations are from this edition.

Herodotus. *The History.* Translated by David Grene. Chicago: University of Chicago Press, 1987.

Hewitt, Andrew. *Political Inversions: Homosexuality, Fascism, and the Modernist Imaginary.* Stanford: Stanford University Press, 1996.

Katz, Wendy R. *Rider Haggard and the Fiction of Empire: A Critical Study of British Imperial Fiction.* Cambridge: Cambridge University Press, 1987.

Pater, Walter. *Greek Studies.* Ed. by Charles L Shadwell. New York: Macmillan, 1903.

Plutarch. *The Life of Lycurgus* in *Plutarch on Sparta.* Trans. with intro. and notes by Richard J. Talbert. New York: Penguin Books, 1988.

Sedgwick, Eve Kosofsky. *Between Men: English Literature and Male Homosocial Desire.* New York: Columbia Univ. Press, 1985.

Sedgwick, Eve Kosofsky. *Epistemology of the Closet.* Berkeley: University of California Press, 1990.

Symonds, John Addington. "A Problem in Modern Ethics," *Male Love: A Problem in Greek Ethics and Other Writings.* New York: Pagan Press, 1983.

Turner, Frank M. "Why the Greeks and Not the Romans in Victorian Britain?" *Rediscovering Hellenism: The Hellenic Inheritance and the English Imagination.* Ed. G. W. Clarke. Cambridge: Cambridge University Press, 1989, 61–81.

Turner, Frank M. *The Greek Heritage in Victorian Britain.* New Haven: Yale University Press, 1981.

Xenophon. "Spartan Society," *Plutarch on Sparta.* Trans. Richard J. A. Talbert. New York: Penguin Books, 1988. Usually translated as "The Constitution of the Lacedæmonians."

NOSTALGIC RIFF ON THE
OLD SEXUAL LIBERATION MOVEMENT
PETER LAMBORN WILSON

Without the Imagination sex would be a very dull Darwinian business indeed — screw & reproduce, screw & reproduce. Luckily this doesn't seem to the case even for animals & birds, much less humans. Probably even plants have their little perversions — you'd certainly think so to look at some of them.

When Erasmus Darwin (grandfather of Charles) meditated on the white cliffs of Dover — & realized they were composed of gazillions of sea shells, each one representing a past sex act — he posited that evolution could be defined as "survival of the happiest."

In his great epic poem *The Botanic Garden* he expresses the whole of Linnaean taxonomy in purely sexual terms — a notion that might've pleased Prince Kropotkin. Anarchist science argues that evolution owes as much to *mutuality* as to competition — in fact maybe more — since without such a concept it's hard to posit any biological excuse for the Social.

Now that we know that Progress itself may turn out to have been counter-evolutionary — & that Social Darwinism was (& still is) a *disaster* — we might want to take a look at some of these "lost paradigms" of Romantic Science — & its precursor, Hermeticism.

Erasmus Darwin was not just a "(grand)father of modern science" — but also a Hermeticist. He expressed "the loves of the vegetables" in a form of Paracelsan alchemical symbolism in which the Four Elements are ruled by "Elemental Spirits"— Earth/Gnomes — Air/Sylphs — Water/Undines — Fire/Salamanders. Darwin borrowed this system from Alexander Pope's *Rape of the Lock* & the weird little anonymous 18th Century occultist novel *Comte de Gabalis*. In more recent times Rudolf Steiner wrote extensively on these Nature Spirits, often called "devas."

Sometimes (like classical nymphs & satyrs) these entities are known to have sex with human beings, as in the tale of *Undine* by Baron de la Motte Fouque. On the esoteric level this interdimensional eroticism both symbolizes & delineates the very form of the Cosmos itself — which (in Hermeticism) is based on Attraction. As Hesiod put it, the first divinities were Chaos, Eros & Gaia — or as a bewildered 20th century chaos scientist once exclaimed, "Matter just seems to love form!"

For the "primitive animist" or Romantic pantheist, all Nature is alive ("even rocks") & therefore all Nature is made up of *personae* — "all our relations" as the American Indians say. Sex with Elementals symbolizes (and "is") the nexus & union of consciousness with Nature. The oldest known human rituals (e.g. "lycanthropy") all involve the Imagination in order to bring about this dialectic dance of union & separation & re-union with Nature as person (*Anima Mundi*) without which for example the hunter can have no success in venery, nor the lover in venery. (These words are supposedly not etymologically related, one meaning art of the hunt & the other art of Venus. Cabalistically however they are the same word.)

Spagyria (Paracelsan alchemy) therefore presupposes an implicit "Tantrik" aspect to sexuality which can only be seen as antinomian in any monotheist moral context. Shamanism

& paganism can afford (& require) a great deal of polymor-pyhous perversion, but without sexual repression no *One True Religion* can channel human energy into a teleology — an ideology — pie in the sky when you die... & above all — how could human fate itself be bound to the emergence of Classical Capitalism (as per Weber) without the mechanism of psychic suppression? (See Wilhelm Reich on this — another German Romantic or mad neo-Hermeticist.)

Obviously then the keynote to any critique of the Civilization of Discontent — as Charles Fourier realized — is sexual liberation. Fourier the "Utopian Socialist" was a left-wing Hermeticist at heart, like Gerard de Nerval or the young Rimbaud. Fourier's "lost" treatise on sexuality turned up & was first published in Paris in 1967 — a curious & poetic fact. His position seemed radical even in 1968, when most of the Left was still suffering from Communist Puritanism. But it perfectly matched the mood & ideals of the non-authoritarian left including Surrealism, Situationism & Psychelicism.

In the dark ages (1950s) sex-lib ideas were mentioned in America only in the tiny newsletters of the Reichean anar-chists — the Mattachine Society — the Daughters of Bilitis — the Sexual Freedom League. (The first was for straights — the second for fags — the third for dykes — the last for all the other pervo's. Years later I met Harry Hay, founder of the Mattachine Society — but I forgot to ask him what "Mattachine" means. Come to think of it who was Bilitis? Harry also founded the Radical Faeries, a pagan anarchist glitter sex-lib communal movement still going on — I hope — somewhere down South on a farm or two.) Suddenly in the 1960s these ideas were "in everybody's heads" as the Sits boasted. Even huge stupid mass media spoke of a "Sexual Revolution." Many readers "alive today" (as the

Bible says) can remember this era, which lasted through the 70s into the mid-80s, when theory & practice so to speak went hand in hand in a paroxysm of sexual freedom unparalleled since pagan antiquity.

I don't know if people had *more* sex in those days — that's not the point. I do know that people *valued* the sex they had as a form of liberation. Their imagination was fired up by liberated desire, & vice versa, in a feedback loop of great intensity (or resonance, or affinity, or attraction).

Gradually however certain world-historical trends began to erode both the rhetoric & reality of liberation. The Triumph of Global Capital was "shadowed" by global plague. Suddenly somewhere in the early 90s one began to hear no more talk of sexual revolution. It was declared "over," sometimes by fatuous liberals ("we won") & sometimes by neo-con puritans ("they won, but we're staging a counter-revolution"). The ubiquity of sex *in media* was cited by both sides as evidence. Erotic imagery in advertising was supposed to represent free speech, proof that "there are no more taboos." Left & Right now agreed that sex *had been* liberated. Consequently all talk of sexual liberation would cease. There is no longer any sex lib movement (not here in the Capitalist Paradise anyway) & the old rhetoric now sounds mawkish & embarrassing.

Queer Liberation talk for example has been superinscribed (& erased) by "gay rights," "gay marriage," etc. Every fetish has its own Website. The *Imaginal Aura* has disappeared from sexuality itself in this age of (post)mechanical (post)reproduction, & been transferred... elsewhere.

So — are people nowadays having more sex — less sex — more or less polymorphous sex? That's not the point. Has or has not Triumphal Capital managed somehow to devalue sexual liberation, or the idea of sex *as* liberation — & replace it with the *Image* of sexuality?

Now why would Kapital want to do such a weird thing? What's in it for Kapital? The answer is so simple it seems stupid: Sex lib argues that eros needs to be liberated & is itself liberating. When the Imagination is thoroughly involved in this (let's call it Love) then it focuses on an *essentially non-commodifiable relation* — the sharing of pleasure in free love as the highest form of human bliss — *instead of shopping*.

The Ponzi-scheme logic of Global Capital requires that every single atomized monad must possess its own full array of Civilization's blessings & not share anything with anyone. Social imagineers can't stop people from fucking — who cares — the important thing is to transfer or transpose their bliss from sexuality to Image of sexuality & thence to *commodity*. This transfer is fraught with magic — Image Magic. As Giordano Bruno said, with magic it's easier to enchain millions of people to Images than to make one person fall in love with you. I'm talking now about the Spectacle as it's morphed (since 1989) into a post-Spectacular state of instantaneity. Hegelian television. I suggest that the holiness of tantrik or liberated sex has been hijacked by the technopathocratic *mecanasm* of what Paul Virilio calls the Global Accident — i.e., the Internet (etc.) as rhizomatic panopticon.

It isn't sex that needs to be liberated. It's liberation that needs to be liberated — like a paradoxical genie in a klein bottle. Imagination needs to be liberated — literally detached from the Image Magic of Corporation/Police/State Power — & re-appropriated by actual human beings in physical bodies — in love.

This neo-luddite revolt of love would make no distinction between "natural" & "unnatural" amatory forms. Even normal hetero-reproductive family-value sexuality will be incompatible with maximal free market functions. Late Late Capitalism is basically a Society of Divorce, of division or "alienation" as Young Marx called it, of *separation* & yet also of *sameness.*

The opposite of sameness would be *difference,* in the French sense too, a kind of "divine" heterogeneity — a *Cauda Pavonis* or array of colors as alchemists say. And the opposite of separation or alienation would be *love.*

The technopathocracy allows for neither true Nietzschean individualism nor true Fourierist collectivity. Rugged individual is replaced by isolated consumer — the Social itself is replaced by its Simulacrum. Therefore the obvious dialectical opposition to PoMo indifference — as well as all other forms of liberal reaction & conservative progressism — would combine both *difference* & *love* (both authentic self & reality of the Other in Attraction) vs. *separation* & *sameness.*

Nietzsche says somewhere something about a person's sexuality being the deepest aspect of one's being. Goethe says "the unnatural is also natural" — or — to put it another way — Natural & Unnatural In Struggle Together against the antibiotic totality. Perverse & normal in solidarity for *bios* vs. *techne.*

Fourier supported — indeed relished — every form of consensual sensuality — he visualized a Society of the Orgy. (Someone once quipped of Fourier that for him lunching alone was the only sin.) But what makes the difference then between the tantrik "peak experience" & the mere scratching of some vaguely (Charles) Darwinian itch? Only the Imagination. All Power to the Imagination.

I apologize for using *Theory* here to explain my ideas. Poetry — or pornography — might be more to the point. Theory has betrayed us — seduced & abandoned us — from the 1970s thru the 90s — & by now is looking pretty shabby. It has the Tieresias/Cassandra Complex — it can explain everything but it can change nothing. When sexual liberation was a *praxis* rather than just a theory, it did indeed succeed in freeing lots of folks from puritan inhibition, gender superstition, psychological repression, sexual selfishness... but it failed to change the Social itself sufficiently to prevent the eventual absorption of sexuality into representation & the reduction of revolt to market niche.

Hypothesis: If any sort of liberational practice is now to be rescued or revived, or even considered, it would have to replace the theoretical with the Imaginal. By this I mean it would have to deal with the Image Magic of Global Mediation with a counter-magic capable of opening up an Outside within the Enclosed space of Capital itself.

Historically, sex-lib ideas have always floated around in occultist circles, from Marsilio Ficino's rediscovery of Platonic Love in the Renaissance to Aleister Crowley's orgiastic Ordo Templi Orientis — William Blake was a Xtian Tantrik (see *Why Mrs Blake Cried*); & 19th-century Paris (of course) blossomed with erotic occultists (Fourier — Sar Peladan the Rosicrucian — de Nerval — Petrus Borel — J.K. Huysmans — to name a few). The idea that sex magic is "dangerous" is both a (post)Xtian superstition & a psychological truism. It's high risk not for health so much as sanity. I agree with Paracelsus, who thought that most Ceremonial Magic rituals "simply attract little devils like flies to rotten meat." I have in mind something more like the magical ("non-ordinary") state of consciousness that both precedes & ensues from a loving erotic experience. Can this state be induced or enhanced by some sort of spiritual practice? The kind of aura lifted by Dante from the Sufis & woven around the figure of Beatrice in his *Vita Nuova* — (*not* in the later & far less interesting *Divine Comedy: Paradiso*).

Really in essence it's all about *Tantra* — that is, worshipping the beloved as divine (or "Elemental") so as to experience eros itself as mystical union in sexual (or even chaste Romantic) bliss — including the re-eroticization of Nature (as Attraction) & a general re-enchantment of the landscape — i.e., the reunification of consciousness & Nature — the ancient goal of Hermeticism — of Romanticism & its prolongations as (for example) Surrealism, Psychedelicism, or Green Anarchy. One needn't be religious to entertain such ideas; Walter Benjamin called this magic "Profane Illumination" (that is, mysticism without religion) & Colin Wilson calls it simply "Peak Experience."

Avicenna believed literally that love makes the world go round — that angels of the planetary spheres are in love with archangels of the celestial heavens just as matter is in love with form; that all motion is Attraction. Ethnography is rife with examples of peoples who believe the world will come to an end unless certain sex acts are performed.

(In 1980 when I was in Surakarta [Solo], I was told that the city's run-down appearance was due to the fact that the Sunan [Sultan] no longer performed ritual intercourse with Loro Kidul the green goddess of the Java Sea, "in that tower over there, once a year, during monsoon." It's true that the electricity in his palace had been turned off for non-payment of bills. On the whole I preferred shabby quiet "unspoiled" Solo to its rival city nearby Yogyakarta, noisy & tourist-ridden.)

Can we say at least that erotic bliss in itself could be an effective act of resistance against the technopathocracy as well as a goal in its own right, a *telos*? If so, then we need a new sexual liberation movement.